Peripheral Arterial Disease

CONTEMPORARY CARDIOLOGY

Christopher P. Cannon, Series Editor

PERIPHERAL ARTERIAL DISEASE

Diagnosis and Treatment

Edited by

JAY D. COFFMAN, MD
ROBERT T. EBERHARDT, MD

Department of Medicine,
Boston University Medical Center,
Boston, MA

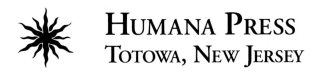

HUMANA PRESS
TOTOWA, NEW JERSEY

© 2003 Humana Press Inc.
999 Riverview Drive, Suite 208
Totowa, New Jersey 07512

humanapress.com

For additional copies, pricing for bulk purchases, and/or information about other Humana titles, contact Humana at the above address or at any of the following numbers: Tel.: 973-256-1699; Fax: 973-256-8341, E-mail: humana@humanapr.com; or visit our Website: http://humanapr.com

Due diligence has been taken by the publishers, editors, and authors of this book to assure the accuracy of the information published and to describe generally accepted practices. The contributors herein have carefully checked to ensure that the drug selections and dosages set forth in this text are accurate and in accord with the standards accepted at the time of publication. Notwithstanding, as new research, changes in government regulations, and knowledge from clinical experience relating to drug therapy and drug reactions constantly occurs, the reader is advised to check the product information provided by the manufacturer of each drug for any change in dosages or for additional warnings and contraindications. This is of utmost importance when the recommended drug herein is a new or infrequently used drug. It is the responsibility of the treating physician to determine dosages and treatment strategies for individual patients. Further it is the responsibility of the health care provider to ascertain the Food and Drug Administration status of each drug or device used in their clinical practice. The publisher, editors, and authors are not responsible for errors or omissions or for any consequences from the application of the information presented in this book and make no warranty, express or implied, with respect to the contents in this publication.

Cover design by Patricia F. Cleary.

This publication is printed on acid-free paper.∞
ANSI Z39.48-1984 (American National Standards Institute) Permanence of Paper for Printed Library Materials.

Photocopy Authorization Policy:
Authorization to photocopy items for internal or personal use, or the internal or personal use of specific clients, is granted by Humana Press Inc., provided that the base fee of US $10.00 per copy, plus US $00.25 per page, is paid directly to the Copyright Clearance Center at 222 Rosewood Drive, Danvers, MA 01923. For those organizations that have been granted a photocopy license from the CCC, a separate system of payment has been arranged and is acceptable to Humana Press Inc. The fee code for users of the Transactional Reporting Service is: [1-58829-052-2/03 $10.00 + $00.25].

Printed in the United States of America.   10 9 8 7 6 5 4 3 2 1

Library of Congress Cataloging-in-Publication Data

Peripheral arterial disease: diagnosis and treatment / edited by Jay D. Coffman, Robert T. Eberhardt
           p.;cm.–(Contemporary cardiology)
      Includes bibliographical references and index.
      ISBN 1-58829-052-2 (alk. paper)
      1. Peripheral vascular diseases. 2. Arteries–Diseases. I. Coffman, Jay D. (Jay Denton), 1928– II. Eberhardt, Robert T., MD. III. Contemporary cardiology (Totowa, N.J.: unnumbered)
      [DNLM: 1. Peripheral Vascular Diseases–diagnosis. 2. Peripheral Vascular Diseases–therapy. 3. Arteries–physiopathology. WG 510 P4404 2002]
      RC694.P473 2002
      616.1'31–dc21   2002024052

DEDICATION

We dedicate this book to two preeminent vascular specialists who died within the last year. Both physicians were prominent in their field and contributed chapters to this book. They were expert clinicians and clinical investigators. Jeff Isner, a professor at Tufts University, was one of the first to apply gene therapy in patients with ischemic limbs and hearts. He was a driving force in therapeutic angiogenesis. Gene Strandness, a professor at the University of Washington, developed ultrasound applications for the extremities and carotid arteries: he was an expert in diagnostic methods for peripheral vascular disease. Gene was a founder and past-president of the American Venous Forum. The death of these investigators was a great loss to vascular medicine that leaves a void in their sphere of expertise. Besides their outstanding scientific achievements, they were gracious and considerate colleagues.

PREFACE

With an aging population owing to our longer life span, peripheral arterial disease will become more common than its already high prevalence. It has usually been assigned a less important role in the education of the lay public and physicians, in contrast to coronary artery and cerebrovascular disease. The importance of peripheral arterial disease, symptomatic and asymptomatic, to the practicing physician and cardiologist is that it predicts disease in other vascular beds—serving as a prognostic factor for myocardial infarction, stroke, and mortality. Furthermore, there is impaired functional capacity and severe disability, particularly in those with critical limb ischemia.

The diagnosis of peripheral arterial disease is often obvious from the history and physical examination, but with the development of noninvasive techniques, especially the Doppler flowmeter, the diagnosis can easily be documented in both symptomatic and asymptomatic patients by all physicians. There are exciting new therapeutic modalities including gene therapy, endovascular interventions, and new pharmaceutical agents.

In *Peripheral Arterial Disease: Diagnosis and Treatment,* we acquaint physicians with all aspects of peripheral arterial disease. Because of the limitations of medical therapy, there is now a special emphasis on prevention of peripheral arterial disease and a special emphasis on risk factors and their treatment. Risks factors are considered from the point of view of the pathophysiologist (Chapter 1), epidemiologist (Chapter 2), and vascular specialist (Chapter 9). The pathogenesis of arteriosclerosis is presented first, followed by a comprehensive treatise on the epidemiology and natural history of the disease. The chapter on the clinical evaluation of intermittent claudication contains the very important differential diagnosis section. A combined chapter on hemodynamics and vascular laboratory testing gives the reader insight into the physiological and pathophysiological basis of the available diagnostic tests. The role of angiography, including newer noninvasive modalities, is discussed.

Regarding treatment, a chapter on risk factors and antiplatelet therapy is especially timely, with a focus on the prevention of myocardial infarctions, strokes, and mortality in peripheral arterial disease patients. Exercise rehabilitation is covered in depth, for it is one of the most effective treatments for peripheral arterial disease. Pharmacotherapy, including new agents for intermittent claudication, and endovascular interventions are the subjects of separate chapters. The intriguing, emerging field of angiogenesis is introduced with appropriate caution. There is a detailed discussion of the time-honored surgical approach to revascularization. For the consultant, a chapter follows on the preoperative evaluation and perioperative management of the vascular disease patient.

There are separate chapters discussing such special problems as peripheral arterial disease in women, management of the diabetic foot, and large vessel vasculitis. Although the concentration is on arteriosclerosis obliterans, two less common causes of peripheral artery disease, arterial embolus and thromboangiitis obliterans, are worthy of separate chapters. Finally a common problem that is often encountered by clinicians involved with catheter-based interventions, atheroembolism, is discussed.

By providing a comprehensive overview and detailed accounting of all aspects of peripheral arterial obstructive disease, we hope to empower the clinician with the skills and knowledge to diagnose and treat this important and often overlooked disorder.

Jay D. Coffman, MD
Robert T. Eberhardt, MD

CONTENTS

CONTRIBUTORS

TIMOTHY BAUER, MS • *Section of Vascular Medicine, University of Colorado Health Sciences Center, Denver, CO*

IRIS BAUMGARTNER, MD • *Swiss Cardiovascular Center, Division of Angiology, University Hospital, Bern, Switzerland*

LISA M. BORDEAUX, RN, MSN, FNP • *Vascular Medicine Program, Cardiovascular Division, Minnesota Vascular Diseases Center, University of Minnesota Medical School, Minneapolis, MN*

JAY D. COFFMAN, MD • *Peripheral Vascular Medicine, Department of Medicine, Boston University School of Medicine, Boston, MA*

ANTHONY J. COMEROTA, MD, FACS • *Section of Vascular Surgery, Department of Surgery, Temple University School of Medicine, Philadelphia, PA*

ROBERT T. EBERHARDT, MD • *Cardiovascular and Peripheral Vascular Medicine, Boston University School of Medicine, Boston, MA*

MARIE GERHARD-HERMAN, MD • *Vascular Diagnostic Laboratory, Brigham and Women's Hospital and Harvard Medical School, Boston, MA*

GARY W. GIBBONS, MD • *Section of Vascular Surgery, Boston University School of Medicine, Boston, MA*

GEOFFREY M. HABERSHAW, DPM • *Department of Podiatry, Foot and Ankle Surgery, Boston University School of Medicine, Boston, MA*

JONATHAN L. HALPERIN, MD • *The Zena and Michael A. Wiener Cardiovascular Institute, Mount Sinai Medical Center, New York, NY*

WILLIAM R. HIATT, MD • *Section of Vascular Medicine, University of Colorado Health Sciences Center, Denver, CO*

ALAN T. HIRSCH, MD • *Vascular Medicine Program, Cardiovascular Division, Minnesota Vascular Diseases Center, University of Minnesota Medical School, Minneapolis, MN*

JEFFREY M. ISNER, MD (DECEASED) • *Department of Medicine, Cardiology, St. Elizabeth's Medical Center, Tufts University School of Medicine, Boston, MA*

JOHN A. KAUFMAN, MD • *Dotter International Institute, Oregon Health Services University, Portland, OR*

EUGENE Y. KISSIN, MD • *Section of Rheumatology, Boston University School of Medicine and Boston Medical Center, Boston, MA*

JAMES O. MENZOIAN, MD • *Section of Vascular Surgery, Division of Surgery, Boston University School of Medicine, Boston, MA*

PETER A. MERKEL, MD, MPH • *Sections of Rheumatology and Clinical Epidemiology Research & Training, Boston University School of Medicine and Boston Medical Center, Boston, MA*

EMILE R. MOHLER III, MD • *Vascular Medicine, Department of Medicine, University of Pennsylvania School of Medicine, Philadelphia, PA*

APRIL NEDEAU, BS • *Boston University School of Medicine, Boston, MA*

JEFFREY W. OLIN, DO • *The Zena and Michael A. Wiener Cardiovascular Institute, Mount Sinai School of Medicine, New York, NY*

JOSEPH D. RAFFETTO, MD • *Section of Vascular Surgery, Division of Surgery, Boston University School of Medicine, Boston, MA*

LAURA M. REICH, DO • *Vascular Medicine Program, Cardiovascular Division, Minnesota Vascular Diseases Center, University of Minnesota Medical School, Minneapolis, MN*

FRANK A. SCHMIEDER, MD • *Section of Vascular Surgery, Department of Surgery, Temple University School of Medicine, Philadelphia, PA*

D. EUGENE STRANDNESS, JR., MD, D MED (HON) (DECEASED) • *Department of Surgery, University of Washington School of Medicine, Seattle, WA*

MARKUS C. STÜHLINGER, MD • *Division of Cardiology, Department of Internal Medicine, University of Innsbruck, Austria*

PHILIP S. TSAO, PhD • *Division of Cardiovascular Medicine, Department of Medicine, Stanford University, Stanford, CA*

CHRISTOPHER J. WHITE, MD • *Department of Cardiology, Ochsner Heart and Vascular Institute, New Orleans, LA*

1   Etiology and Pathogenesis of Atherosclerosis

Markus C. Stühlinger, MD and Philip S. Tsao, PhD

CONTENTS

INTRODUCTION

The World Health Organization defines atherosclerosis as a chronic vascular disease of medium and large arteries that includes thickening and remodeling of the vessel wall leading to reduction or obstruction of blood flow through plaque formation and thrombosis *(1)*. It is characterized by a variable combination of intimal changes—patchy subintimal deposition of lipid substances, complex carbohydrates, blood components, connective tissue, and calcium—and changes in the media. Atherosclerosis is the most common and serious vascular disease, which can affect the heart, brain, kidneys, and other vital organs as well as the extremities. It is the leading cause of morbidity and mortality in the United States and in the Western hemisphere *(2)*. In 1994, for example, approximately 1 million deaths in the United States were attributable to vascular, twice as many as from cancer and 10 times as many as from accidental causes *(3)*. Atherosclerosis is a progressive disease process that generally begins in childhood and has clinical manifestations in middle to late adulthood *(4)*.

MORPHOLOGY OF THE NORMAL ARTERY

The wall of the normal artery consists of three concentric layers: the innermost intima, the middle layer called the media, and the outermost adventitia. The three layers are

From: *Contemporary Cardiology: Peripheral Arterial Disease: Diagnosis and Treatment*
Edited by: J. D. Coffman and R. T. Eberhardt © Humana Press Inc., Totowa, NJ

separated by concentric rings of elastin, known as the internal elastic lamina (which separates the intima from the media) and the external elastic lamina (which separates the media from the adventitia).

The luminal surface of arteries (intima) is lined by a single layer of endothelial cells situated on a basement membrane of extracellular matrix and bordered by the internal elastic lamina. Endothelial cells are attached to each other by a series of interconnections known as junctional complexes. The endothelium forms a dynamic barrier between the luminal surface of the artery and the stroma of the arterial wall and also serves as a connecting tissue layer between the vessel wall and the circulating blood. It was thought that endothelial cells were quite passive in their function, acting only as a smooth, nonthrombogenic surface. However, research over the past two decades has demonstrated that the endothelium regulates a wide array of functions in the arterial wall including vascular tone, leukocyte adhesion, and trafficking within the arterial wall as well as thrombosis. The media consists of multiple layers of a single cell type, the vascular smooth muscle cells. These cells produce and are held together by an extracellular matrix, consisting mainly of elastic fibers, collagen, and proteoglycans. The number of smooth muscle cell layers and therefore the thickness of the media depends on the location, size, and function of the artery. The adventitia, the outermost layer of the arterial wall, typically consists of a loose matrix of smooth muscle cells, fibroblasts, collagen, and elastin *(5)*.

PATHOLOGY OF THE ATHEROSCLEROTIC LESION

The initial lesion (type I) occurs in the absence of tissue damage and consists of intimal accumulation of lipoproteins and some lipid-laden macrophages. These macrophages have migrated as monocytes from the circulation into the subendothelial layer of the intima. Soon this lesion develops into the early lesion or "fatty-streak" lesion (type II), which is characterized by the abundance of "foam cells." Foam cells are filled with vacuoles containing predominantly cholesteryl oleate and are localized in the intima immediately underlying the endothelium. Type II lesions may quickly progress into the so-called preatheromic lesion (type III), which is defined by increased quantities of extracellular lipid and minor localized tissue damage. The atheroma (type IV) exhibits extensive structural damage to the intima and may be either silent or overt. The next more advanced lesion is the developing lesion or fibroatheroma (type V). It appears macroscopically as a dome shaped, firm, and pearly white plaque. The fibroatheroma is usually composed of the necrotic core—usually localized at the base of the lesion near the internal elastic lamina, composed of extracellular lipid and extensive cell debris—and the fibrotic cap, consisting of collagen and surrounding smooth muscle cells. Indeed, the term "atherosclerosis" is derived from *athero*, the Greek word for gruel and corresponding to the necrotic core, and from *sclerosis*, the Greek word for hard, corresponding to the fibrous cap. The complicated lesion (type VI) is used to describe a variety of advanced atherosclerotic lesions that exhibit special characteristics not found in classic fibroatheroma, such as an ulcerated lesion (formed by the erosion of the cap), a hemorrhagic lesion (characterized by a hemorrhage in the necrotic core), or a thrombotic lesion (carrying thrombotic deposition). The type VII lesion is a calcified lesion, also characterized by the lay description "hardening of the arteries," and the type VIII lesion is a fibrotic lesion, composed predominantly of collagen *(6)*.

ETIOLOGY OF ATHEROSCLEROSIS

Atherosclerosis is the most common cause of arterial disease of the lower extremities. Major nonreversible risk factors of atherosclerosis include age, male sex, and family history of premature atherosclerosis. Major reversible risk factors for the development and progression of atherosclerotic disease include smoking, dyslipidemia, diabetes mellitus, hypertension, and hyperhomocysteinemia.

Cigarette Smoking

The risk of developing intermittent claudication is at least two-fold higher for smokers than for nonsmokers *(7–10)*. Moreover, continued cigarette smoking greatly enhances the risk of progression from stable claudication to severe limb ischemia and amputation. Nicotine and other tobacco-derived chemicals are toxic to the vascular endothelium. Cigarette smoking increases low-density lipoprotein (LDL), and decreases high-density lipoprotein (HDL) levels, raises blood carbon monoxide (and could thereby produce endothelial hypoxia), and promotes vasoconstriction of already atherosclerotic artery segments. Cigarette smoke also increases platelet reactivity, which may favor platelet thrombus formation, and increases plasma fibrinogen concentration and hematocrit, resulting in increased blood viscosity.

Diabetes Mellitus

Diabetes mellitus is associated with a three-fold excess risk of intermittent claudication *(9–11)*. The severity and extent of peripheral atherosclerosis are often more severe and the tibial and peroneal arteries are involved more frequently in diabetic patients than in nondiabetic individuals *(12)*. The prognosis is poor for patients with diabetes who have claudication, as 30–40% develop critical limb ischemia over a 6-yr period. By comparison, approx 10–20% of nondiabetic patients with claudication develop critical limb ischemia within 6 yr *(13,14)*.

Dyslipidemia

Dyslipidemia, particularly hypercholesterolemia, is present in 40% of patients with peripheral atherosclerosis. Patients with cholesterol levels > 270 mg/dL have more than a two-fold increase in risk of developing claudication. In addition, unusual forms of dyslipidemia are associated with peripheral atherosclerosis, especially Fredrickson type III hyperlipoproteinemia, which is characterized by increased intermediate-density lipoproteins and an abnormal apolipoprotein E level *(7)*.

Hypertension

Epidemiological studies have established an association between hypertension and a greater prevalence of atherosclerosis and occlusive vascular disease *(15,16)*. Moreover, hypertension increases the risk of claudication by at least two-fold in men and four-fold in women *(7)*. The Framingham Heart Study determined that the incidence of heart disease rises progressively with increasing levels of either systolic or diastolic blood pressure *(16)*. A meta-analysis of nine major prospective observational studies indicated a "direct, continuous and apparently independent association" between diastolic blood pressure and the incidence of stroke (34%) and coronary heart disease (CHD) (21%) *(17)*. Individuals with hypertension also demonstrate increased rate of restenosis after angioplasty *(18)*. This is thought to be due to exaggerated neointimal hyperplasia rather than altered vessel remodeling. Furthermore, congestive heart failure is twice as common in middle-aged hypertensive men and five times as common in women with hypertension, as compared to the normotensive population. The importance of hypertension to cardiovascular disease was further emphasized by the Veterans Administration Cooperative Study Group *(19)*. Their findings indicated that pharmacological treatment of hypertension resulted in reduced cardiovascular morbidity and mortality. As such, there was a significant decrease in deaths directly related to and associated with hypertension.

NEW POTENTIAL RISK FACTORS
Insulin Resistance Syndrome (Syndrome X)

There is general consensus that resistance to insulin-mediated glucose disposal is a characteristic finding in patients with type 2 diabetes *(20)*. In addition, insulin resistance and/or compensatory hyperinsulinemia (a surrogate marker for insulin resistance) can be discerned in first-degree relatives of patients with type 2 diabetes *(21)*. Finally, insulin resistance and/or compensatory hyperinsulinemia are highly significant predictors of type 2 diabetes in nondiabetic individuals *(22–24)*.

Although insulin-resistant individuals can prevent gross decompensation of glucose tolerance if they are able to maintain the degree of hyperinsulinemia needed to overcome the defect in insulin action, they are at greatly increased risk to develop atherosclerosis. Initial evidence linking insulin resistance to cardiovascular disease (CVD) was derived from the results of prospective epidemiologic studies in which plasma insulin concentrations were used as surrogate measures of insulin resistance *(25–27)*. Although controversy exists as to the meaning of the association between hyperinsulinemia and CVD *(25–27)*, epidemiologic results describing this relationship continue to be published *(28,29)*. Indeed, specific measurements of insulin resistance have been shown in cross-sectional studies to be associated with CVD *(26–28)*. More recently, the first prospective study showing that insulin resistance predicts CVD has been published *(30)*. Whether insulin resistance or compensatory hyperinsulinemia, or both, are responsible for the increased risk of atherosclerosis is still being debated. Insulin resistance and/or compensatory hyperinsulinemia are also highly significant predictors of the development of hypertension in normotensive individuals *(31,32)*. It has also been shown that the risk of CVD in hypertensive individuals is significantly increased in patients with insulin resistance/hyperinsulinemia or the cluster of abnormalities associated with these changes in insulin metabolism *(33)*.

In addition to the role it plays as a fundamental abnormality in the genesis of hyperglycemia and hypertension, insulin resistance/hyperinsulinemia greatly increases the likelihood of developing a cluster of abnormalities, initially designated in 1988 as syndrome X, that increase risk of CVD *(34)*. For example, insulin resistance and compensatory hyperinsulinemia are independent predictors of a high plasma triglyceride and a low HDL concentration *(35)*, the characteristic dyslipidemia in patients with type 2 diabetes *(34)*. Studies done by Reaven and colleagues have also been able to show that the remaining components of the atherogenic lipoprotein profile present in patients with type 2 diabetes, small dense LDL particles and an enhancement of postprandial lipemia (accumulation of remnant lipoprotein), are also present in insulin resistant/hyperinsulinemic, nondiabetic individuals *(36,37)*. The growing list of abnormalities associated with insulin resistance and compensatory hyperinsulinemia has steadily increased since the notion of syndrome X was introduced and now includes hyperuricemia, elevated plasma concentrations of plasminogen activator inhibitor-1 and fibrinogen, increased sympathetic nervous system activity, and enhanced sodium retention.

Hyperhomocysteinemia

Elevated plasma homocysteine has emerged as an important new risk factor for cardiovascular diseases *(38)*. Prospective and case-controlled studies have demonstrated that elevations in plasma homocysteine levels are associated with a two- to fourfold increased risk in cardiovascular diseases *(39,40)*, including peripheral atherosclerosis *(41)* and myocardial infarction *(42)*. This may be an issue of significant clinical relevance, as elevations in plasma homocysteine are common, affecting approx 10% of the general population, and more than 40–50% of individuals with coronary artery disease *(39,41–43)*.

ATHEROGENESIS: THE "RESPONSE TO INJURY" HYPOTHESIS

The development and the progression of atherosclerosis is a complex process. Atherosclerotic lesions result from time-dependent interactions of gene products of multiple biological pathways and environmental factors. Although there are similarities between patients regarding presentation and final outcome of atherosclerosis—such as stroke, heart attack, or peripheral arterial disease—there is heterogeneity in the factors that initiate and drive the progression of this disease within each individual. Thus multiple hypotheses have been proposed to explain the development of atherosclerosis. As early as 1856, Virchow hypothesized that atherogenesis included the infiltration of lipids from the plasma into arterial walls *(44)*. The mechanism by which lipid accumulated in the subendothelial space has been the topic of much debate since that time. Ross and colleagues *(45)* were the first to postulate that lesions of atherosclerosis could arise as a result of chronic injury to the arterial endothelium. This hypothesis is based on the idea that various mechanisms (Fig. 1) could alter the endothelial–intercellular attachment or endothelial cell–connective tissue attachment, so that mechanical forces derived from blood flow result in focal desquamation of the endothelium. The latter process is followed by adherence, aggregation, and adhesion of platelets and leukocytes at the sites of focal injury and could subsequently cause intima proliferation, synthesis of new connective tissue matrix proteins, and deposition of extracellular and intracellular lipids.

THE ENDOTHELIUM

The vascular endothelium constitutes approximately 1% of the human body mass; it is fivefold heavier than the heart and is a large endocrine organ with a total surface area of approx 5000 m^2 *(46)*. A single layer of endothelial cells covers the luminal surface of the entire vascular tree. Once thought to be a lifeless, nonthrombogenic surface, the endothelium is now recognized to be an active organ that is constantly reacting to metabolic factors, physical forces initiated by fluid flow, and concentration changes in vasoactive substances. The numerous functions ascribed to the endothelium include maintaining vascular tone as well as blood fluidity and providing homeostasis in the

Table 1
Major Substances Generated and Released by the Endothelium

Vasodilators	*Cellular adhesion molecules*	*Coagulants/fibrinolytics*
Nitric oxide	VCAM-1	von Willebrand factor
EDHF	ICAM-1	Tissue type plasminogen activator
Prostacyclin	E-selectin	Plasminogen activator inhibitor-1
Adrenomodulin	Thrombomodulin	
Natriuretic peptide		
Vasoconstrictors	*Growth factors*	*Chemokines*
Endothelin	VEGF	MCP-1
Angiotensin II	PDGF	IL-8
Thromboxane A2	TGF-β	

VCAM-1, vascular cell adhesion molecule 1; EDHF, endothelium-derived hyperpolarizing factor; ICAM-1, intracellular adhesion molecule 1; VEGF, vascular endothelial growth factor; PDGF, platelet-derived growth factor; TGF-β, transforming growth factor β; MCP-1, monocyte chemoattractant protein 1; IL-8, interleukin 8.

event of endothelial injury. Specifically, endothelial functions include control of vascular tone, modulation of vascular structure by regulation of angiogenesis and proliferation, maintenance of a selective permeability barrier, regulation of lipid oxidation, and mediation of immune responses. In addition, given its strategic location, the endothelium plays a major role in interactions between circulating blood and the vessel wall by responding to hemodynamic influences as well as neurohumoral and inflammatory factors. Thus the adherence of leukocytes to the endothelium, aggregation and adhesion of platelets, and coagulation and fibrinolysis are regulated by the endothelium *(47,48)*. Endothelial cells are able to fulfill all these functions by generating a number of paracrine substances, including vasodilators and constrictors, coagulants and fibrinolytics, adhesion molecules, growth factors, and chemokines (Table 1).

Functions of the Endothelium

The healthy endothelium normally functions to maintain vascular homeostasis by inhibiting smooth muscle cell contraction, intimal proliferation, thrombosis, and monocyte adhesion. Although Ross and colleagues initially surmised frank endothelial injury (i.e., desquamation) as the initial insult involved with atherogenesis, it has become clear that the endothelium can now undergo more subtle, but chronic, dysfunction that can ultimately participate in lesion development. A dysfunctional endothelium can stimulate leukocyte infiltration, smooth muscle cell migration from the media to the intima, smooth muscle cell proliferation, and the formation of foam cells. A large body of accumulated evidence indicates that endothelial dysfunction is associated with most of the known risk factors for cardiovascular disease, thereby offering a central mechanism for atherogenesis.

The normal endothelium provides an antithrombotic surface that inhibits platelet aggregation and facilitates blood flow. Also, the endothelium regulates thrombosis through the release of nitric oxide (NO) (which inhibits platelet activation, adhesion, and aggregation) and other mediators with antithrombotic activities (Table 1). Finally, the endothelium plays an important role in the regulation of inflammation within blood

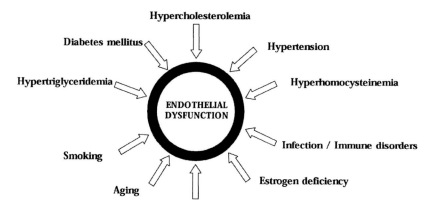

Fig. 1. Endothelial antagonists.

vessels. The antiinflammatory properties of the healthy endothelium are essential in the prevention of atherosclerosis development. The adhesion of leukocytes to the endothelial surface is important in the early development of an atherosclerotic plaque and is also responsible for the plaque rupture and instability that occur later in the atherogenesis process.

Endothelial Dysfunction

Because modulation of vasomotor tone was one of the first physiological functions ascribed to endothelial cells, it is often used as an indication of the general health of the endothelium *(47,48)*. As such, decrements in endothelium-derived vasodilatation have been associated with all known risk factors for cardiovascular disease (Fig. 1). In fact, endothelial dysfunction usually precedes the development of coronary atherosclerotic lesions and thrombotic events (e.g., acute myocardial infarction and unstable angina).

Mechanisms of Endothelial Dysfunction

As illustrated by the panoply of vasoactive agents produced by the endothelium (Table 1), vasomotor tone is eventually determined by the profile of factors produced at any given time. Arguably, the most important substance responsible for endothelium-dependent vascular relaxation is NO. NO not only is involved in relaxation of vascular smooth muscle, but also partially mediates inhibition of platelet activation, adhesion, and aggregation; prevention of vascular smooth muscle proliferation; and adhesion of leukocytes to the endothelium. Notably other endothelium-derived substances are also known to cause relaxation including prostacyclin and endothelium-derived hyperpolarizing factor (EDHF) (Table 1).

NITRIC OXIDE

Furchgott and Zawadzski *(49)* were the first to report that acetylcholine-induced vasodilatation occurs only in the presence of an intact endothelium. Indeed, once the endothelial cell layer was removed, acetylcholine paradoxically induced contractions of rabbit aortic rings. Through a series of elegant studies they determined that acetylcholine binds to its muscarinic receptor on the endothelial cell, and the endothelium, in turn, releases a substance that caused vasorelaxation that they termed "endothelium-derived relaxing factor (EDRF)." Originally they speculated that this factor was a prostanoid metabolite of lipoxygenase. EDRF is now known to be NO *(50)*. NO is the most potent endogenous vasodilator known and it exerts its actions in the same manner as other nitrovasodilators such as nitroglycerin *(51)*. However, in physiologic conditions, the NO radical has a half-life of just fractions of seconds, unless it is bound to a carrier molecule, such as a thiol. Indeed some evidence indicates that EDRF/NO may be released in the form of a nitrosothiol *(52)*. Free NO is rapidly oxidized to nitrite and nitrate by oxygenated hemoglobin before being excreted into the urine. Endothelium-derived NO can also diffuse from the endothelium into vascular smooth muscle cells and is there able to activate soluble guanylate cyclase, leading to the production of cyclic guanosine monophosphate (cGMP). Accumulation of c-GMP activates cGMP-dependent proteins within the smooth muscle cell that mediate vascular relaxation *(53)*.

Endogenous NO is generated by the five-electron oxidation of L-arginine, an essential amino acid, to citrulline catalyzed by the enzyme NO synthase (NOS) *(54)*. There are three isoforms of NOS: Neuronal NOS (nNOS, NOS-1) is predominantly expressed in neuronal tissue, endothelial NOS (eNOS, NOS-3) is constitutively expressed in endothelial cells (but also in cardiomyocytes and thrombocytes), and inducible NOS (iNOS, NOS-2) is present only if stimulated by lipopolysaccharides or inflammatory cytokines. All three isoforms of NOS require L-arginine as a substrate for the enzymatic reaction as well as several cofactors for NO biosynthesis, which include NADPH, tetrahydrobiopterin (BH_4), calmodulin, and others.

Expression and activation of endothelial NOS is a highly regulated process. The major physiological stimulus for NO generation and release is shear stress, the tangential drag produced by flowing blood over the endothelial surface *(55)*. Furthermore a number of vasoconstrictors, for example, endothelin, norepinephrine, or serotonin, can bind to specific endothelial receptors and induce release of NO. Therefore the increasing NO diffusion from the endothelium into vascular smooth muscle cells can overcome any direct vasoconstrictor effects by these substances on the smooth muscle. Along the same lines, acetylcholine triggers the release of NO and subsequently leads to vasodilatation by binding to muscarinic receptors on the surface of healthy endothelial cells. On the other hand, if the endothelial cell layer is removed (e.g., by endothelial denudation) or if the endothelial cells undergo chronic injury and are dysfunctional, the direct effect of acetylcholine on the smooth muscle is unmasked and leads to paradoxical vasoconstriction *(56)*. Therefore endothelial vasodilator function is typically assessed as the ability of a vessel to dilate in response to an endothelial stimulus. In epicardial coronary arteries endothelial function can be determined by measuring dilatation in response to acetylcholine by angiography. Furthermore, noninvasive methods have recently been developed to allow measurements of endothelial function in larger populations in peripheral arteries.

PLEIOTROPIC EFFECTS OF NO

NO diffuses freely across membranes but has a short half-life because it is highly reactive. Hence, NO is well suited to serve as a transient signal molecule within cells and between adjacent cells. NO also opposes several atherogenic processes (Fig. 2). NO inhibits platelet aggregation *(57)*, monocyte adherence *(58)*, and the proliferation of vascular smooth muscle *(59)*. Flow-stimulated endothelial cells are less adhesive for

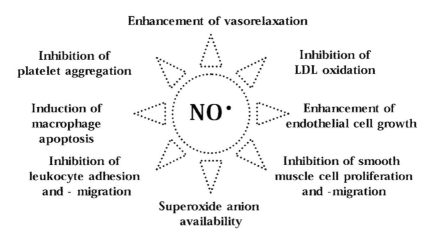

Fig. 2. Pleiotropic effects of endothelium-derived NO.

monocytes *(60)* (Fig. 2). This antiatherogenic effect is due to the release of NO, and is related to the suppression by NO of adhesion molecules and chemokines mediating monocyte adherence and entry into the vessel wall *(61–63)*. In hypercholesterolemic animals, the enhancement of NO synthesis markedly reduces the progression of atheroma, and can even induce regression of vascular lesions *(64)*. Conversely, inhibition of NO accelerates diet-induced atherosclerosis *(65,66)*.

MECHANISMS OF IMPAIRMENT OF THE NO SYNTHASE PATHWAY

Mechanisms of the impairment of the NOS pathway leading to endothelial dysfunction are likely to be multifactorial (Fig. 3). They depend on type, localization, and size of the artery as well as on the disease state causing endothelial dysfunction. In general, the reduced availability of NO in established vascular disease or in metabolic disorders preceding atherosclerosis can be due to reduced NO production (through reduced NOS expression or reduced NOS activity), increased degradation (by superoxide anion), or reduced NO sensitivity by inactivation of soluble guanylate cyclase (Fig. 3).

PROSTACYCLIN

Notably prostacyclin, the most abundantly produced prostaglandin, was recognized for its ability to relax bovine coronary arteries. In addition, examples of other arteries and vascular beds do exist in which the production of prostacyclin accounts for at least part of the vasodilator influence of stimulated endothelial cells *(67)*.

Endothelial Dysfunction in Established Peripheral Arterial Disease

Impaired endothelium-dependent vasorelaxation in response to acetylcholine has been demonstrated in several experimental animal models of atherosclerosis. In the same studies, however, relaxation to endothelium-independent NO donors (e.g., glyceryl trinitrate, sodium nitroprusside) was unaffected, indicating that the impairment of endothelial function in atherosclerotic vessels is mainly due to impaired activity of the endothelium-derived vasodilators NO and prostacyclin *(67)*. Thus prostaglandin E_1 (PGE_1), which activates prostacyclin receptors and thereby induces endothelium-independent vasodilatation, has been used successfully for the pharmacologic treatment of patients with critical limb ischemia and severe peripheral arterial disease (PAD) for over a decade *(68,69)*.

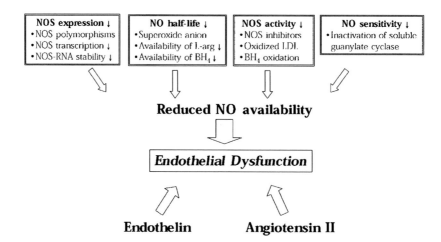

Fig. 3. Multifactorial mechanisms of endothelial dysfunction.

On the other hand, the biological activity of NO is impaired in patients with atherosclerotic vascular disease of the coronary *(70)* and the peripheral vasculature *(71)*. This has been assessed in vivo by measurements of endothelium-dependent vascular dilatations in coronary *(56)* and forearm conduit vascular beds *(72,73)* in patients with atherosclerotic disease. Decreased systemic NO formation in atherosclerosis may be due to reduced NOS protein expression or to reduced NOS enzyme activity. Impaired NOS activity is due to decreased intracellular L-arginine availability and/or increased concentrations of endogenous NOS inhibitors. Indeed, Boger and colleagues observed reduced urinary nitrite excretion rates—a surrogate marker of systemic NO formation—in patients with PAD, dependent on the severity of disease *(71)*. Furthermore, the decrement of urinary NO metabolites was associated with increased plasma concentrations of the endogenous competitive NOS inhibitor asymmetric dimethylarginine (ADMA). The authors conclude that decreased NO formation in patients with PAD may be at least partly due to increased plasma concentrations of ADMA *(71)*.

This hypothesis is supported by studies by the same group and others, which show that endothelial dysfunction observed in patients with coronary or peripheral atherosclerosis can be reversed by L-arginine. Egashira and colleagues showed that the vasodilator response to acetylcholine in coronary arteries was significantly improved after intracoronary L-arginine infusions in patients with microvascular angina and normal coronary angiograms *(74)*. Moreover, improvement of coronary endothelial function by L-arginine seems to be more prominent in stenosed coronary arteries than in healthy vessel segments *(75)*. In patients with severe PAD, an acute intravenous infusion of 30 g of L-arginine can increase femoral arterial blood flow by 43%, as determined by duplex ultrasonography *(76)*. Intermittent therapy with intravenous L-arginine significantly increased urinary NO metabolite excretion rates in patients with chronic stable intermittent claudication and improved flow-induced, endothelium-dependent vasodilatation in the diseased leg of these patients *(77)*.

In patients with established coronary artery disease, endothelial function is significantly compromised *(78)*. However, in patients with early coronary artery disease, abnormal responses to acetylcholine were found even in angiographically normal segments of vessels. Therefore, experimental data suggest that endothelial dysfunction precedes overt atherosclerosis in experimental models of hypercholesterolemia and that endothelial dysfunction may represent an important early event predisposing conduit vessels to vasospasm and vasoconstriction *(79)*.

Endothelial Dysfunction in Hypercholesterolemia

Given the strong association between hypercholesterolemia and coronary artery disease, and the hypothesis that endothelial function could play a dramatic role in vascular homeostasis, it was natural to investigate the relationship between cholesterol and endothelium-dependent vasorelaxation. Early experiments in predictive animal models demonstrated reduced endothelial function associated with atherosclerosis *(80,81)*. Observations with earlier time points indicated that this endothelial dysfunction preceded the development of lipid-engorged lesions, arguing for a possible causative role *(82)*. Moreover, even modest elevations in serum cholesterol levels could depress endothelium-dependent vasodilation *(83)*. Soon after, investigations in humans showed that endothelial function was directly related to cholesterol metabolism. Excess LDL cholesterol leads to selective impairment of NO-dependent vasodilation. This is true even in young adults with familial hypercholesterolemia who do not yet have evidence of vascular disease *(84)*. On the other hand, HDL cholesterol, long considered a protective factor for cardiovascular disease, has opposing effects on endothelial function. Endothelial dysfunction is prevented by high endogenous levels of HDL *(85)* and is reversed by therapies that elevate HDL *(86)*.

Pharmacological therapies that reduce cholesterol levels also enhance endothelial function *(87–89)* In addition, HMG-CoA reductase inhibitors, or statins, are recognized to have lipid-independent effects on endothelial function. Liao and colleagues *(90)* have recently demonstrated that some statins can directly affect the vascular wall. Specifically, they have shown that both lovastatin and simvastatin can stabilize the gene responsible for NO production, endothelial NOS. In addition, the ability of statins to reduce the number of intermediates involved in cholesterol synthesis may have other effects on atherogenesis. For example, one such intermediate, geranylgeranyl pyrophosphate, affects signaling molecules involved with diverse processes including reactive oxygen species generation *(91)*, vascular smooth muscle calcium sensitivity *(92)*, and expression of the potent vasoconstrictor endothelin-1 *(93)*.

Endothelial Dysfunction in Diabetes and Insulin Resistance

Increasing evidence indicates that endothelial dysfunction may also be involved in the pathogenesis of vascular disease in diabetic patients. Numerous groups could show that endothelial-dependent relaxation of conduit and resistance vessels is impaired in patients with diabetes mellitus type-1 (DM-1) *(94)* and type-2 (DM-2) *(95)*. The mechanisms for endothelial dysfunction in DM-1, however, seem to differ from those that occur in DM-2.

Local infusions of NOS inhibitors into the brachial artery of DM-1 patients leads to vasoconstriction, suggesting that basal release of NO release is reduced in these patients compared to healthy controls. In addition, whereas relaxation in response to acetylcholine was not different in patients with DM-1, nitroglycerin-induced vasodilatation was blunted in the study *(96)*. These results could indicate that endothelial dysfunction in DM-1 is due to reduced NO sensitivity of vascular smooth muscle cells.

In individuals with DM-2, however, endothelial dysfunction seems to be based on reduced bioavailability of NO *(97)*. Specifically increased production of superoxide radicals not only leads to enhanced inactivation of NO, but also increases the synthesis of vasoconstricting prostanoids by formation of hydrogen peroxide (H_2O_2) and hydroxyl radicals *(98,99)*. It is, however, yet to be determined if hyperglycemia, hyperinsulinemia, or insulin resistance is the culprit mechanism of endothelial dysfunction in DM-2. Acute hyperglycemia (induced by intravenous infusions of glucose) has been shown to reduce endothelium-dependent relaxation in healthy humans *(100)*. This effect is likely due to inactivation of NO by oxygen-derived free radicals such as superoxide anions *(98)*.

In addition, the tight association between insulin resistance and impaired endothelial dysfunction has been studied extensively throughout the last decade. Several groups have recently provided evidence for NO-dependent, endothelium-mediated vasodilator dysfunction of the coronary *(101)* and mesenteric arteries *(102)* as well as in aortic strips *(103)* in rat models of fructose-diet-induced insulin resistance. In humans, results are often limited by the strong association of insulin resistance with secondary metabolic changes such as obesity, hypertension, and dyslipidemia, which also impair endothelial function independently of insulin resistance. Reduced maximal blood flow in response to methacholine has been shown in a small study with obese insulin-resistant patients *(104)* and an impairment of NO-dependent, flow-mediated vasodilatation of the brachial artery was observed in hypertensive patients with impaired glucose tolerance *(105)*. The best evidence for an impairment of NO-dependent, but not NO-independent vasorelaxation in insulin-resistant subjects was published in a recent study comparing healthy normotensive insulin-sensitive and insulin-resistant first-degree relatives of patients with DM-2. Furthermore, a significant direct correlation between NO-dependent endothelial function and insulin sensitivity was found in this latter study *(106)*. The mechanisms for endothelial dysfunction in insulin resistance are still unclear. Increased production of superoxide radicals was observed in rat models of fructose-diet-induced insulin resistance and increased degradation of NO by superoxide anion due to hyperinsulinemia has been postulated *(103)*. Finally, we have recently demonstrated that ADMA levels are elevated in insulin resistant, nondiabetic individuals and that ADMA concentrations are directly related to the degree of insulin resistance (*107*).

Endothelial Dysfunction in Hypertension

NO plays a major role in the regulation of systemic vascular resistance. It is therefore conceivable that endothelial vasodilator dysfunction could precipitate hypertension. Indeed, an endothelial abnormality is associated with hypertension in animal models *(108)*. Depending on the experimental model, the reduction in endothelium-dependent relaxation is due to an attenuation of endothelium-mediated, NO-dependent activity or to the augmented elaboration of an endothelium-derived contracting factor. Whether endothelial dysfunction is primary in the initiation of hypertension, or is merely an epiphenomenon, is not clear. Treatment of the elevated blood pressure normalizes endothelium-dependent relaxation, suggesting that the endothelial abnormality is secondary in the hypertensive process *(108,109)*. Conversely, infusions of NOS antagonists produce marked increases in blood pressure in experimental animals *(110)*. These inhibitors have been considered nonspecific and the effect on blood pressure could conceivably be due to an effect on the neuronal NOS. However, more definitive data for a primary role of NO in the regulation of blood pressure were provided by Huang and colleagues *(111)*. They found that inactivation of the mouse endothelial NOS gene by homologous recombination produced mice that were significantly hypertensive.

There is extensive evidence for endothelial vasodilator dysfunction in hypertensive humans *(112,113)*. The most direct evidence has come from measurements of forearm blood flow by strain-gauge plethysmography in response to intraarterial infusions of endothelium-dependent and -independent vasodilators. In young patients with mild essential hypertension, endothelium-independent vasodilation is relatively undisturbed. By contrast, cholinergic-induced vasodilation (presumably endothelium-dependent) is attenuated. Whether this is a primary or secondary phenomenon is not known. The impairment of endothelium-dependent vasodilation is likely multifactorial and may involve abnormalities of signal transduction, NO activity, or NO biosynthesis. There is preliminary evidence that, at least in some cases, the endothelial deficit may precede the appearance of essential hypertension *(112,113)*. In young normotensive individuals with hypertensive parents cholinergic-induced forearm vasodilation is impaired; by contrast, endothelium-independent vasodilation is normal.

Endothelial Dysfunction in Hyperhomocysteinemia

Hyperhomocysteinemia also impairs vascular function. Specifically, endothelium-dependent, flow-mediated dilatation of the brachial artery was found to be impaired in humans with chronically elevated total plasma homocysteine *(114)* and with experimental hyperhomocysteinemia induced by oral L-methionine, the precursor of homocysteine *(115)*. As mentioned above, flow-mediated vasodilatation of the brachial artery is largely due to the release of endothelium-derived NO *(116)*. The mechanisms for diminished NO bioavailability observed in hyperhomocysteinemia and subsequent endothelial dysfunction, however, remain incompletely defined. Hyperhomocysteinemia has a direct cytotoxic effect on endothelial cells, and patchy denudation of vascular endothelium has been observed during infusions of homocysteine *(117)*, but these toxic effects occur at levels of homocysteine that are not relevant to human disease. A more plausible mechanism may be that homocysteine increases oxidative degradation of NO via formation of disulfides and generation of hydrogen peroxide *(118)* and superoxide anion *(119)*. Other potential effects of homocysteine may be to decrease NO synthesis *(120)*. This observation would be most consistent with a dysregulation of NOS activity, as protein expression is not affected by homocysteine *(121)*.

One mechanism that might be responsible for a reduced NOS activity is an elevation of ADMA. Indeed ADMA plasma concentrations are threefold elevated in hyperhomocysteinemic monkeys and ADMA plasma concentrations strongly correlate with endothelium-dependent relaxation of the carotid artery of these animals *(122)*. Furthermore, in humans an acute increase in plasma homocysteine levels due to oral methionine loading is associated with a significant increase in plasma levels of ADMA, and impairment of endothelial function after methionine loading correlates with ADMA levels in those individuals. These results suggest that ADMA may also mediate impaired endothelium-dependent vasodilation during experimental hyperhomocysteinemia in humans *(123)*.

CONCLUSION

Atherosclerosis is the most common cause of arterial disease of the lower extremities. The major risk factors of atherosclerosis include advancing age, male sex, family history of premature atherosclerosis, smoking, dyslipidemia, diabetes mellitus, hypertension, and hyperhomocysteinemia. Multiple hypotheses have been proposed to explain the development of atherosclerosis but recent developments have focused on the role of endothelium. It is now clear that the endothelium can undergo subtle dysfunction that can ultimately participate in lesion development. A dysfunctional endothelium can stimulate leukocyte infiltration, smooth muscle cell migration from the media to the intima, smooth muscle cell proliferation, and the formation of foam cells. Each of the major risk factors for atherosclerosis has been associated with endothelial dysfunction in predictive animal models as well as in humans. In many circumstances, endothelial dysfunction precedes evidence of frank lesions. Moreover, therapies targeted to specific risk factors reverse decrements in endothelial activity. Thus, a greater understanding of the underlying mechanisms of endothelial dysfunction will lead to new therapeutic strategies for atherosclerosis, restenosis, and other vascular disorders.

REFERENCES

1. WHO. Classification of atherosclerotic lesions: report of a study group. WHO Techn Rep Ser 1958:1–20.
2. Tunstall-Pedoe H, Kuulasmaa K, Amouyel P, Arveiler D, Rajakangas AM, Pajak A. Myocardial infarction and coronary deaths in the World Health Organization MONICA Project: registration procedures, event rates, and case-fatality rates in 38 populations from 21 countries in four continents. Circulation 1994;90:583–612.
3. Lam JYT. Cardiovascular Disorders. In: Beers MH, Berkow R, eds. The Merck Manual, 17th ed. Whitehouse Station, NJ: Merck, 1999, pp. 1654–1656.
4. Zipes DB, Libby P. Heart Disease: A Textbook of Cardiovascular Medicine. Philadelphia: WB Saunders, 2001.
5. Keaney JFJ. Atherosclerosis: from lesion formation to plaque activation and endothelial dysfunction. Mol Aspects Med 2000;21:99–166.
6. Stary HC. The Evolution of Human Atherosclerotic Lesions. Philadelphia: Merck&Co, 1993.
7. Kannel WB, McGee DL. Update on some epidemiologic features of intermittent claudication: the Framingham Study. J Am Geriatr Soc 1985;33:13–18.
8. Fowkes FG. Epidemiology of atherosclerotic arterial disease in the lower limbs. Eur J Vasc Surg 1988; 2:283–291.
9. Newman AB, Siscovick DS, Manolio TA, et al. Ankle-arm index as a marker of atherosclerosis in the Cardiovascular Health Study: Cardiovascular Heart Study (CHS) Collaborative Research Group. Circulation 1993;88:837–845.
10. Murabito JM, D'Agostino RB, Silbershatz H, Wilson WF. Intermittent claudication: a risk profile from the Framingham Heart Study. Circulation 1997;96:44–49.
11. Brand FN, Abbott RD, Kannel WB. Diabetes, intermittent claudication, and risk of cardiovascular events: the Framingham Study. Diabetes 1989;38:504–509.
12. Strandness DE, Jr, Priest RE, Gibbons GE. Combined clinical and pathologic study of diabetic and nondiabetic peripheral arterial disease. Diabetes 1964;13:366.
13. Jonason T, Ringqvist I. Diabetes mellitus and intermittent claudication: relation between peripheral vascular complications and location of the occlusive atherosclerosis in the legs. Acta Med Scand 1985;218:217–221.
14. McDaniel MD, Cronenwett JL. Basic data related to the natural history of intermittent claudication. Ann Vasc Surg 1989;3:273–277.
15. Perloff D, Sokolow M, Cowan R. The prognostic value of ambulatory blood pressures. JAMA 1983; 249:2792–2798.

16. Levy D, Wilson PW, Anderson KM, Castelli WP. Stratifying the patient at risk from coronary disease: new insights from the Framingham Heart Study. Am Heart J 1990;119:712–717.
17. MacMahon S, Peto R, Cutler J, et al. Blood pressure, stroke, and coronary heart disease: part 1. Prolonged differences in blood pressure: prospective observational studies corrected for the regression dilution bias. Lancet 1990;335:765–774.
18. Gurlek A, Dagalp Z, Oral D, et al. Restenosis after transluminal coronary angioplasty: a risk factor analysis. J Cardiovasc Risk 1995;2:51–55.
19. Veterans Administration Cooperative Study Group on Antihypertensive Agents. Effects of treatment on morbidity in hypertension. Results in patients with diastolic blood pressures averaging 115 through 129 mm Hg. JAMA 1967;202:1028–1034.
20. Reaven GM. Insulin resistance and its consequences: type 2 diabetes mellitus and coronary heart disease. In: LeRoith D, Taylor SI, Olefsky JM, eds. Diabetes Mellitus, 2nd edit. Philadelphia: Lippincott-Raven, 2000, pp. 604–615.
21. Chen YD, Swami S, Skowronski R, Coulston A, Reaven GM. Differences in postprandial lipemia between patients with normal glucose tolerance and noninsulin-dependent diabetes mellitus. J Clin Endocrinol Metab 1993;76:172–177.
22. Haffner SM, Stern MP, Mitchell BD, Hazuda HP, Patterson JK. Incidence of type II diabetes in Mexican Americans predicted by fasting insulin and glucose levels, obesity, and body-fat distribution. Diabetes 1990;39:283–288.
23. Lillioja S, Mott DM, Spraul M, et al. Insulin resistance and insulin secretory dysfunction as precursors of non-insulin-dependent diabetes mellitus: prospective studies of Pima Indians. N Engl J Med 1993;329:1988–1992.
24. Warram JH, Martin BC, Krolewski AS, Soeldner JS, Kahn CR. Slow glucose removal rate and hyperinsulinemia precede the development of type II diabetes in the offspring of diabetic parents. Ann Intern Med 1990;113:909–915.
25. Welborn TA, Wearne K. Coronary heart disease incidence and cardiovascular mortality in Busselton with reference to glucose and insulin concentrations. Diabetes Care 1979;2:154–160.
26. Pyorala K. Relationship of glucose tolerance and plasma insulin to the incidence of coronary heart disease: results from two population studies in Finland. Diabetes Care 1979;2:131–141.
27. Ducimetiere P, Eschwege E, Papoz L, Richard JL, Claude JR, Rosselin G. Relationship of plasma insulin levels to the incidence of myocardial infarction and coronary heart disease mortality in a middle-aged population. Diabetologia 1980;19:205–210.
28. Despres JP, Lamarche B, Mauriege P, et al. Hyperinsulinemia as an independent risk factor for ischemic heart disease. N Engl J Med 1996;334:952–957.
29. Burchfiel CM, Sharp DS, Curb JD, et al. Hyperinsulinemia and cardiovascular disease in elderly men: the Honolulu Heart Program. Arterioscler Thromb Vasc Biol 1998;18:450–457.
30. Yip J, Facchini FS, Reaven GM. Resistance to insulin-mediated glucose disposal as a predictor of cardiovascular disease. J Clin Endocrinol Metab 1998;83:2773–2776.
31. Lissner L, Bengtsson C, Lapidus L, Kristjansson K, Wedel H. Fasting insulin in relation to subsequent blood pressure changes and hypertension in women. Hypertension 1992;20:797–801.
32. Raitakari OT, Porkka KV, Ronnemaa T, et al. The role of insulin in clustering of serum lipids and blood pressure in children and adolescents: the Cardiovascular Risk in Young Finns Study. Diabetologia 1995;38:1042–1050.
33. Jeppesen J, Hein HO, Suadicani P, Gyntelberg F. High triglycerides and low HDL cholesterol and blood pressure and risk of ischemic heart disease. Hypertension 2000;36:226–232.
34. Reaven GM, Chen YD. Role of insulin in regulation of lipoprotein metabolism in diabetes. Diabetes Metab Rev 1988;4:639–652.
35. Laws A, Reaven GM. Evidence for an independent relationship between insulin resistance and fasting plasma HDL-cholesterol, triglyceride and insulin concentrations. J Intern Med 1992;231: 25–30.
36. Reaven GM, Chen YD, Jeppesen J, Maheux P, Krauss RM. Insulin resistance and hyperinsulinemia in individuals with small, dense low density lipoprotein particles. J Clin Invest 1993;92:141–146.
37. Abbasi F, McLaughlin T, Lamendola C, et al. Fasting remnant lipoprotein cholesterol and triglyceride concentrations are elevated in nondiabetic, insulin-resistant, female volunteers. J Clin Endocrinol Metab 1999;84:3903–3906.
38. McCully KS. Vascular pathology of homocysteinemia: implications for the pathogenesis of arteriosclerosis. Am J Pathol 1969;56:111–128.

39. Malinow MR. Hyperhomocyst(e)inemia: a common and easily reversible risk factor for occlusive atherosclerosis. Circulation 1990;81:2004–2006.

40. Stubbs PJ, Al-Obaidi MK, Conroy RM, et al. Effect of plasma homocysteine concentration on early and late events in patients with acute coronary syndromes. Circulation 2000;102:605–610.

41. Clarke R, Daly L, Robinson K, et al. Hyperhomocysteinemia: an independent risk factor for vascular disease. N Engl J Med 1991;324:1149–1155.

42. Nygard O, Nordrehaug JE, Refsum H, Ueland PM, Farstad M, Vollset SE. Plasma homocysteine levels and mortality in patients with coronary artery disease. N Engl J Med 1997;337:230–236.

43. Selhub J, Jacques PF, Bostom AG, et al. Association between plasma homocysteine concentrations and extracranial carotid-artery stenosis. N Engl J Med 1995;332:286–291.

44. Virchow R. Gesammelte Abhandlungen zur Wissenschaftlichen Medizin. Frankfurt: Meidinger Sohn & Co., 1856, pp. 219–732.

45. Ross R, Glomset J, Harker L. Response to injury and atherogenesis. Am J Pathol 1977;86:675–684.

46. Jaffe EA. Biology of the Endothelial Cell. New York: Martinus Nijhoff, 1984.

47. Cooke JP. The endothelium: a new target for therapy. Vasc Med 2000;5:49–53.

48. Cooke JP, Tsao P. Endothelium-derived relaxing factor: an overview. In: Sowers JR, ed. Contemporary Endocrinology: Endocrinology of the Vasculature. Totowa, NJ: Humana Press, 1996, 3–19.

49. Furchgott RF, Zawadzki JV. The obligatory role of endothelial cells in the relaxation of arterial smooth muscle by acetylcholine. Nature 1980;288:373–376.

50. Palmer RM, Ferrige AG, Moncada S. Nitric oxide release accounts for the biological activity of endothelium-derived relaxing factor. Nature 1987;327:524–526.

51. Ignarro LJ, Byrns RE, Buga GM, Wood KS. Endothelium-derived relaxing factor from pulmonary artery and vein possesses pharmacologic and chemical properties identical to those of nitric oxide radical. Circ Res 1987;61:866–879.

52. Myers PR, Minor RL, Jr, Guerra R, Jr, Bates JN, Harrison DG. Vasorelaxant properties of the endothelium-derived relaxing factor more closely resemble S-nitrosocysteine than nitric oxide. Nature 1990;345:161–163.

53. Ignarro LJ. Introduction and overview. In: Ignarro LJ, ed. Nitric Oxide-Biology and Pathobiology. San Diego: Academic Press, New York, 2000, pp. 3–19.

54. Palmer RM, Ashton DS, Moncada S. Vascular endothelial cells synthesize nitric oxide from L-arginine. Nature 1988;333:664–666.

55. Cooke JP, Rossitch E, Jr, Andon NA, Loscalzo J, Dzau VJ. Flow activates an endothelial potassium channel to release an endogenous nitrovasodilator. J Clin Invest 1991;88:1663–1671.

56. Ludmer PL, Selwyn AP, Shook TL, et al. Paradoxical vasoconstriction induced by acetylcholine in atherosclerotic coronary arteries. N Engl J Med 1986;315:1046–1051.

57. Radomski MW, Palmer RM, Moncada S. Comparative pharmacology of endothelium-derived relaxing factor, nitric oxide and prostacyclin in platelets. Br J Pharmacol 1987;92:181–187.

58. Bath PM, Hassall DG, Gladwin AM, Palmer RM, Martin JF. Nitric oxide and prostacyclin: divergence of inhibitory effects on monocyte chemotaxis and adhesion to endothelium in vitro. Arterioscler Thromb 1991;11:254–260.

59. Garg UC, Hassid A. Nitric oxide-generating vasodilators and 8-bromo-cyclic guanosine monophosphate inhibit mitogenesis and proliferation of cultured rat vascular smooth muscle cells. J Clin Invest 1989;83:1774–1777.

60. Tsao PS, Lewis NP, Alpert S, Cooke JP. Exposure to shear stress alters endothelial adhesiveness: role of nitric oxide. Circulation 1995;92:3513–3519.

61. Tsao PS, Buitrago R, Chan JR, Cooke JP. Fluid flow inhibits endothelial adhesiveness: nitric oxide and transcriptional regulation of VCAM-1. Circulation 1996;94:1682–1689.

62. Tsao PS, Wang B, Buitrago R, Shyy JY, Cooke JP. Nitric oxide regulates monocyte chemotactic protein-1. Circulation 1997;96:934–940.

63. De Caterina R, Libby P, Peng HB, et al. Nitric oxide decreases cytokine-induced endothelial activation: nitric oxide selectively reduces endothelial expression of adhesion molecules and proinflammatory cytokines. J Clin Invest 1995;96:60–68.

64. Cooke JP, Singer AH, Tsao P, Zera P, Rowan RA, Billingham ME. Antiatherogenic effects of L-arginine in the hypercholesterolemic rabbit. J Clin Invest 1992;90:1168–1172.

65. Cayatte AJ, Palacino JJ, Horten K, Cohen RA. Chronic inhibition of nitric oxide production accelerates neointima formation and impairs endothelial function in hypercholesterolemic rabbits. Arterioscler Thromb 1994;14:753–759.

66. Naruse K, Shimizu K, Muramatsu M, et al. Long-term inhibition of NO synthesis promotes atherosclerosis in the hypercholesterolemic rabbit thoracic aorta. PGH2 does not contribute to impaired endothelium-dependent relaxation. Arterioscler Thromb 1994;14:746–752.

67. Cohen RA. The role of nitric oxide and other endothelium-derived vasoactive substances in vascular disease. Prog Cardiovasc Dis 1995;38:105–128.

68. Diehm C, Balzer K, Bisler H, et al. Efficacy of a new prostaglandin E1 regimen in outpatients with severe intermittent claudication: results of a multicenter placebo-controlled double-blind trial. J Vasc Surg 1997;25:537–544.

69. Scheffer P, de la Hamette D, Leipnitz G. Therapeutic efficacy of intravenously applied prostaglandin E1. Vasa 1989;28S:19–25.

70. Drexler H, Zeiher AM, Meinzer K, Just H. Correction of endothelial dysfunction in coronary microcirculation of hypercholesterolaemic patients by L-arginine. Lancet 1991;338:1546–1550.

71. Boger RH, Bode-Boger SM, Thiele W, Junker W, Alexander K, Frolich JC. Biochemical evidence for impaired nitric oxide synthesis in patients with peripheral arterial occlusive disease. Circulation 1997; 95:2068–2074.

72. Creager MA, Cooke JP, Mendelsohn ME, et al. Impaired vasodilation of forearm resistance vessels in hypercholesterolemic humans. J Clin Invest 1990;86:228–234.

73. Casino PR, Kilcoyne CM, Quyyumi AA, Hoeg JM, Panza JA. The role of nitric oxide in endothelium-dependent vasodilation of hypercholesterolemic patients. Circulation 1993;88:2541–2547.

74. Egashira K, Hirooka Y, Kuga T, Mohri M, Takeshita A. Effects of L-arginine supplementation on endothelium-dependent coronary vasodilation in patients with angina pectoris and normal coronary arteriograms. Circulation 1996;94:130–134.

75. Tousoulis D, Davies GJ, Tentolouris C, et al. Effects of changing the availability of the substrate for nitric oxide synthase by L-arginine administration on coronary vasomotor tone in angina patients with angiographically narrowed and in patients with normal coronary arteries. Am J Cardiol 1998;82:1110–1113.

76. Bode-Boger SM, Boger RH, Alfke H, et al. L-Arginine induces nitric oxide-dependent vasodilation in patients with critical limb ischemia: a randomized, controlled study. Circulation 1996;93:85–90.

77. Boger RH, Bode-Boger SM, Thiele W, Creutzig A, Alexander K, Frolich JC. Restoring vascular nitric oxide formation by L-arginine improves the symptoms of intermittent claudication in patients with peripheral arterial occlusive disease. J Am Coll Cardiol 1998;32:1336–1344.

78. Anderson TJ. Oxidative stress, endothelial function and coronary atherosclerosis. Cardiologia 1997; 42:701–714.

79. Drexler H. Nitric oxide and coronary endothelial dysfunction in humans. Cardiovasc Res 1999;43: 572–579.

80. Verbeuren TJ, Coene MC, Jordaens FH, Van Hove CE, Zonnekeyn LL, Herman AG. Effect of hypercholesterolemia on vascular reactivity in the rabbit. II: Influence of treatment with dipyridamole on endothelium-dependent and endothelium-independent responses in isolated aortas of control and hypercholesterolemic rabbits. Circ Res 1986;59:496–504.

81. Harrison DG, Freiman PC, Armstrong ML, Marcus ML, Heistad DD. Alterations of vascular reactivity in atherosclerosis. Circ Res 1987;61 (Suppl II):74–80.

82. McLenachan JM, Williams JK, Fish RD, Ganz P, Selwyn AP. Loss of flow-mediated endothelium-dependent dilation occurs early in the development of atherosclerosis. Circulation 1991;84: 1273–1278.

83. Merkel LA, Rivera LM, Bilder GE, Perrone MH. Differential alteration of vascular reactivity in rabbit aorta with modest elevation of serum cholesterol. Circ Res 1990;67:550–555.

84. Preik M, Kelm M, Schoebel F, Schottenfeld Y, Leschke M, Strauer BE. Selective impairment of nitric oxide dependent vasodilation in young adults with hypercholesterolaemia. J Cardiovasc Risk 1996;3:465–471.

85. Zeiher AM, Schachlinger V, Hohnloser SH, Saurbier B, Just H. Coronary atherosclerotic wall thickening and vascular reactivity in humans: elevated high-density lipoprotein levels ameliorate abnormal vasoconstriction in early atherosclerosis. Circulation 1994;89:2525–2532.

86. Evans M, Anderson RA, Graham J, et al. Ciprofibrate therapy improves endothelial function and reduces postprandial lipemia and oxidative stress in type 2 diabetes mellitus. Circulation 2000;101: 1773–1779.

87. Dupuis J, Tardif JC, Cernacek P, Theroux P. Cholesterol reduction rapidly improves endothelial function after acute coronary syndromes: the RECIFE (reduction of cholesterol in ischemia and function of the endothelium) trial. Circulation 1999;99:3227–3233.

88. Rosenson RS, Tangney CC. Antiatherothrombotic properties of statins: implications for cardiovascular event reduction. JAMA 1998;279:1643–1650.
89. Vita JA, Yeung AC, Winniford M, et al. Effect of cholesterol-lowering therapy on coronary endothelial vasomotor function in patients with coronary artery disease. Circulation 2000;102:846–851.
90. Laufs U, La Fata V, Plutzky J, Liao JK. Upregulation of endothelial nitric oxide synthase by HMG CoA reductase inhibitors. Circulation 1998;97:1129–1135.
91. Di-Poi N, Faure J, Grizot S, Molnar G, Pick E, Dagher MC. Mechanism of NADPH oxidase activation by the Rac/Rho-GDI complex. Biochemistry 2001;40:10014–10022.
92. Kandabashi T, Shimokawa H, Miyata K, et al. Inhibition of myosin phosphatase by upregulated rho-kinase plays a key role for coronary artery spasm in a porcine model with interleukin-1beta. Circulation 2000;101:1319–1323.
93. Hernandez-Perera O, Perez-Sala D, Soria E, Lamas S. Involvement of Rho GTPases in the transcriptional inhibition of preproendothelin-1 gene expression by simvastatin in vascular endothelial cells. Circ Res 2000;87:616–622.
94. Johnstone MT, Creager SJ, Scales KM, Cusco JA, Lee BK, Creager MA. Impaired endothelium-dependent vasodilation in patients with insulin-dependent diabetes mellitus. Circulation 1993;88: 2510–2516.
95. McVeigh GE, Brennan GM, Johnston GD, et al. Impaired endothelium-dependent and independent vasodilation in patients with type 2 (non-insulin-dependent) diabetes mellitus. Diabetologia 1992;35: 771–776.
96. Calver A, Collier J, Vallance P. Inhibition and stimulation of nitric oxide synthesis in the human forearm arterial bed of patients with insulin-dependent diabetes. J Clin Invest 1992;90:2548–2554.
97. Williams SB, Cusco JA, Roddy MA, Johnstone MT, Creager MA. Impaired nitric oxide-mediated vasodilation in patients with non-insulin-dependent diabetes mellitus. J Am Coll Cardiol 1996;27: 567–574.
98. Tesfamariam B, Brown ML, Deykin D, Cohen RA. Elevated glucose promotes generation of endothelium-derived vasoconstrictor prostanoids in rabbit aorta. J Clin Invest 1990;85:929–932.
99. Tesfamariam B, Cohen RA. Role of superoxide anion and endothelium in vasoconstrictor action of prostaglandin endoperoxide. Am J Physiol 1992;262:H1915–1919.
100. Williams SB, Goldfine AB, Timimi FK, et al. Acute hyperglycemia attenuates endothelium-dependent vasodilation in humans in vivo. Circulation 1998;97:1695–1701.
101. Miller AW, Katakam PV, Ujhelyi MR. Impaired endothelium-mediated relaxation in coronary arteries from insulin-resistant rats. J Vasc Res 1999;36:385–392.
102. Katakam PV, Ujhelyi MR, Hoenig ME, Miller AW. Endothelial dysfunction precedes hypertension in diet-induced insulin resistance. Am J Physiol 1998;275:R788–792.
103. Kashiwagi A, Shinozaki K, Nishio Y, Okamura T, Toda N, Kikkawa R. Free radical production in endothelial cells as a pathogenetic factor for vascular dysfunction in the insulin resistance state. Diabetes Res Clin Pract 1999;45:199–203.
104. Steinberg HO, Chaker H, Leaming R, Johnson A, Brechtel G, Baron AD. Obesity/insulin resistance is associated with endothelial dysfunction. Implications for the syndrome of insulin resistance. J Clin Invest 1996;97:2601–2610.
105. Tomiyama H, Kimura Y, Okazaki R, et al. Close relationship of abnormal glucose tolerance with endothelial dysfunction in hypertension. Hypertension 2000;36:245–249.
106. Balletshofer BM, Rittig K, Enderle MD, et al. Endothelial dysfunction is detectable in young normotensive first-degree relatives of subjects with type 2 diabetes in association with insulin resistance. Circulation 2000;101:1780–1784.
107. Stülhlinger MC, Abbasi F, Chu JW, Lamendola C, McLaughlin TL, Cooke JP, Reaven GM, Tsao PS. Relationship between insulin resistance and an endogenous nitric oxide synthase inhibitor. JAMA 2002; 287:1420–1426.
108. Luscher TF, Vanhoutte PM, Raij L. Antihypertensive treatment normalizes decreased endothelium-dependent relaxations in rats with salt-induced hypertension. Hypertension 1987;9(Suppl III): 193–197.
109. Shultz PJ, Raij L. Effects of antihypertensive agents on endothelium-dependent and endothelium-independent relaxations. Br J Clin Pharmacol 1989;28:151S–157S.
110. Ribeiro MO, Antunes E, de Nucci G, Lovisolo SM, Zatz R. Chronic inhibition of nitric oxide synthesis: a new model of arterial hypertension. Hypertension 1992;20:298-303.
111. Huang PL, Huang Z, Mashimo H, et al. Hypertension in mice lacking the gene for endothelial nitric oxide synthase. Nature 1995;377:239–242.

112. Linder L, Kiowski W, Buhler FR, Luscher TF. Indirect evidence for release of endothelium-derived relaxing factor in human forearm circulation in vivo: blunted response in essential hypertension. Circulation 1990;81:1762–1767.
113. Panza JA, Quyyumi AA, Brush JE, Jr., Epstein SE. Abnormal endothelium-dependent vascular relaxation in patients with essential hypertension. N Engl J Med 1990;323:22–27.
114. Tawakol A, Omland T, Gerhard M, Wu JT, Creager MA. Hyperhomocyst(e)inemia is associated with impaired endothelium-dependent vasodilation in humans. Circulation 1997;95:1119–1121.
115. Chambers JC, McGregor A, Jean-Marie J, Obeid OA, Kooner JS. Demonstration of rapid onset vascular endothelial dysfunction after hyperhomocysteinemia: an effect reversible with vitamin C therapy. Circulation 1999;99:1156–1160.
116. Joannides R, Haefeli WE, Linder L, et al. Nitric oxide is responsible for flow-dependent dilatation of human peripheral conduit arteries in vivo. Circulation 1995;91:1314–1319.
117. Harker LA, Ross R, Slichter SJ, Scott CR. Homocystine-induced arteriosclerosis: the role of endothelial cell injury and platelet response in its genesis. J Clin Invest 1976;58:731–741.
118. Starkebaum G, Harlan JM. Endothelial cell injury due to copper-catalyzed hydrogen peroxide generation from homocysteine. J Clin Invest 1986;77:1370–1376.
119. Lang D, Kredan MB, Moat SJ, et al. Homocysteine-induced inhibition of endothelium-dependent relaxation in rabbit aorta: role for superoxide anions. Arterioscler Thromb Vasc Biol 2000;20:422–427.
120. Eberhardt RT, Forgione MA, Cap A, et al. Endothelial dysfunction in a murine model of mild hyperhomocyst(e)inemia. J Clin Invest 2000;106:483–491.
121. Upchurch GR, Jr., Welch GN, Fabian AJ, et al. Homocyst(e)ine decreases bioavailable nitric oxide by a mechanism involving glutathione peroxidase. J Biol Chem 1997;272:17012–17017.
122. Boger RH, Bode-Boger SM, Sydow K, Heistad DD, Lentz SR. Plasma concentration of asymmetric dimethylarginine, an endogenous inhibitor of nitric oxide synthase, is elevated in monkeys with hyperhomocyst(e)inemia or hypercholesterolemia. Arterioscler Thromb Vasc Biol 2000;20:1557–1564.
123. Boger RH, Lentz SR, Bode-Boger SM, Knapp HR, Haynes WG. Elevation of asymmetrical dimethylarginine may mediate endothelial dysfunction during experimental hyperhomocyst(e)inaemia in humans. Clin Sci (Colch) 2001;100:161–167.

2

The Epidemiology and Natural History of Peripheral Arterial Disease

Lisa M. Bordeaux, RN, MSN, FNP,
Laura M. Reich, DO, and Alan T. Hirsch, MD

CONTENTS

INTRODUCTION

Peripheral arterial disease (PAD) is a manifestation of systemic atherosclerosis, and is defined by progressive stenosis or occlusion within the arteries of the lower extremities. Although PAD is the currently accepted international term for this clinical syndrome *(1)*, historically, other names have been used interchangeably, including peripheral arterial occlusive disease (PAOD), arteriosclerosis obliterans (ASO), lower extremity occlusive disease (LEAD), and peripheral vascular disease (PVD). Widely prevalent, it has been estimated that more than 8.4 million people are afflicted with this disease in the United States *(2,3)*. As with other clinical atherosclerotic syndromes, the etiology of PAD is due to both modifiable (diabetes, smoking, hypertension, and hypercholesterolemia) and nonmodifiable (e.g., age, gender, family history) risk factors.

The decreased blood flow to the legs caused by PAD may be mild or severe, resulting in a broad range of symptoms. Patients may not suffer recognizable limb symptoms, or they may experience intermittent claudication (IC), or manifest symptoms of severe limb ischemia. IC, the most common symptom of PAD, is defined as fatigue, cramping,

From: *Contemporary Cardiology: Peripheral Arterial Disease: Diagnosis and Treatment*
Edited by: J. D. Coffman and R. T. Eberhardt © Humana Press Inc., Totowa, NJ

or frank pain of the gluteal, thigh, or calf muscles that is consistently provoked by exercise and that is reproducibly relieved by rest. Patients with IC are often limited in their daily activities owing to this walking impairment and in turn experience a diminished quality of life. With continued exposure to atherosclerotic risk factors, PAD may progress to critical limb ischemia (CLI), which portends a severe diminution in quality of life, and is associated with a high rate of amputation and a marked increase in short-term mortality. Thus, PAD is a common manifestation of atherosclerosis that is associated with a range of symptoms, a variable impact on quality of life, and a heightened risk of cardiovascular ischemic events.

Whereas the clinical diagnosis of PAD is dependent on the vascular history, the physical examination, and selective use of noninvasive vascular laboratory and invasive angiographic criteria, the epidemiologic definition of PAD is based on measurement of the ankle–brachial index (ABI). The ABI serves as a simple and accurate noninvasive tool to objectively assess lower extremity blood flow, and any ABI value < 0.90 defines the presence of PAD. This dependence on the ABI is based on data demonstrating that an abnormal pulse examination alone underestimates the true prevalence of PAD, and may specifically underestimate small-vessel PAD *(4)*. These data from Criqui and colleagues demonstrated that the sensitivity and specificity of an abnormal pulse detecting PAD were 77% and 86%, respectively, while the positive and negative predictive values (PPV) were 40% and 97%, respectively. Other surveys have suggested that the sensitivity of an absent pulse to predict the presence of PAD may be only 5% and the positive predictive value as low as 20% *(5)*. In contrast, the ABI has high sensitivity and specificity for angiographically defined PAD *(6,7)*. It should be noted that an abnormal ABI is not only diagnostic of PAD, but is also a predictor of cardiovascular morbidity and mortality *(8)*.

CLASSICAL ATHEROSCLEROTIC RISK FACTORS AND THE DEVELOPMENT OF PAD

Specific risk factors have been associated with the development of peripheral arterial, coronary artery, and cerebrovascular disease. These traditional risk factors include smoking, diabetes, family history, hypertension, and hyperlipidemia *(9,10)*. The relative risk (RR) of developing PAD is most closely associated with diabetes (RR 4.05), current smoking (RR 2.55), increasing age (in 5-yr increments, RR 1.54), hypertension (RR 1.51), hyperhomocystinemia (RR 1.44), and elevated total cholesterol (RR 1.10 per 10 mg/dL increment) (Fig. 1). Compared to the impact of these risk factors on coronary artery disease (CAD) prevalence rates, smoking and diabetes are particularly prominent factors in the development of PAD.

Tobacco Smoking

Smoking is one of the primary risk factors for developing PAD, especially in young individuals. Smoking causes damage to the vascular endothelium, promotes coagulation, and accelerates the progression of atherosclerosis *(11)*. In the Cardiovascular Health Study, the relative risk of developing PAD was 2.5 for current smokers *(12)*. Another study found that the relative risk of developing PAD was increased as much as sevenfold in ex-smokers and as much as 16-fold in current smokers, as compared to those who had never smoked *(13)*. Just as PAD prevalence is known to be directly related

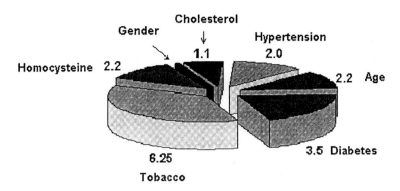

Fig. 1. The relative risk of developing PAD associated with each atherosclerosis risk factor. Tobacco use and diabetes confer the highest relative risk for PAD. PAD is a "gender neutral" atherosclerotic syndrome, although the onset of PAD is delayed in women until after menopause. (Modified from Newman AB, Siscovick DS, Manolio TA, et al. Ankle–arm index as a marker of atherosclerosis in the Cardiovascular Health Study. Cardiovascular Health Study (CHS) Collaborative Research Group. Circulation. 1993; 88:837–845.)

to population-based smoking rates, so too has the prevalence of PAD been shown to decrease with a decline in current smoking rates. The landmark Reykjavik Study *(14)* prospectively observed Icelandic males for 18 yr and identified smoking and serum cholesterol level as the only significant risk factors, other than age, that predicted the incidence of IC in this defined population. Smoking was shown to increase the risk of IC eight- to tenfold. More importantly, the prevalence and incidence of IC in the male Icelandic population fell sharply after 1970, as lifestyle-derived exposure to atherosclerotic risk factors improved in the population at risk. The relationship between tobacco use and claudication prevalence was also noted in the Framingham Study. In this American cohort of 5209 individuals, aged 30–62 yr at enrollment and followed for 34 yr, there was a direct correlation between the amount of cigarette smoking in the population and the incidence of IC. A similar relationship was noted between tobacco use and the incidence of stroke and transient ischemic attacks and the population-based burden of total cardiovascular disease *(15)*.

Smoking not only has been shown to cause a more rapid development of PAD with long-term use, but is also associated with the development of "premature atherosclerosis" and a particular syndrome of PAD in young women who are heavy smokers. These young women may develop an atherosclerotic "hypoplastic aortoiliac syndrome" in their third and fourth decades of life, causing both claudication and/or CLI *(16)*. The morbidity associated with this syndrome can be significant, because a high fraction may progress to severe limb ischemia that may require aorto-bifemoral bypass surgery *(16)*. The impact of continued tobacco use on PAD progression has also been demonstrated by the work of Jonason and colleagues, who demonstrated that patients with PAD who continue to smoke face a markedly increased risk of developing CLI, with as many as 18% of a PAD population developing CLI with continued tobacco use *(17)*. Furthermore, the mortality rate within a 5-yr period is approx 40–50% due to myocardial infarction (MI) or stroke *(18,19)*. Patients with PAD who undergo limb bypass who continue to smoke suffer lower patency rates and higher amputation rates than those who quit *(20,21)*.

Diabetes Mellitus

Another common risk factor, diabetes mellitus, promotes acceleration of the athero-sclerotic process, resulting in a higher incidence of peripheral, coronary, and cere-brovascular disease. The exact pathophysiologic relationship of diabetes to development of PAD is unclear, as there are both direct effects of hyperglycemia as well as an increased frequency of hypertension and hyperlipidemia in patients with diabetes. Patients with the metabolic syndrome (defined by insulin resistance, increased trigly-cerides, decreased high-density lipoprotein [HDL], and small dense low-density lipoprotein [LDL] particles) seem to have an especially elevated risk for developing PAD (9). In the Cardiovascular Health Study, the relative risk for developing PAD was increased more than fourfold for those with diabetes (12). The high prevalence of PAD in individuals with diabetes has been demonstrated in the Hoorn Study, in which almost 21% of those elderly individuals with diabetes had an ABI < 0.9, and in which almost 42% had either an abnormal ABI, diminished ankle pulse, or history of prior limb bypass surgery (22).

Diabetes serves as a powerful risk factor for development of atherosclerosis of the large- and medium-sized muscular conduit arteries that supply the lower extremity and it is this effect that leads to the greatest burden of PAD in diabetic patients. However, diabetes is also associated with multisegmental and more distal arterial stenoses, and may damage the microvascular circulation, which makes revascularization difficult. The diffuse anatomic arterial disease, magnitude of small vessel disease, associated neu-ropathy, propensity for infection, and impaired wound healing common in diabetics may together contribute to the higher incidence of amputation among them (23). Whether this particularly adverse PAD natural history can be altered by aggressive glycemic con-trol has not yet been demonstrated in prospective clinical trials (24,25).

Hyperlipidemia

Hyperlipidemia alters the endothelial cells of the arterial wall, which leads to the for-mation of atherosclerotic lesions. Endothelial cells play a key role in preventing this process. They produce nitric oxide, which inhibits monocytes, leukocytes, and platelet adhesion to the arterial lining; decrease LDL permeability; and prevent smooth muscle cell proliferation (26). LDL cholesterol is one of the major causes of endothelial dys-function and smooth muscle injury. It is this initial alteration to the endothelium that allows lipoprotein to enter the arterial wall, become oxidized, and promote the develop-ment of the fatty streak, which is the earliest lesion in atherosclerosis. This in turn leads to a more complex lesion causing arterial stenosis or occlusion (27). Elevated levels of LDL cholesterol pose an increased risk of developing cardiovascular disease and PAD (28). In the Framingham Heart Study, individuals with total cholesterol levels > 270 mg/dL had twice the incidence of developing IC (29). In addition, people with IC had a higher mean cholesterol level (10).

Hypertension

Twenty-four percent of the U.S. population has hypertension, and thus the impact of this common vascular risk factor on PAD prevalence rates is high (30). Hypertension causes complex alterations in the structure of the arterial wall. Endothelial function is impaired, collagen may replace elastin in arterial walls, and there is medial hypertrophy (31). All these factors contribute to decreasing vascular compliance (31). Hypertension leads to more aggressive atherosclerosis in all circulations, and is a recognized risk factor for cerebrovascular and coronary disease. Hypertension is now also recognized as a major risk factor for developing PAD *(32)*.

One clinical investigation that evaluated the association between hypertension, cardiovascular event rates, and PAD, the Systolic Hypertension in the Elderly Program (SHEP), demonstrated a 27% reduction in coronary ischemic events in patients actively treated for their systolic hypertension *(33)*. A subgroup of the SHEP cohort with peripheral atherosclerotic disease was shown to experience significantly fewer cardiovascular ischemic events and less mortality when systolic hypertension was actively treated vs placebo (the relative risk of a cardiac event in the placebo group vs active treatment was 2.2) *(33)*. This supports the need for aggressive hypertensive management in patients with PAD to decrease rates of mortality and ischemic events. Although the treatment of hypertension would be expected to impact beneficially the prognosis of PAD symptoms or limb outcomes, there have been no investigations to address this hypothesis.

Newer Risk Factors for the Development of PAD

There is increasing interest in the association between the development of PAD and selected newer risk factors, such as hyperhomocystinemia *(34,35)*. Recent studies have also shown that markers of vascular inflammation, such as an elevated C-reactive protein (CRP) value, may predict the future risk of developing PAD *(36)*.

HYPERHOMOCYSTINEMIA

Elevated homocysteine has been shown to be an independent risk factor associated with development of premature atherosclerosis or atherothrombosis *(37)*. A genetic mutation of the enzyme involved with homocysteine metabolism or a deficiency of essential B vitamins leads to elevated homocysteine levels. Homocysteine is a highly reactive amino acid that is known to cause endothelial cell dysfunction and injury resulting in platelet activation, thrombosis, and increased vascular smooth muscle proliferation leading to more aggressive atherogenesis *(38)*.

INFLAMMATION AND INFECTION

The formation and progression of atherosclerosis are presumed to be due to the complex interplay of classical risk factors, in association with an intravascular inflammatory process *(39)*. A fatty streak, which is the earliest lesion of atherosclerosis, is a pure inflammatory lesion consisting of monocyte-derived macrophages and T lymphocytes *(40)*. One marker that may prove useful to detect this inflammatory process is the CRP. In the Physicians' Health Study and the Women's Health Study, individuals with the highest CRP levels at baseline showed a two- to sevenfold higher risk of stroke, three- to sevenfold higher risk of MI, and four- to fivefold higher risk of severe PAD or vascular events compared to the control group *(41,42)* (Fig. 2). In addition, the Monitoring Trends and Determinants in Cardiovascular Disease Augsburg Cohort (MONICA) also showed that CRP is a predictor of cardiovascular disease *(43)*.

The possibility that chronic infection and inflammation due to atypical organisms may contribute to the pathogenesis of atherosclerosis in coronary, cerebral, and peripheral vessels has recently been a subject of investigation. The infectious microorganisms that have been linked to atherosclerotic plaque formation include cytomegalovirus (CMV), the herpes viruses, *Chlamydia pneumoniae*, and *Helicobacter pylori (44)*.

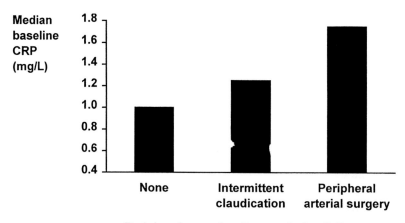

Fig. 2. C-reactive protein (CRP) is an inflammatory marker of atherosclerosis and is elevated in patients with PAD. High-sensitivity CRP levels are elevated in individuals with claudication, and are highest in those patients with PAD who required vascular surgical intervention, as compared to individuals with no PAD. (Modified from: Ridker PM, Cushman M, Stampfer MJ, Tracy RP, Hennekens, CH. Plasma concentration of C-reative protein and risk of developing peripheral arterial disease. Circulation 1998;97: 425-428.)

These microorganisms have been found in high serum concentrations and/or within the arterial wall plaque of individuals with atherosclerosis. It has been hypothesized that such infectious agents could enter vascular endothelial cells and promote plaque formation or rupture. In addition, the leukocytes, macrophages, and lymphocytes within the evolving atheroma may also be infected by these organisms, and this may further promote lesion progression. Although this infection-mediated hypothesis is under active investigation as a cause of coronary artery disease, it is not yet known whether these putative infectious causes of atherosclerosis are important risk factors for PAD.

THE HIGH PREVALENCE OF PAD

PAD is a common syndrome that affects a large proportion of most adult populations worldwide. Claudication is the symptomatic expression of PAD and therefore defines a subset of the total population with PAD. The landmark Framingham Heart Study initially described the high prevalence of PAD. This large cohort study has followed 2336 men and 2873 women between the ages of 28 and 62 at standardized examinations every 2 yr since 1948 *(29)*. The Rose claudication questionnaire was utilized to define the prevalence of IC as a marker of PAD. This study demonstrated that the annual incidence of PAD increased with age and in relation to the previously described risk factors *(29)*. The age-specific annual incidence of IC for ages 30–44 was 6 per 10,000 men and 3 per 10,000 women, and this incidence increased to 61 per 10,000 men and 54 per 10,000 women within the ages of 65–74. In this initial Framingham cohort, the investigators noted that IC was twice as prevalent among men as compared to women *(45)*. A risk profile of age, sex, serum cholesterol, hypertension, cigarette smoking, diabetes, and CAD were all associated with an increased risk of developing claudication. Male sex, increasing age, and smoking conferred a 1.5-fold increased risk for developing IC. Diabetes and stage 2 (or greater) hypertension were associated with a more than twofold increase in IC, while clinical evidence of CAD almost tripled the risk *(10)*.

In another population study, Criqui and colleagues evaluated the prevalence of PAD among an older defined population of 613 men and women in Southern California, utilizing a battery of four noninvasive tests—the Rose questionnaire, the pulse examination, the ABI, and the pulse wave velocity (PWV)—to assess the prevalence of PAD *(46)*. Use of the Rose questionnaire severely underestimated the prevalence of PAD demonstrating the insensitivity of this tool to assess true population rates for PAD. Basing the diagnosis solely on history and physical examination also showed low sensitivity for detecting PAD *(9)*. PAD detection increased two to seven times over the detection rate of the Rose questionnaire when the ABI and pulse wave velocity techniques were applied. On the other hand, an abnormal limb pulse examination overestimated the prevalence by twofold. Using the objective noninvasive ABI and PWV techniques, the prevalence of PAD in this population was 2.5% among individuals < 60 yr of age, 8.3% among those between 60 and 69 yr, and 18.8% among those older than 70 yr *(9)* (Fig. 3).

The San Luis Valley Diabetes Study evaluated the prevalence of PAD among diabetics in a Hispanic and a white population *(5)*. The diagnostic tool used in this study was an ABI of 0.94 at rest, 0.73 post-exercise, and 0.78 after reactive hyperemia. The prevalence of PAD was 13.7% using this diagnostic criteria. Notably, a history of IC or an absent pulse exam were uncommon findings within this population (5).

The Edinburgh Artery Study in 1988 randomly selected 1592 individuals ages 55–74 with IC determined by the World Health Organization questionnaire, the ABI, and the hyperemia test. These participants were followed prospectively for 5 yr for subsequent cardiovascular events and death *(47)*. The prevalence of IC was 4.5% and the incidence was 15.5 per 1000 person-years *(47,48)*. In individuals who were symptomatic initially, 28.8% continued to have pain after 5 yr, 8.2% underwent revascularization or amputation, and 1.4% developed ischemic ulcers *(47)*. Of those individuals who were asymptomatic, 8.0% had advanced PAD with significant blood flow impairment *(48)*.

The relevance of these epidemiologic data to current medical practice has been assessed most recently in the PAD Awareness, Risk and Treatment: New Resources for Survival (PARTNERS) program *(49)*. This was a large prospective survey designed to determine the prevalence of PAD in American primary care practices by applying the ABI to a targeted cohort of 6979 patients evaluated in 350 large volume primary care practices in 25 American cities. In this study, patients older than 70 yr of age or between 50 and 69 yr old with a history of cigarette smoking or diabetes were evaluated prospectively during the course of routine office practice. The diagnosis of PAD was established by either a prior chart diagnosis or by demonstration of an ABI of ≤ 0.90 during the study screening. Using this technique, PAD was detected in a high fraction (29%) of the study population. Within this population, 13% of these patients had PAD only, and 16% had both PAD and another form of atherosclerotic cardiovascular disease (a clinical manifestation of CAD, cerebrovascular disease, or aortic aneurysmal disease). Although PAD was obviously prevalent in this targeted population, the diagnosis was new in 55% of those patients with "PAD only" and in 35% of patients who had both PAD and CVD. As anticipated, the prevalence of tobacco use (23% current, 37%

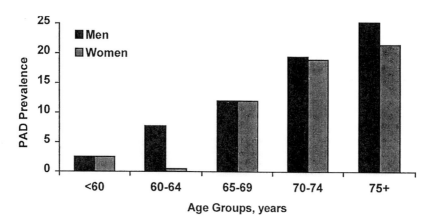

Fig. 3. The increased prevalence of PAD in men and women with advancing age. (Modified from: Criqui MH, Fronek A, Barrett-Connor E, Klauber MR, Gabriel S, Goodman D. The prevalence of peripheral arterial disease in a defined population. Circulation. 1985;71:510-515.)

former), hypertension (69%), hyperlipidemia (47%), and diabetes (38%) was elevated in the PAD-only cohort.

Thus, current epidemiologic and community survey data demonstrate a high prevalence of PAD in individuals in the United States and Europe that increases with advancing age and with increasing exposure to atherosclerosis risk factors.

RELATIONSHIP OF PAD TO OTHER ATHEROSCLEROTIC SYNDROMES

Atherosclerosis is a systemic disease that may affect multiple arteries throughout the body. The diagnosis of PAD should be considered a marker for increased risk of coexistent atherosclerosis involving other vascular territories regardless of whether the patient is asymptomatic or suffers claudication symptoms. It has been shown that individuals diagnosed with PAD have a higher coprevalence of CAD and cerebrovascular disease *(29,32,49)*. Patients found to have lower extremity arterial occlusive disease should undergo a focused physical examination to ascertain if there is coexistent coronary or carotid disease, or an aortic aneurysm.

In a large study by Hertzer and colleagues, severe CAD was found angiographically in 36% of patients with an abdominal aortic aneurysm and in 28% of patients with lower extremity occlusive disease *(50)*. In a separate report, carotid bruits were noted in 11% of patients with abdominal aortic aneurysm and 25% of patients with PAD, while a significant number of patients (44%) proved to have high-grade (> 75%) carotid stenoses or occlusions *(51)*.

In a study of coprevalence of atherosclerotic syndromes by Aronow and Ahn in a long-term care facility, 25% of patients over 62 yr of age had at least two manifestations of atherosclerosis *(52)*. Of patients with CAD, 33% also had PAD and 32% had experienced an ischemic stroke. Of patients with a history of ischemic stroke, 53% also had CAD and 33% also had PAD. Conversely, of those patients with PAD, 58% had CAD and 34% had suffered an ischemic stroke *(52)*.

The clinical overlap of PAD with other atherosclerotic vascular disease was also well defined in the recent Minnesota Regional PAD Screening Program *(53)*. This population, defined by age and presence of exertional limb pain, segregated an elderly (mean age 73 yr) community population into PAD and non-PAD subjects. Of the subjects with PAD, a history of cerebrovascular disease was present in 14% and a history of CAD was present in 56.5%. Non-PAD subjects had much less disease burden—only 2% had cerebrovascular disease and only 26% had CAD.

PAD AS A MARKER OF INCREASED RISK FOR VASCULAR ISCHEMIC EVENTS

Individuals with PAD suffer an increased risk of developing angina, congestive heart failure, fatal and nonfatal MI, fatal and nonfatal stroke, and death. Individuals with PAD suffer a 20–40% increased risk of nonfatal MI *(47)*, 60% risk of developing congestive heart failure *(8)*, and a two- to sevenfold increased risk of death *(2,47)*. The 5-yr longitudinal survey performed in the Edinburgh Artery Study demonstrated an equivalent increased risk for coronary ischemic events and death in both symptomatic and asymptomatic patients with PAD *(47)*. The ABI was shown to be a predictor of cardiovascular events among patients with PAD in the Edinburgh Artery Study, as well as an independent risk factor in the Cardiovascular Health Study *(8)*. The lower the ABI, the greater the occurrence of a fatal or nonfatal MI *(54)*. McKenna and colleagues have documented a 5-yr mortality of approx 30% and 50% in patients with an ABI of 0.70 and 0.40, respectively *(55)*. Even minimal decrements in ABI portend a heightened mortality *(56)*. As noted above, most data suggest that this increased risk of cardiovascular ischemic events and increased mortality is comparable, whether the PAD itself is associated with limb symptoms or not. However, those patients with the most severe limb symptoms or CLI do suffer a magnified short-term risk of ischemic events and death *(2)* (Fig. 4).

The clinical overlap between PAD and cerebrovascular disease also underlies the increased risk of brain ischemic events in those with PAD of any severity. It has also been shown that there is a correlation between symptomatic and asymptomatic PAD and increased intima–media thickness within the carotid arteries *(57)*. The ABI has been shown to be a potent predictor for cerebrovascular events *(54)* and an independent risk factor in the Cardiovascular Health Study *(8)*. Individuals with an ABI < 0.9 had a relative risk of 1.05–3.77 for subsequent stroke *(54)*. In the Edinburgh Artery Study, asymptomatic PAD patients were found to have an increased risk of a nonfatal stroke, although this was not demonstrated for fatal strokes *(47)*. In the study of Ness and colleagues, 42% of elderly patients with PAD (mean age 80) had a coexistent stroke *(58)*.

THE NATURAL HISTORY OF PAD

PAD causes significant morbidity and mortality because of its systemic manifestations. The epidemiology of PAD has been assessed in a number of international investigations that are reviewed in this chapter. However, whereas most clinicians consider patients with claudication to represent the primary clinical presentation, the Rotterdam Study of 7715 patients demonstrated that the vast majority of patients with PAD reported no symptoms of claudication *(59)*.

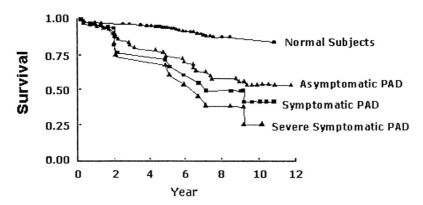

Fig. 4. The survival of all patients with PAD is significantly decreased compared to normal subjects. For patients with severe PAD, 5-yr survival is approx 30%, compared with an approx 80% survival in normal subjects. For patients with asymptomatic or symptomatic PAD, 5-yr survival is only slightly better than for those with severe PAD. (Modified from Criqui MH, Langer RD, Fronek A, Feigelson HS, Klauber MR, McCann TJ, Browner D. Mortality over a period of 10 years in patients with peripheral arterial disease. New Engl J Med 1992;326:381-386. With permission ©1999 Massachusetts Medical Society.)

CLI occurs when PAD progresses to critical impairment of blood flow to the limb due to arterial stenosis or occlusion and may be considered the end stage of the disease. Individuals afflicted by CLI develop rest pain in the affected limb that worsens with elevation and improves with dependency. Dormandy and colleagues reviewed the data from 10 trials that followed patients with IC for 5–18 yr and who did not undergo surgical treatment *(60)*. The general consensus from these studies was that most patients with IC (75%) experience stabilization of their symptoms. Overall, in a population of patients with claudication, only 15–20% ever develop CLI and only 10% require amputation *(61)* (Fig. 5). But as iterated earlier in this chapter, this prognosis is not entirely favorable because the risk of ischemic events and death due to systemic atherosclerotic disease remains formidable, and, unlike that for some patients with PAD, does not improve over time.

THE MODERN ERA: MEDICAL TREATMENT OF PAD MODIFIES THE NATURAL HISTORY

In past decades, the natural history of PAD was defined by the inexorable anatomic progression of arterial stenoses, both within limb arteries and other systemic arteries, with adverse clinical consequences. Past paradigms recounted this natural history with a fatalism that was based on the reality that atherosclerotic risk factors would cause damage that was unlikely to be affected by medical therapies or by vascular surgical interventions. This paradigm no longer applies to the natural history of PAD in modern health care systems, and it is likely that prevalence rates and cardiovascular ischemic event rates are now, more than ever, within the control of the patient and his or her clinician. "Modifiable" risk factors, when modified successfully during long-term care, lead to a more benign natural history and improved clinical outcomes. A comprehensive approach to the medical treatment of PAD is beyond the scope of this chapter; however, risk factor modification and antiplatelet therapies that may alter the natural history of PAD merit careful review (*see* Chapter 9).

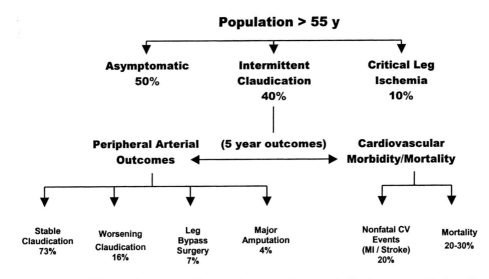

Fig. 5. The natural history of patients with PAD, demonstrating the relative frequency of limb and systemic cardiovascular ischemic events during 5 yr of follow-up. The rates of fatal and nonfatal cardiovascular ischemic events and death are higher than rates of severe limb ischemia. (Modified from Weitz JI, Byrne J, Clagett P, et al. Diagnosis and treatment of chronic arterial insufficiency of the lower extremities: a critical review. Circulation. 1996; 94:3026-3049.)

SUMMARY

PAD is a manifestation of systemic atherosclerosis that is defined by progressive stenosis or occlusion of the arteries of the lower extremities. PAD affects approx 8.4 million Americans and both PAD prevalence and rates of progression increase in association with exposure to atherosclerosis risk factors. The relative risk of developing PAD is most closely associated with diabetes (RR 4.05), current smoking (RR 2.55), increasing age (in 5-yr increments, RR 1.54), hypertension (RR 1.51), hyperhomocystinemia (RR 1.44), and elevated total cholesterol (RR 1.10 per 10 mg/dL increment). Although diabetes and a history of tobacco use are most predictive of PAD risk, hypertension and hypercholesterolemia are highly prevalent in individuals with PAD and serve as potent therapeutic targets that can modify the systemic risk of PAD. PAD severity is also associated with increased levels of high-sensitivity C-reactive protein.

The clinical presentation of PAD includes a spectrum that spans individuals with no apparent lower extremity ischemic symptoms, those who experience IC (discomfort in the limb muscles with exertion), and those with symptoms of severe limb ischemia (pain at rest, nonhealing wounds, or gangrene). Patients with IC are often limited in their daily activities as a result of this walking impairment and in turn experience a diminished quality of life. In a population of patients with claudication, only 15–20% ever develop CLI and only 10% require amputation, yet all face a high risk of systemic cardiovascular ischemic events. With continued exposure to atherosclerotic risk factors, the progression of PAD to critical limb ischemia portends a severe diminution in quality of life, and is associated with a high rate of amputation and a marked short-term increase in mortality.

The diagnosis of PAD should be considered a marker for increased risk of coexistent atherosclerosis regardless of whether the patient is asymptomatic or symptomatic and is most closely predicted by diminution of the ABI. The lower the ABI, the greater the occurrence of a fatal or nonfatal myocardial infarction and death. Individuals with PAD have a higher coprevalence of CAD and cerebrovascular disease. In elderly patients with PAD, as many as 58% may have coexistent CAD and 34% may have a past history of ischemic stroke. This coprevalence of atherosclerotic syndromes in patients with PAD underpins a markedly increased rate of cardiovascular ischemic events in this population. Individuals with PAD suffer a 20–40% increased risk of nonfatal MI, 60% risk of developing congestive heart failure, and a two- to sevenfold increased risk of death.

Thus, PAD is a common manifestation of atherosclerosis that is associated with a range of symptoms, a variable impact on quality of life, and a heightened risk of cardiovascular ischemic events. Poor control of atherosclerosis risk factors is associated with more rapid progression of the PAD natural history, more severe limb symptoms, increased rates of limb loss, and increased mortality. Despite limitations in the treatment database, medical therapies are known to improve the natural history of PAD.

REFERENCES

1. TransAtlantic Inter-Society Consensus (TASC) Working Group. Management of peripheral arterial disease (PAD). J Vasc Surg 2000;31:S1–S296.
2. Criqui MH, Langer RD, Fronek A, et al. Mortality over a period of 10 years in patients with peripheral arterial disease. N Engl J Med 1992;326:381–386.
3. Hiatt WR, Hoag S, Hamman RF. Effect of diagnostic criteria on the prevalence of peripheral arterial disease: the San Luis Valley Diabetes Study. Circulation 1995;91:1472–1479.
4. Criqui MH, Fronek A, Klauber MR, Barrett-Connor E, Gabriel S. The sensitivity, specificity, and predictive value of traditional clinical evaluation of peripheral arterial disease: results from noninvasive testing in a defined population. Circulation 1985;71:516–522.
5. Hiatt WR, Marshall JA, Baxter J, et al. Diagnostic methods for peripheral arterial disease in the San Luis Valley Diabetes Study. J Clin Epidemiol 1990;43:597–606.
6. Carter SA. Indirect systolic pressures and pulse waves in arterial occlusive disease of the lower extremities. Circulation 1968;37:624–637.
7. Fowkes FG. The measurement of atherosclerotic peripheral arterial disease in epidemiological surveys. Int J Epidemiol 1988;17:248–254.
8. Newman AB, Shemanski L, Manolio TA, et al. Ankle-arm index as a predictor of cardiovascular disease and mortality in the cardiovascular health study. Arterioscler Thromb Vasc Biol 1999;19:539–545.
9. Criqui MH, Denenberg JO, Langer RD, Fronek A. The epidemiology of peripheral arterial disease: importance of identifying the population at risk. Vasc Med 1997;2:221–226.
10. Murabito JM, D'Agostino RB, Silbershatz H, Wilson PW. Intermittent claudication: a risk profile from the Framingham Heart Study. Circulation 1997;96:44–49.
11. Hirsch AT, Treat-Jacobson D, Lando HA, Hatsukami DK. The role of tobacco cessation, antiplatelet and lipid-lowing therapies in the treatment of peripheral arterial disease. Vasc Med 1997;2:243–251.
12. Newman AB, Sutton-Tyrrell K, Vogt MT, Kuller LH. Morbidity and mortality in hypertensive adults with a low ankle/arm blood pressure index. JAMA 1993;270:487–489.
13. Cole CW, Hill GB, Farzad E, et al. Cigarette smoking and peripheral arterial disease. Surgery 1993; 114:753–756.
14. Ingolfsson IÖ, Sigurdsson G, Sigvaldason H, Thorgeirsson G, Sigfusson N. A marked decline in the prevalence and incidence of intermittent claudication in Icelandic men 1968–1986: a strong relationship to smoking and serum cholesterol—the Reykjavik Study. J Clin Epidemiol 1994;47:1237–1243.
15. Freund KM, Belanger AJ, D'Agostino RB, Kannel WB. The health risks of smoking: the Framingham Study: 34 years of follow-up. Ann Epidemiol 1993;3:417–424.
16. Jernigan WR, Fallat ME, Hatfield DR. Hypoplastic aortoiliac syndrome: an entity peculiar to women. Surgery 1983;94:752–757.
17. Jonason T, Bergstrom R. Cessation of smoking in the patients with intermittent claudication: effects on the risk of peripheral vascular complications, myocardial infarction and mortality. Acta Med Scand 1987;21:253–260.

18. Faulkner KW, House AK, Castleden WM. The effect of cessation of smoking on the accumulative survival rates of patients with symptomatic peripheral vascular disease. Med J Aust 1983;1:217–219.
19. Reunanen A, Takkunen H, Aromaa A. Prevalence of intermittent claudication and its effect on mortality. Acta Med Scand 1982;211:249–256.
20. Ameli FM, Stein M, Provan JL, Prosser R. The effect of postoperative smoking on femoropopliteal bypass grafts. Ann Vasc Surg 1989;3:20–25.
21. Lassila R, Lepantalo M. Cigarette smoking and the outcome after lower limb arterial surgery. Acta Chir Scand 1988;154:635–640.
22. Beks PJ, Mackaay AJ, de Neeling JN, et al. Peripheral arterial disease in relation to glycaemic level in an elderly Caucasian population: the Hoorn Study. Diabetologia 1995;38:86–96.
23. Tierney S, Fennessy F, Hayes DB. Secondary prevention of peripheral vascular disease. Br Med J 2000; 320:1262–1265.
24. The Diabetes Control and Complications Trial (DCCT) Research Group. Effect of intensive diabetes management on macrovascular events and risk factors in the Diabetes Control and Complications Trial. Am J Cardiol 1995;75:894–903.
25. UK Prospective Diabetes Study (UKPDS) Group. Intensive blood-glucose control with sulphonylureas or insulin compared with conventional treatment and risk of complications in patients with type 2 diabetes (UKPDS 33). Lancet 1998;352:837–853.
26. Greenland P, Abrams J, Aurigemma GP, et al. Prevention Conference V: beyond secondary prevention: identifying the high-risk patient for primary prevention: noninvasive tests of atherosclerotic burden: writing group III. Circulation 2000;101:e16.
27. Steinberg D. Low density lipoprotein oxidation and its pathobiological significance. J Biol Chem 1997;272:20963–20966.
28. Stamler J, Wentworth D, Neatone JD. Is there a relationship between serum cholesterol and risk of premature death from coronary heart disease continuous and graded? Findings in 356,222 primary screenees of the Multiple Risk Factor Intervention Trial (MRFIT). JAMA 1986;256:2823–2828.
29. Kannel WB, Skinner JJ, Schwartz MJ, Shurtleff D. Intermittent claudication: incidence in the Framingham Study. Circulation 1970;41:875–883.
30. Burt VL, Whelton P, Roccella EJ, et al. Prevalence of hypertension in the US adult population: results from the third national health and nutrition examination survey, 1988–1991. Hypertension 1995;25: 305–313.
31. Izzo JL, Levy D, Black HR. Importance of systolic blood pressure in older Americans. Hypertension 2000;35:1021–1024.
32. Hiatt WR. Medical treatment of peripheral arterial disease and claudication. N Eng J Med 2001;344: 1608–1621.
33. Frost PH, Davis BR, Burlando AJ, et al. Coronary heart disease risk factors in men and women aged 60 years and older. Circulation 1996;94:26–34.
34. Molgaard J, Malinow MR, Lassvik C, Holm AC, Upson B, Olsson AG. Hyperhomocyst(e)inemia: an independent risk factor for intermittent claudication. J Intern Med 1992;231:273–279.
35. Robinson K, Arheart K, Refsum H, et al. Low circulating folate and B6 concentrations: risk factors for stroke, peripheral vascular disease, and coronary artery disease. European COMAC Group. Circulation 1998;97;437–443.
36. Ridker PM, Cushman M, Stampfer MJ, Tracy RP, Hennekens CH. Plasma concentrations of c-reactive protein and risk of developing peripheral vascular disease. Circulation 1998;97:425–428.
37. Evans RW, Shaten J, Hempel JD, Cutler JA, Kuller LH. Homocysteine and risk of cardiovascular disease in the Multiple Risk Factor Intervention Trial. Arterioscler Thromb Vasc Biol 1997;17: 1947–1953.
38. Welch, GN, Loscalzo J. Homocysteine and atherothrombosis. N Engl J Med 1998;338:1042–1050.
39. Ross R. Atherosclerosis: an inflammatory disease. N Engl J Med 1999;340:115–126.
40. Stary HC, Chandler AB, Glagov S, et al. A definition of initial, fatty streak, and intermediate lesions of atherosclerosis: a report from the Committee on Vascular Lesions of the Council on Arteriosclerosis, American Heart Association. Circulation 1994;89:2462–2478.
41. Ridker PM, Cushman M, Stampfer MJ, Tracy RP, Hennekens CH. Inflammation, aspirin, and the risk of cardiovascular disease in apparently healthy men. N Engl J Med 1997;336:973–979.
42. Ridker PM, Buring JE, Shih J, Matias M, Hennekens CH. Prospective study of C-reactive protein and the risk of future cardiovascular events among apparently healthy women. Circulation 1998;98: 731–733.

43. Koenig W, Sund M, Frohlich M, et al. C-reactive protein, a sensitive marker of inflammation, predicts future risk of coronary heart disease in initially healthy middle-aged men: results from the MONICA (Monitoring Trends and Determinants in Cardiovascular Disease) Augsburg Cohort Study, 1984 to 1992. Circulation 1999;99:237–242.

44. Libby P, Egan D, Skarlatos S. Roles of infectious agents in atherosclerosis and restenosis. Circulation 1997;96:4095–4103.

45. Kannel WB. The demographics of claudication and the aging of the American population. Vasc Med 1996;1:60–64.

46. Criqui MH, Fronek A, Barrett-Connor E, Klauber MR, Gabriel S, Goodman D. The prevalence of peripheral arterial disease in a defined population. Circulation 1985;71:510–515.

47. Leng GC, Lee AJ, Fowkes FGR, et al. Incidence, natural history and cardiovascular events in symptomatic and asymptomatic peripheral arterial disease in the general population. Int J Epidemiol 1996; 25:1172–1181.

48. Fowkes FG, Housley E, Cawood EH, Macintyre CC, Ruckley CV, Prescott RJ. Edinburgh Arterial Study: prevalence of asymptomatic and symptomatic peripheral arterial disease in the general population. Int J Epidemiol 1991;20:384–392.

49. Hirsch AT, Criqui MH, Treat-Jacobson D, et al. Peripheral arterial disease, detection, awareness, and treatment in primary care. JAMA 2001;286:1317–1324.

50. Hertzer NR, Beven EG, Young JR, et al: Coronary artery disease in peripheral vascular patients: a classification of 1000 coronary angiograms and results of surgical management. Ann Surg 1984;199: 223–233.

51. Kramer JR, Hertzer NR. Coronary atherosclerosis in patients undergoing elective abdominal aortic aneurysm resection. Cardiovasc Clin 1981;12:143–152.

52. Aronow WS, Ahn C. Prevalence of coexistence of coronary artery disease, peripheral arterial disease, and atherothrombotic brain infarction in men and women > or = 62 years of age. Am J Cardiol 1994; 74:64–65.

53. Hirsch AT, Halverson S, Treat-Jacobson D, et al. The Minnesota Regional Peripheral Arterial Disease Screening Program: toward a definition of community standards of care. Vasc Med 2001;6:87–96.

54. Leng GC, Fowkes FGR, Lee AJ, Dunbar J, Housley E, Ruckley CV. Use of ankle brachial pressure index to predict cardiovascular events and death: a cohort study. Br Med J 1996;313:1140–1443.

55. McKenna M, Wolfson S, Kuller L. The ratio of ankle and arm blood pressure as an independent risk factor of mortality. Atherosclerosis 1991;87:119–128.

56. Vogt MT, Cauley JA, Newman AB, Kuller LH, Hulley SB. Decreased ankle/arm blood pressure index and mortality in elderly women. JAMA 1993;270:465–469.

57. Allan PL, Mowbray PI, Lee AJ, Fowkes FGR. Relationship between carotid intima-media thickness and symptomatic and asymptomatic peripheral arterial disease: the Edinburgh Artery Study. Stroke 1997;28:348–353.

58. Ness J, Aronow WS. Prevalence of coexistence of coronary artery disease, ischemic stroke, and peripheral arterial disease in older persons, mean age 80 years, in an academic hospital-based geriatrics practice. J Am Geriatr Soc 1999;47:1255–1256.

59. Meijer WT, Hoes AW, Rutgers D, Bots ML, Hofman A, Grobbee DE: Peripheral arterial disease in the elderly: the Rotterdam Study. Arterioscler Thromb Vasc Biol 1998;18:185–192.

60. Dormandy J, Mahir M, Ascady G, et al. Fate of the patient with chronic leg ischaemia. J Cardiovasc Surg 1989;30:50–57.

61. Weita JI, Byrne J. Clagett P, et al. Diagnosis and treatment of chronic arterial insufficiency of the lower extremities: a critical review. Circulation 1996:94:3026–3049.

3   Clinical Evaluation of Intermittent Claudication

Robert T. Eberhardt, MD and
Jay D. Coffman, MD

CONTENTS

HISTORY
PHYSICAL EXAMINATION
DIFFERENTIAL DIAGNOSIS
NATURAL HISTORY
EVALUATING DISEASE SEVERITY AND IMPACT
SUMMARY
REFERENCES

INTRODUCTION

The word *claudication* is derived from the Latin word *claudico* meaning "to limp." The current definition of intermittent claudication (IC) is pain or discomfort of the lower extremity brought on by walking and relieved by rest—hence the intermittent nature. It is often described as pain, cramping, aching, numbness, fatigue, or weakness in the muscles of the leg, thigh, or buttocks that occurs during exercise and abates in a short time with rest.

In > 90% of patients, IC is due to stenosis or occlusion of the artery supplying the lower extremity caused by arteriosclerosis obliterans. At rest, the stenosis may have minimal hemodynamic effect on limb blood pressure or blood flow. During exercise, however, the hemodynamic effects of the stenosis may result in a pressure gradient, and attenuation of the increase in blood flow to the muscle group supplied by this vessel; the demands of exercise for an increase in blood flow cannot be met (*see* Chapter 4). Limb perfusion may be further compromised due to extravascular compressive forces from muscle contraction that may even transiently stop blood flow during exercise. Although ischemia occurs in muscle groups with supply–demand mismatch, the precise cause of the pain or fatigue is not known. Some have suggested that the discomfort may result from activation of local chemoreceptors due to accumulation of lactate or other metabolites. However, infusion of lactate does not cause pain and bicarbonate

From: *Contemporary Cardiology: Peripheral Arterial Disease: Diagnosis and Treatment*
Edited by: J. D. Coffman and R. T. Eberhardt © Humana Press Inc., Totowa, NJ

infusions attenuate the pain *(1)*. Furthermore, patients with McArdle's disease cannot produce lactate but still have claudication.

IC is the most common symptomatic manifestation of peripheral arterial disease (PAD) (Table 1). It is estimated that in the United States 5% of the adult population above the age of 55 yr suffers from IC *(2)*. Establishing the diagnosis of IC as the cause of exertional leg pain is important to initiate appropriate therapy including modification of atherosclerosis risk factors (*see* Chapter 9). This chapter reviews the clinical presentation of IC with emphasis on the differential diagnosis.

HISTORY

Patients with IC complain of pain or discomfort in the buttocks, thighs, or legs with exercise, typically while walking. The discomfort is often described as aching, tightness, cramping, heaviness, or numbness, as well as weakness or fatigue. These symptoms are relieved with the cessation of exercise within 1–5 min. The symptoms are remarkably reproducible, precipitated by the same walking duration and distance with a given speed and grade. If a patient exercises to the point of claudication and then recovers, he or she can exercise to the same extent again. The constant nature is an important feature that helps to distinguish arteriosclerosis obliterans from some of the alternative etiologies of exertional leg pain (Table 2). Some patients are able to walk through their claudication, perhaps because they slow their pace or shift work to other muscle groups. Patients with claudication do not have muscle pain without exercise or on prolonged stationary standing. Pain that occurs at rest is either a result of severe PAD or due to another disorder.

The location of the discomfort with exercise may help localize the site of the stenosed or obstructed artery. Symptoms typically occur in the muscle groups immediately distal to the diseased vessel. Obstruction at the level of the superficial femoral artery, the most common site of atherosclerosis in the lower limbs, causes calf muscle symptoms. However, as during walking the gastrocnemius musculature has the greatest workload and highest oxygen consumption of any muscle group in the leg, calf pain is common even with more proximal disease. Patients with proximal disease, such as aortoiliac occlusive disease, may develop claudication in a buttock, thigh, or even lower back. The classic presentation of aortoiliac disease, termed Leriche syndrome, is bilateral "high" claudication accompanied by impotency and atrophy of the lower extremity muscles. Obstruction in the tibial or peroneal arteries may cause discomfort in the ankle or foot, which in diabetics may be difficult to distinguish from diabetic neuropathy.

PHYSICAL EXAMINATION

A complete vascular examination should be performed on all patients suspected to have claudication. This examination includes an inspection of the lower extremity for signs of chronic ischemia such as subcutaneous atrophy, hair loss, pallor, dependent rubor, coolness, or deformed or hypertrophied toenails. These trophic signs in the lower extremity are often present but are nonspecific. Profound tissue ischemia may produce edema, ulceration, and gangrene. Patients with rest pain often alleviate the discomfort by placing the leg in the dependent position, which increases the edema. Patients with aortoiliac disease may also have global atrophy of the limb musculature.

All pulses in the lower extremities should be palpated including the femoral, popliteal, dorsalis pedis, and posterior tibial pulsations. The strength and quality of each

Table 1
Signs and Symptoms of Peripheral Arterial Disease

Exertional leg pain and relief with rest
Cool or cold feet to palpation
Nocturnal and rest pain relieved with dependency
Absent pulses
Blanching or pallor on elevation
Delayed venous filling after elevation
Dependent rubor
Atrophy of subcutaneous fatty tissue
Shiny skin
Loss of hair on foot and toes
Thickened nails, often with fungal infections
Gangrene or nonhealing ulcer

Table 2
Causes of Exertional Leg Pain

Atherosclerotic arterial occlusive disease
Nonatherosclerotic arterial occlusive disease
   Entrapment syndromes (popliteal)
   Fibrodysplasia
   Cystic adventitial disease
   External iliac endofibrosis
   Spontaneous popliteal dissection
   Vasculitis (Takayasu's disease, giant cell arteritis)
   Thromboangiitis obliterans
   Arterial embolism
Neurogenic claudication
Venous claudication
McArdle's disease
Arthritis

pulse should be noted with comparison to the contralateral side. Each site is often assigned a subjective rating using one of several grading schemes. One such scheme is to grade the pulses as 0 if absent, 1+ if diminished, and 2+ if normal. The characteristic finding of PAD is a diminished or absent pulse in the affected limb. It should be noted that the dorsalis pedis pulse cannot be palpated in 8%, the posterior tibial pulse in 2%, and both pulses in 0.5% of normal subjects. Originally this was thought to be due to congenital absence; however, the vessels are present but pursue an aberrant course or divide into smaller branches at a proximal level.

The vascular examination includes auscultation for bruits created by turbulence as blood flows through a stenotic lesion. A systolic bruit is common when there is obstructive disease proximal to the site auscultated. When a diastolic component is also present, it means the collateral circulation is inadequate to even allow diastolic pressure distal to the diseased area to rise to the systemic diastolic pressure and thus stop flow during diastole. Bruits may be heard in the abdominal, femoral, carotid, subclavian, and even popliteal locations.

In conjunction auscultation and palpation may help to localize the level of arterial obstruction. In patients with aortoiliac disease the femoral pulses will typically be absent or diminished and there may be a bruit over the femoral arteries or abdomen. However, in the occasional patient with significant aortoiliac disease the pedal pulses may be normal. In patients with calf claudication due to superficial femoral artery disease the femoral pulse is usually normal without a bruit but the popliteal and distal pulses are diminished or absent. In patients with ankle or foot symptoms due to tibial–peroneal disease the popliteal artery may have a strong pulse in the absence of distal pulses; diabetes mellitus should be suspected in these patients. Only one pedal vessel needs to be present (with a normal systolic blood pressure) to make the diagnosis of claudication less likely. A patient with a normal pulse examination and a typical history of claudication should undergo further evaluations, such as treadmill exercise testing. This may disclose the presence of disease without a hemodynamically significant gradient at rest but with a gradient with exercise.

Other vascular territories need to be examined in detail for evidence of atherosclerotic disease. Measurement of the arm blood pressures and palpation of the brachial, radial, and ulnar pulses should be obtained bilaterally. A discrepancy of the blood pressures between the arms (of > 15 mmHg) often indicates the presence of subclavian or innominate artery disease. A systolic bruit is often present in the supraclavicular area or over the axillary artery in the axilla. Some patients with a lower blood pressure and diminished upper extremity pulsations will have "claudication" of the arm. A carotid examination includes palpation of the carotid pulse low in the neck and auscultation for cervical bruits, especially under the angle of the jaw. Bilateral simultaneous palpation of the carotid arteries should never be performed. As most carotid lesions are at the bifurcation, the carotid pulses are either normal or increased. The abdominal aorta should also be examined with careful palpation, as an unsuspected aneurysm may be found. If the aorta is enlarged on physical examination, then further imaging is warranted to evaluate for an aneurysm.

Simple tests may be performed in the office to gauge the collateral circulation. Cutaneous perfusion can be estimated by assessing the color and temperature of the feet with positional changes. The feet or toes should remain normal in color with the lower extremities raised above the level of the heart while supine. This is true even with exercise, which can unmask perfusion abnormalities due to collateral insufficiency. Pallor of the feet or toes at rest or with exercise indicates inadequate collateral circulation. If blanching of the feet does not occur at a 30° angle, then the ankle blood pressure is usually > 80 mmHg (3). If blanching occurs at this angle, then the ankle pressure is usually < 65 mmHg. After the seated position is resumed with the legs dependent, the time for color return of the skin of the feet and filling of the veins on the dorsum of the feet is measured. A normal response in a warm room is for flushing to occur within 10 s and venous refilling to occur within 20 s. With an inadequate collateral circulation these times are usually > 30 s. It is important to note that the use of venous refilling time is not valid if venous insufficiency is present. The capillary filling time is performed by pressing on the skin to cause blanching and observing the time of return of color. The color returns immediately except in severe ischemia. Although rather crude tests, these bedside maneuvers provide a dependable index of the adequacy of blood flow in physiologic terms.

More sophisticated tests using bedside instruments can be utilized to confirm the diagnosis of arterial obstructive disease, to assess its severity, and to follow the course of the disease (*see* Chapter 4). If a Doppler device to detect flow is available, the ankle blood pressure can be measured and an ankle to brachial index (ABI) calculated (Fig. 1). The ABI has an excellent sensitivity and specificity for the detection of PAD as validated by angiography *(4)*. It is important to remember that angiography provides visual images of the luminal anatomy but not hemodynamic information. To measure the ankle pressure, a standard-sized blood pressure cuff is placed around the ankle and the pressure raised to obliterate the arterial signal. As a rough guide palpation of the pedal pulses can be used if present without a Doppler, but the use of a Doppler is preferred. Then the cuff is slowly deflated to record the pressure at which there is a return of the Doppler signal (or the systolic pressure). The pressures at the ankle should be equal to or greater than the arm pressure. The ABI for each foot is calculated by dividing the higher pressure obtained at the ankle, both the dorsalis pedis and posterior tibial arteries, by the higher pressure in the two brachial arteries. Although extremely valuable the ABI is limited if there is resistance to compressiblity of the blood vessels due to medial calcification that can lead to false elevation of the value. In such an instance, measurement of the pressure in the great toe is often helpful. Perhaps the most informative procedure is measurement of the ankle pressures in each foot before and after exercise. Calf muscle exercise, with heel raises/toe stands, is often used as the mode of exercise in the office. This has been shown to correlate well with the treadmill exercise findings *(5)*. Another method infrequently used today is aneroid oscillometry, which provides an index of arterial pulse pressure. Diminished pulsatility is seen in arterial obstructive disease and this technique is not limited by calcifications. These tests can be performed in the office but are often done in a diagnostic vascular laboratory under standardized conditions (*see* Chapter 4).

DIFFERENTIAL DIAGNOSIS

Neurogenic Claudication

Neurogenic claudication is a form of lumbosacral radiculopathy, due to narrowing of the vertebral canal, manifested by symptoms of claudication provoked by ambulation *(6)*. The pathophysiology involves compression of intraspinal neurovascular structures with ischemia of the spinal cord, cauda equina, or nerve roots during exercise. The compression of the lower spinal cord or cauda equina due to lumbosacral spinal stenosis impairs venous drainage with venous pooling even at rest. With further compression, there is impairment of arterial vasodilation and blood flow, creating ischemia. Proof of this concept is the motor conduction abnormalities seen following the onset of neurogenic claudication *(7)*. Pathologic features include narrowing of the spinal canal, degenerative bone and soft tissue pathology, and/or vertebral displacement.

Neurogenic claudication more commonly affects men beyond their 50s with a male to female ratio of 8:1. It is manifested by discomfort of the buttocks, thighs, calves, or feet on walking that is usually bilateral. The symptoms are not typically present at rest but with walking there is progressive discomfort, often described as weakness, tiredness, or heaviness, that requires a rest. This is often quite difficult to distinguish from claudication from arterial obstructive disease; however, several features are helpful (Table 3). The distance walked prior to the onset of symptoms is variable in neurogenic claudication and may even occur with prolonged standing. Many find walking downhill worse in neurogenic claudication than with arterial insufficiency. During ambulation afflicted

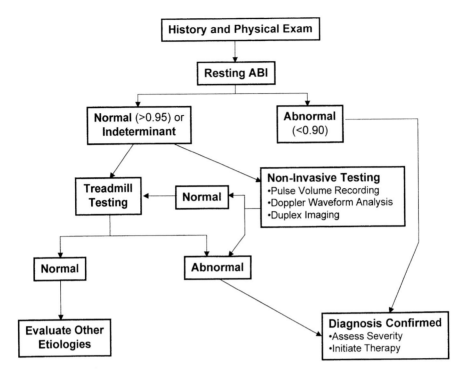

Fig. 1. Establishing the diagnosis of intermittent claudication.

persons will lean forward progressively until they stoop forward with hyperextension of the back. Relief of the discomfort is not achieved simply by stopping walking but requires a change in position. Other important clues to neurogenic claudication include back pain especially upon lifting, standing, coughing, sneezing, or at night in bed; a history of back injury; and paresthesias or weakness of the legs *(8,9)*.

The examination is often remarkable for a lack of gross abnormalities. The heavily emphasized straight leg raise maneuver is generally normal and frequently neurologic signs are absent. However, examination may reveal an absence of reflexes in the lower limbs before or after exercise, nerve distribution sensory loss, motor root weakness, and a positive leg raising test. Peripheral pulses and pedal artery systolic blood pressures should be normal, except with coexistent arterial disease. However, another problem is that vasospasm of blood vessels may be present with spinal canal stenosis or prolapsed intervertebral disc leading to diminished or absent distal pulses and cool limbs; the pedal artery systolic blood pressures should be normal in this instance.

Plain radiographs may raise the suspicion of a narrow vertebral canal and perhaps show degenerative changes. A computed tomography (CT) scan can demonstrate the cross-sectional area of the canal and may reveal a stenosis, but in limited sections. Because the disease is often multilevel, magnetic resonance imaging (MRI) is considered the best diagnostic modality *(10)*. Conventional CT or MR myelography can reveal the extent of stenosis and root impingement at rest or with dynamic motion *(11)*. This provides useful information that is predictive of the postoperative outcome *(12)*. Others have advocated the use of treadmill testing for both diagnostic and prognostic information as well as functional capacity *(13–15)*.

Table 3
Distinguishing Arterial Claudication from Neurogenic Claudication

Feature	Arterial claudication	Pseudoclaudication
Onset	Walking	Walking or prolonged standing
Character	Cramping or aching	Tingling or numbness
Bilateral	+/−	+
Distance	Fairly constant	More variable
Cause	Atherosclerosis	Spinal stenosis
Relief	Standing still	Sitting down or leaning forward

Conservative management is advocated as the first line of therapy, but in those with severe debility it rarely improves functional status and quality of life *(16)*. Surgical decompression provides good results if used as an initial therapy for those with severe symptoms, as well as delayed therapy in those with moderate symptoms failing conservative management *(17)*. A laminectomy to decompress the narrow canal is the treatment of choice; vertebral fusions or foraminotomy may also be necessary.

It is important to emphasize that this is a difficult differential diagnosis with clinical features similar to IC due to PAD *(18)*. It is made more challenging to determine the cause of the claudication when both lumbosacral spinal stenosis and obstructive arterial disease coexist. A mistaken diagnosis as to the cause of the symptoms is not uncommon and occasionally both problems may contribute. Such patients often undergo surgery for both diseases sequentially to relieve their symptoms.

Arthritis

Arthritis, including inflammatory and degenerative forms, is characterized by inflammation and/or destruction of the joint space. Involvement of the large joints of the lower extremities with arthritis may result in exertional leg discomfort. This is described as an aching or a pain that is worse with weight bearing and relieved with rest; however, it is localized to the joints, rather than the muscles. The onset of the discomfort is more variable and symptoms improve with the use of antiinflammatory agents. Physical examination may reveal evidence of joint inflammation with effusions and joint destruction with deformity. Radiographic examination with plain films will often confirm the diagnosis. Although this diagnosis needs to be considered for the cause of exertional leg discomfort, clinical features typically allow arthritis to be easily differentiated from IC.

Thromboangiitis Obliterans

Thromboangiitis obilterans (or Buerger's disease) is characterized by segmental inflammation and occlusion of small and medium-sized arteries and veins of the extremities. The occlusive lesion of the vessels of the leg may result in symptoms of IC of the feet or even calves. The diagnosis should be considered in younger male smokers who develop claudication. A detailed description of the disorder and its management are discussed elsewhere (*see* Chapter 18).

Entrapment Syndromes

The popliteal artery is particularly susceptible to entrapment with compression by the gastrocnemius or other calf muscles during exercise, leading to ischemia and causing typical symptoms of IC. There are many developmental variations with an anomalous relationship between the popliteal artery and neighboring muscular structures that cause this syndrome *(19)*. The most common abnormalities are a lateral attachment of the medial head of the gastrocnemius muscle with medial displacement of the popliteal artery, or an aberrant medial head of the muscle. Overtraining in athletes may cause a similar syndrome due to hypertrophy of the soleus and plantaris muscles *(20)*.

In this syndrome the popliteal artery is traumatized by repeated compression leading to segmental stenosis, thrombosis, and occlusion (Fig. 2). Pathologic features include fibrous intimal thickening, destruction of smooth muscle, and proliferation of connective tissue. Turbulent blood flow may cause poststenotic dilatation and aneurysm formation, which can result in thromboembolic complications.

This syndrome should be considered in young adults presenting with claudication. It is typically found prior to the age of 40, although it has been reported in the sixth decade of life. There is male predominance attributed to the larger muscular development. The symptoms of the syndrome may be vague and slowly progressive but in up to two thirds of patients they consist of claudication with calf cramping after intense physical activity that is often unilateral *(21)*. Although bilateral symptoms are present in only about one third of patients, the anatomical abnormality is present in both extremities in up to two thirds of patients. Other symptoms such as numbness, coolness, or paresthesias of the affected limb may be the only manifestation. Infrequently, patients present with an acutely ischemic limb due to popliteal artery thrombosis.

The examination of the affected limb is usually normal; however, ischemic signs and absent pedal pulses may occur with occlusion of the popliteal artery. Collateral blood flow is usually excellent as there are normal vessels proximal and distal to the affected artery. Disappearance of the pedal pulses during plantar (or dorsi-) flexion of the foot against resistance has been used as the hallmark physical finding but is unreliable *(22)*. This finding, even confirmed by Doppler examination, may be seen in normal subjects. However, when this sign is present, it should lead to more definitive studies. Other findings on physical examination may include a pulsatile mass in the popliteal fossa if an aneurysm is present, edema after exercise, and varicose veins if the popliteal vein is compressed.

Numerous imaging modalities have been employed to assist in establishing the diagnosis of popliteal entrapment syndrome. Digital subtraction angiography may reveal details of vascular luminal anatomy but overlook the underlying cause of the arterial stenosis or occlusion. Provocative maneuvers such as dorsiflexion of the foot may disclose the dynamic obstruction during angiography. Similarly, duplex ultrasonography has been used to document provokable compression of the popliteal artery with forced plantar flexion *(23)*. However, ultrasonography yields many false-positive results with even complete occlusion or arterial diameter reduction during plantar flexion in some unaffected individuals. MRI appears to be the single most useful technique, providing anatomic details of the vascular and surrounding structures in the region *(24)*. CT angiography may also provide information on the relationship of the arterial abnormalities to adjacent structures *(25)*.

Early diagnosis and intervention provides superior long-term results *(26,27)*. This approach allows for an essentially curative popliteal artery release by the musculotendinous section without vascular reconstruction *(28)*. For the same reason, the opposite extremity should be treated even if the anatomic abnormality is asymptomatic. Arterial bypass with autologous interposition vein graft is the procedure of choice if

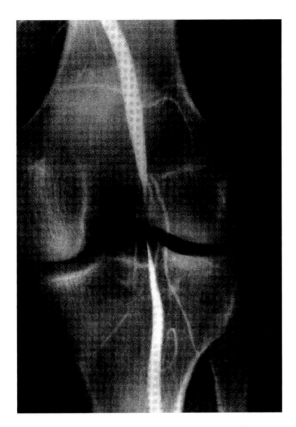

Fig. 2. Angiographic appearance of popliteal artery entrapment syndrome complicated by arterial occlusion. The popliteal artery is normal in appearance proximally but tapers with an occlusion in the popliteal fossa behind the knee joint. (Courtesy of Dr. Bruce H. Gray, Greenville Memorial Hospital System, Greenville, SC 29681.)

reconstruction is needed due to extensive intimal damage or occlusion of the popliteal artery *(29)*. Although endarterectomy or vein patch angioplasty are attractive alternatives, these procedures seem to provide inferior long-term results. For acute thrombosis of the popliteal artery, transluminal thrombectomy followed by thrombolytic therapy has been successful but must be followed by surgery to resect the musculotendinous abnormality *(30)*. Endovascular intervention with stenting may be feasible but should be approached with caution given the anatomic considerations and skepticism regarding long-term results *(31)*. In patients with muscle hypertrophy only, symptoms are usually relieved by surgical release of the soleus muscle from its tibial attachments, resection of its fascial band, and resection of the plantaris muscle.

Cystic Adventitial Disease

Adventitial cysts within the arterial wall of peripheral arteries may cause localized stenosis or occlusion by compression of the vessel lumen. This most commonly involves the popliteal artery, accounting for 85% of cases, but may involve the femoral or external iliac arteries *(32,33)*. It is a rare cause of IC, estimated as 1 in 1200 cases. Cystic adventitial disease more commonly affects men, predominately in the fourth or fifth decade of life, with a male to female ratio of at least 5:1 *(34)*.

The origin of these adventitial cysts is uncertain. However, it has been speculated that this involves developmental inclusion or extension and invasion of a mucin-secreting cystic structure, perhaps of ganglion or synovial origin. The developmental theory postulates that mesenchymal cells that are destined to form joint tissue are incorporated into the developing vessel adventitia. It has also been postulated that the pathogenesis may involve repetitive trauma. The cysts are located between the medial and adventitial layers of the arterial wall and contain gelatinous material under tension. The intima and media may undergo necrosis by compression and lead to luminal thrombus formation.

The clinical presentation is typically sudden onset of unilateral claudication; however, symptoms may wax and wane. Other symptoms including paresthesias may occur distal to the knee. The physical examination is usually normal but flexion of the knee may cause disappearance of pedal pulses. If thrombosis of the popliteal artery has occurred, the popliteal and pedal pulses will be absent although ischemic signs do not usually appear due to collateral blood flow. It is important to suspect this disorder when there is an abrupt onset of unilateral claudication without evidence of occlusive vascular disease in other territories or embolic manifestations.

Traditionally, contrast angiography to establish the diagnosis has been regarded as the definitive imaging modality. An hourglass or "scimitar" sign may be seen owing to cystic compression narrowing the arterial lumen; the outline of the stenotic area is smooth (Fig. 3). However, if the artery is thrombosed, then the cyst cannot be diagnosed. This is not true of duplex ultrasonography, which can assess vessel patency and provide details of the cyst and surrounding structures. Duplex ultrasonography followed by MRI is considered the modality of choice (34).

The simplest treatment is complete excision of the cyst, but only if the artery is patent (33). Open cyst aspiration and aspiration guided by radiographic imaging has been used but is limited by a high recurrence rate. The best results for the occluded artery is an interposition graft with autologous vein graft (34,35). Percutaneous techniques with local thrombolysis and/or thrombus aspiration to restore vessel patency and radiographically-guided aspiration have been used (36).

Fibrodysplasia

Fibrodysplasia (fibromuscular dysplasia) often involves the renal and carotid arteries, but in the lower extremity it most commonly involves the external iliac arteries (37). Only rarely does it affect the infrainguinal arteries, but it has been reported in the superficial femoral, deep femoral, and popliteal arteries (38–42). Women are affected more often than men. Pathologically, there are various forms including intimal fibroplasia, medial fibrodysplasia or hyperplasia, or periarterial fibroplasia. The most common form, medial fibroplasia, is characterized by destruction of elastic and muscle fibers of the media.

IC is only one of a spectrum of clinical presentations that have been reported with involvement of the peripheral circulation. External iliac artery fibroplasia often presents with unilateral thigh or calf claudication due to stenotic narrowing of the vessel. In addition acute occlusion, embolism, aneurysm, and dissection may be seen (43–46). On physical examination pedal pulses are diminished or absent and Doppler systolic blood pressures are abnormal. The diagnosis is typically made by arteriography with specific magnification views. Medial fibroplasia gives a classic "string of beads" appearance on angiography. Treatment with intraluminal dilation by percutaneous transluminal angio-

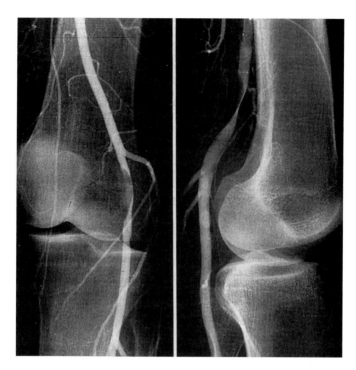

Fig. 3. Angiographic appearance of cystic adventitial disease. There is a smooth, concentric narrowing with an hourglass appearance of the popliteal artery due to extrinsic cystic compression. (Courtesy of Dr. Bruce H. Gray, Greenville Memorial Hospital System, Greenville, SC 29681.)

plasty is often sufficient and durable if the arterial lumen is patent. However, arterial bypass with autologous vein is the favored treatment if the artery is occluded.

Iliac Artery Endofibrosis

Arterial endofibrosis is a rare disorder usually affecting the external iliac arteries in highly trained athletes, often cyclists (47). Clinically this needs to be suspected in young athletes complaining of exercise-related lower extremity pain that may be unilateral or bilateral. It is characterized pathologically by progressive thickening of the arterial intima with fibrotic tissue that leads to stenosis (48). The etiology is uncertain but involves repetitive motion with trauma to the vessel. The pathophysiology involves the development of a gradient across a stenotic lesion with vigorous exercise that limits limb perfusion. The diagnosis is established with the measurement of the ankle pressure before and after heavy-load exercise. The relative limb pressure is usually normal at rest but reduced following exercise as demonstrated by a reduction in the ankle–brachial index at 1 min following exercise (49). Digital subtraction or magnetic resonance angiography may reveal a "moderate" lesion that has minimal or no gradient at rest. Treatment is individualized based on the patient's desires. Long-term follow-up suggests that the lesions stabilize when intense training stops (50). Intervention is not required if there are no symptoms during daily activities or submaximal exercise. However, surgery (with an autologous vein graft or endarterectomy with patch angioplasty) may allow an early return to competition (51). The use of endoluminal techniques is uncertain at this time (52).

Spontaneous Arterial Dissection

Spontaneous arterial dissection of a peripheral artery is a rare event. This has been reported in the external iliac artery, femoral artery (with or without extension), and popliteal artery. Spontaneous peripheral artery dissection more commonly affects persons prior to the fifth decade with a slight male preponderance. Dissection is associated with hypertension in 90% of affected patients but this is often mild. The pathologic hallmark is cystic medial degeneration. The clinical feature includes severe pain of sudden onset that is localized to the affected area. Patients may have ischemia distal to the affected vessel with progressive claudication or a more dramatic presentation with acute limb ischemia *(53)*. The latter has been reported to occur following strenuous exercise including running *(54)*. The diagnosis is often difficult to establish preoperatively but angiography may reveal a long segmental lesion of the affected vessel with minimal disease proximal or distal. The preferred treatment is vascular reconstruction with a bypass graft and resection or ligation of the diseased segment.

Venous Claudication

Intermittent venous claudication most commonly results from chronic iliofemoral venous obstruction. The venous obstruction may be due to an iliofemoral thrombus or may be iatrogenic after surgical interruption of the common femoral vein. The pathophysiology described involves high venous pressure in the limb, due to inadequate venous collateral circulation and high venous resistance, with exercise with a progressive increase in limb volume and intramuscular pressure that result in the discomfort *(55,56)*. There is also an impediment to arteriolar blood flow and increase in lactate production with exercise in the obstructed limb *(57)*.

The description is severe thigh pain and a sensation of tightness with exercise. This discomfort requires 15–20 min to subside after stopping exercise and is facilitated by leg elevation. Physical examination reveals obvious swelling of the limb, collateral superficial veins in the thigh and inguinal region, and distended pedal veins even with elevation of the limb above heart level. Arterial examination, including the femoral, popliteal, and pedal pulses, is usually normal. The diagnosis can be supported with the finding of venous obstruction by ultrasonography or occasionally venography; however, these do not provide physiologic information. Assessing venous drainage by plethysmography during treadmill work or ambulatory venous pressure monitoring may provide objective confirmation, but are not used clinically *(56)*. Treatment has generally been disappointing. Venous reconstruction of the iliac vein with a vein bypass graft, from below the venous obstruction to the opposite iliac vein, has been successful in some cases *(58)*. Percutaneous techniques, especially endoluminal stenting, can be performed if there is reconstitution of a lumen after thrombolysis or venous thrombectomy. Venous thrombectomy alone is usually followed by reocclusion without some other intervention.

Arterial Embolus

Although typically causing acute limb ischemia, IC may ensue as consequence of an arterial embolus to a peripheral artery (*see* Chapter 7). This is most common if there is good collateral circulation from a preexisting stenosis, so that there is no ischemia of the limb at rest. The history is typically that of sudden onset of claudication. However, many patients develop claudication even following embolectomy after an acute presentation. In these limbs, the pedal pulses are diminished or absent and the ankle systolic blood pressure is abnormal. Normal pulses and ankle systolic blood pressures in the opposite limb are helpful to distinguish an embolus from atherosclerotic obstructions. Such a history and findings should prompt an investigation for the source for the embolus. The treatment is thrombolysis, embolectomy, or a bypass graft preferably with autologous vein.

Vasculitis

Large vessel vasculitis may cause vessel narrowing and rarely lead to symptoms of IC. These disorders, including giant cell arteritis, Takayasu's arteritis, and others, are discussed in detail in Chapter 19.

McArdle's Disease and Other Exercise Intolerance Syndromes

McArdle's disease, due to muscle phosphorylase deficiency, is one of a number of "exercise myopathies" characterized by exercise intolerance *(59,60)*. The main clinical feature is typical IC with muscle fatigue and cramping, especially during strenuous exercise. Muscle glycogen normally is the primary oxidative fuel during vigorous exercise (requiring > 75% of maximal oxygen uptake) *(61)*. However, deficiency of muscle glycogen phosphorylase in McArdle's disease impairs the ability to utilize glycogen as an energy source, thus impairing oxidative metabolism *(61)*. There is no accumulation of lactate or pyruvate with exercise in McArdle's disease. There is a decline in phosphocreatine and accumulation of inorganic phosphate and adenosine diphosphate that contribute to the muscle fatigue and cramping *(62,63)*. Symptoms of McArdle's disease usually occur at a very young age but the onset of claudication has been described in the fifth decade. The lack of a rise in venous lactate following vigorous exercise is the basis for a diagnostic test rather than muscle biopsy, which has been used in the past.

NATURAL HISTORY

Reviewing the natural history of IC requires consideration of both limb- and cardiovascular-related outcomes. The progression of symptoms and complications of IC are due to the pathophysiology of the underlying disorder, atherosclerosis. Most patients with IC have atherosclerotic involvement in one or more arterial segments supplying the lower extremity; however, the limbs are not typically in jeopardy because of adequate collateral circulation *(64)*. Progression of atherosclerotic disease in the lower extremity may lead to worsening symptoms or the development of critical limb ischemia, but only in a minority of patients. It is readily recognized that peripheral arterial disease and IC are markers of coronary artery disease and risk factors for future coronary events. Treatments focused at altering this process are critical to prevent or delay the progression of arterial stenoses and occlusions, not only in the peripheral circulation but also in the coronary circulation (*see* Chapter 9).

Peripheral Outcomes and Functional Status

Most patients with IC have stable symptoms over a 5-yr period. In fact at the onset of claudication, symptoms may improve for several months because of the development of collateral blood vessel prior to stabilizing. It has been suggested that during this time treatment, except for exercise, should not be started. However, it is estimated that over 5 yr worsening claudication occurs in 16%, lower extremity bypass surgery is required in 7%, and primary major amputation is required in 4% of those with IC *(2)*. Of those requiring lower extremity bypass surgery, 26% require repeat revascularization and up to 20% require subsequent amputation. In those with IC approx 1.4% per year develop critical limb ischemia with rest pain and/or gangrene, accounting for the majority of these procedures. This rate of progression is higher among those with a history of diabetes mellitus and current tobacco use *(65,66)*. The risk of developing rest pain and/or gangrene over 6 yr was 40% in diabetic patients with IC compared 18% in nondiabetic patients *(66)*. In patients with IC who continued to smoke 16% developed rest pain over a 7-yr period compared to none of those who stopped smoking *(65)*.

There is a gradual loss of mobility and decline in functional status as a consequence of chronic ischemia of the limb. Acute ischemia due to impaired limb perfusion impairs the ability to walk because of claudication. However, chronic ischemia leads to changes in skeletal muscle fibers and diminished strength of the limb musculature. The hip abductor and knee extension force is reduced in peripheral arterial disease. On the microscopic level, the number and size of the muscle fibers are decreased. There is a reduction in the number of muscle fibers by > 50% and atrophy of the remaining fibers with severe impaired limb perfusion *(67)*. This involves fibers responsible both for short bursts of energy and prolonged exertion and walking endurance *(68)*. Diminished muscle strength and function leads to further decline in the ambulatory ability and creates a cycle of decline that is difficult to terminate.

Poor limb perfusion and IC impairs walking performance and ability as demonstrated by objective testing as well as questionnaires. The walking distance and duration on exercise testing is decreased in patients with IC. Walking velocity, during a paced 4-m walk, and walking endurance, during a 6-min walk test, is less in PAD. This poorer walking ability has a detrimental impact on the ability to engage in daily activities. In one study, elderly persons with PAD were less likely to leave the home at least once daily, as only 73% of those with limb arterial disease did so compared to 84% of controls *(69)*.

Mortality and Coronary Outcomes

More important than the limb-related complications is an impaired survival in persons with IC *(70)*. The 10-yr mortality in those with symptomatic PAD is > 60% in men and 30% in women *(71)*. This resulted in a relative risk of dying from coronary artery disease of 6.6, from cardiovascular disease of 5.9, and all-cause mortality of 3.1 compared to a similarly matched group without PAD. The frequent involvement of the coronary arteries with atherosclerosis in patients with symptomatic PAD has been demonstrated by multiple methodologies including angiography *(72)*. In a group of patients undergoing elective lower extremity revascularization at the Cleveland Clinic, normal coronary arteries were found in only 10%. Significant coronary artery disease with at least a 50% stenosis was found in nearly 60%, with single-vessel disease in 21%, double-vessel disease in 20%, and triple-vessel disease in 18%. Another important finding was impaired left ventricular function in 34% of those with PAD requiring revascularization *(72)*.

EVALUATING DISEASE SEVERITY AND IMPACT

Hemodynamic and Anatomic Assessment

Measurement of the ankle pressure, especially before and during exercise, in thought to be the most valuable information to assess disease severity. Lower limb perfusion can be gauged by measuring the resting ankle pressure and calculating the ABI (see Chapter 4). This has very high sensitivity and specificity for confirming the presence of disease as validated by angiography. Furthermore, the ABI is a useful guide to determine the severity of disease, providing prognostic information about limb complications. This simple office test is often performed serially over time to monitor for disease progression. It is important to emphasize that this is only a guide to disease severity, as the degree of symptoms and level of debility can vary considerably even with the same value.

Other noninvasive modalities typically provide physiologic information that can help to determine the severity of disease and localize the level of involvement (see Chapter 4). These include Doppler segmental pressures and waveform analysis, pulse volume recording, and duplex ultrasonography. Imaging techniques, such as angiography, provide a detailed anatomic assessment of disease severity but no physiologic information. Generally imaging techniques are reserved for patients in whom revascularization options are being considered.

Exercise testing is generally considered the test with the greatest clinical utility. The ankle pressures are measured before and after exercise; a drop in systolic ankle pressure > 20% is considered significant (*see* Chapter 4). This is valuable to help establish the diagnosis of PAD with subcritical stenosis at rest by "unmasking" the lesion. This is also useful to determine the severity of disease and its impact on functional capacity. The duration of exercise, the magnitude of the drop in the ankle systolic pressure, and the recovery time are parameters that may be used.

Assessment of Limitation

Evaluating the impact of IC on functional status in the community setting is strongly encouraged both during clinical trials and in clinical practice *(73)*. The use of the Rose questionnaire and its variations has served as a standard to assess leg pain in patients with PAD *(74)*. The responses to the questions confirm the clinical diagnosis of IC in a standardized way. Other community-based measures are used to assess functional status and quality of life. The functional status is evaluated looking at aspects of walking and activity levels. Measures of quality of life assess the perceived well being in physical, emotional, and social terms. Persons with IC have been shown to have impaired functional capacity and reduced quality of life.

The walking impairment questionnaire (WIQ) is a subjective assessment of the walking ability reported by the patient. This includes aspects of walking speed, distance, and difficulty as well as stair climbing ability. The test has been validated against more objective tests of walking performance such as treadmill testing and the 6-min walk test *(75)*. This is being used in most claudication trials assessing the response to therapy as well as in clinical practice. Measures of physical activity are useful to determine the functional impact of claudication. Questionnaires such as the low-level physical activity recall assess the total energy expenditure at work and during home and leisure time activities. Actual measurement of energy expenditure of physical activity by radiolabeled techniques can be used to determine the free-living daily physical activity *(76,77)*.

More objective testing of walking ability and performance is also utilized. The standard is treadmill exercise testing performed using one of several standardized protocols *(73)*. The protocols geared toward evaluating PAD have a reduced speed and grade compared to the standard protocols used for coronary artery disease. Such testing is useful to determine claudication distances and time as well as functional capacity, and estimated or measured maximal oxygen uptake. Persons with IC have poorer functional capacity with maximal oxygen uptake reduced by about half *(78)*. This is similar to the functional capacity encountered in severe heart failure. Another useful test that is gaining popularity is the 6-min walk test, which measures the distance walked during this time using two points 100 ft apart in a marked corridor *(79)*. This test is well suited for use in clinical practice as it does not require special equipment and is a reproducible, objective measure of walking performance.

SUMMARY

IC, the most common symptomatic manifestation of PAD, is characterized by discomfort of the lower extremity brought on by walking and relieved by rest. The differential diagnosis of exertional leg discomfort includes arterial obstructive disease due to atherosclerosis and nonatherosclerotic disorders, neurogenic claudication, venous claudication, exercise intolerance syndromes, and other disorders such as arthritis. Historical information and physical examination findings provide clues to help differentiate IC due to arteriosclerosis obilterans from other etiologies. Further studies are often required but bedside evaluation and testing is often sufficient. Evaluating the impact of IC on functional capacity is important and may be performed using various assessment instruments and exercise testing.

REFERENCES

1. Katz LN, Lindner E, Landt H. On the nature of the substances producing pain in contracting skeletal muscle: its bearing on the problems of angina pectoris and intermittent claudication. J Clin Invest 1935;14:807.
2. Weitz JI, Byrne J, Clagett GP, et al. Diagnosis and treatment of chronic arterial insufficiency of the lower extremities: a critical review. Circulation 1996;94:3026–3049.
3. Lorentsen E. The significance of the plantar ischemic test in the clinical diagnosis of peripheral arterial disease. Scand J Clin Lab Invest 1972;30:163–168.
4. Yao ST, Hobbs JT, Irvine WT. Ankle systolic pressure measurements in arterial disease affecting the lower extremities. Br J Surg 1969;56:676-679.
5. Amirhamzeh MM, Chant HJ, Rees JL, Hands LJ, Powell RJ, Campbell WB. A comparative study of treadmill tests and heel raising exercise for peripheral arterial disease. Eur J Vasc Endo Surg 1997;13: 301–305.
6. Porter RW. Spinal stenosis and neurogenic claudication. Spine 1996;21:2046–2052.
7. Baramki HG, Steffen T, Schondorf R, Aebi M. Motor conduction alterations in patients with lumbar spinal stenosis following the onset of neurogenic claudication. Eur Spine J 1999;8:411–416.
8. Heath JM. The clinical presentation of lumbar spinal stenosis. Ohio Med 1989;85:484–487.
9. Jonsson B, Stromqvist B. Symptoms and signs in degeneration of the lumbar spine: a prospective, consecutive study of 300 operated patients. J Bone Joint Surg 1993;75:381–385.
10. Jinkins JR, Runge VM. The use of MR contrast agents in the evaluation of disease of the spine. Topics Mag Reson 1995;7:168–180.
11. Wildermuth S, Zanetti M, Duewell S, et al. Lumbar spine: quantitative and qualitative assessment of positional (upright flexion and extension) MR imaging and myelography. Radiology 1998;207: 391–398.
12. Herno A, Airaksinen O, Saari T, Miettinen H. The predictive value of preoperative myelography in lumbar spinal stenosis. Spine 1994;19:1335–1338.
13. Deen HG, Zimmerman RS, Lyons MK, McPhee MC, Verheijde JL, Lemens SM. Measurement of exercise tolerance on the treadmill in patients with symptomatic lumbar spinal stenosis: a useful indicator of functional status and surgical outcome. J Neurosurg 1995;83:27–30.
14. Deen HG, Zimmerman RS, Lyons MK, McPhee MC, Verheijde JL, Lemens SM. Use of the exercise treadmill to measure baseline functional status and surgical outcome in patients with severe lumbar spinal stenosis. Spine 1998;23:244–248.

15. Fritz JM, Delitto A, Welch WC, Erhard RE. Lumbar spinal stenosis: a review of current concepts in evaluation, management, and outcome measurements. Arch Physical Med 1998;79:700–708.

16. Onel D, Sari H, Donmez C. Lumbar spinal stenosis: clinical/radiologic therapeutic evaluation in 145 patients: conservative treatment or surgical intervention? Spine 1993;18:291–298.

17. Amundsen T, Weber H, Nordal HJ, Magnaes B, Abdelnoor M, Lilleas F. Lumbar spinal stenosis: conservative or surgical management? A prospective 10-year study. Spine 2000;25:1424–1435.

18. Stanton PE, Jr., Rosenthal D, Clark M, Vo N, Lamis P. Differentiation of vascular and neurogenic claudication. Am Surgeon 1987;53:71–76.

19. Lambert AW, Wilkins DC. Popliteal artery entrapment syndrome. Br J Surg 1999;86:1365–1370.

20. Turnipseed WD, Pozniak M. Popliteal entrapment as a result of neurovascular compression by the soleus and plantaris muscles. J Vasc Surg 1992;15:285–293.

21. Persky JM, Kempczinski RF, Fowl RJ. Entrapment of the popliteal artery. Surg Gynecol Obst 1991; 173:84–90.

22. Hoffmann U, Vetter J, Rainoni L, Leu AJ, Bollinger A. Popliteal artery compression and force of active plantar flexion in young healthy volunteers. J Vasc Surg 1997;26:281–287.

23. Akkersdijk WL, de Ruyter JW, Lapham R, Mali W, Eikelboom BC. Colour duplex ultrasonographic imaging and provocation of popliteal artery compression. Eur J Vasc Endo Surg 1995;10:342–345.

24. Atilla S, Akpek ET, Yucel C, Tali ET, Isik S. MR imaging and MR angiography in popliteal artery entrapment syndrome. Eur Radiol 1998;8:1025–1029.

25. Beregi JP, Djabbari M, Desmoucelle F, Willoteaux S, Wattinne L, Louvegny S. Popliteal vascular disease: evaluation with spiral CT angiography. Radiology 1997;203:477–483.

26. Zund G, Brunner U. Surgical aspects of popliteal artery entrapment syndrome: 26 years of experience with 26 legs. Vasa 1995;24:29–33.

27. Marzo L, Cavallaro A, Mingoli A, Sapienza P, Tedesco M, Stipa S. Popliteal artery entrapment syndrome: the role of early diagnosis and treatment. Surgery 1997;122:26–31.

28. Ohara N, Miyata T, Oshiro H, Shigematsu H. Surgical treatment for popliteal artery entrapment syndrome. Cardiovasc Surg 2001;9:141–144.

29. Hoelting T, Schuermann G, Allenberg JR. Entrapment of the popliteal artery and its surgical management in a 20-year period. Br J Surg 1997;84:338–341.

30. Ring DH, Jr, Haines GA, Miller DL. Popliteal artery entrapment syndrome: arteriographic findings and thrombolytic therapy. J Vasc Intervent Radiol 1999;10:713–721.

31. Burger T, Meyer F, Tautenhahn J, Halloul Z, Fahlke J. Initial experiences with percutaneous endovascular repair of popliteal artery lesions using a new PTFE stent-graft. J Endovasc Surg 1998;5:365–372.

32. Flanigan DP, Burnham SJ, Goodreau JJ, Bergan JJ. Summary of cases of adventitial cystic disease of the popliteal artery. Ann Surg 1979;189:165–175.

33. Miller A, Salenius JP, Sacks BA, Gupta SK, Shoukimas GM. Noninvasive vascular imaging in the diagnosis and treatment of adventitial cystic disease of the popliteal artery. J Vasc Surg 1997;26: 715–720.

34. Tsolakis IA, Walvatne CS, Caldwell MD. Cystic adventitial disease of the popliteal artery: diagnosis and treatment. Eur J Vasc Endovasc Surg 1998;15:188–194.

35. Hierton T, Karacagil S, Bergqvist D. Long-term follow-up of autologous vein grafts: 40 years after reconstruction for cystic adventitial disease. Vasa 1995;24:250–252.

36. Samson RH, Willis PD. Popliteal artery occlusion caused by cystic adventitial disease: successful treatment by urokinase followed by nonresectional cystotomy. J Vasc Surg 1990;12:591–593.

37. Sauer L, Reilly LM, Goldstone J, Ehrenfeld WK, Hutton JE, Stoney RJ. Clinical spectrum of symptomatic external iliac fibromuscular dysplasia. J Vasc Surg 1990;12:488–495.

38. Schneider PA, LaBerge JM, Cunningham CG, Ehrenfeld WK. Isolated thigh claudication as a result of fibromuscular dysplasia of the deep femoral artery. J Vasc Surg 1992;15:657–660.

39. Tisnado J, Barnes RW, Beachley MC, Vines FS, Amendola MA. Fibrodysplasia of the popliteal arteries. Angiology 1982;33:1–5.

40. van den Dungen JJ, Boontje AH, Oosterhuis JW. Femoropopliteal arterial fibrodysplasia. Br J Surg 1990;77:396–399.

41. Neukirch C, Bahnini A, Delcourt A, Kieffer E. Popliteal aneurysm due to fibromuscular dysplasia. Ann Vasc Surg 1996;10:578–581.

42. Vertruyen M, Garcez JL. Fibromuscular dysplasia of the superficial femoral artery: an unusual localization. Acta Chir Belg 1993;93:249–251.

43. Burri B, Fontolliet C, Ruegsegger CH, Mosimann R. External iliac artery dissection due to fibromuscular dysplasia. Vasa 1983;12:76–78.
44. Herpels V, de Van V, Wilms G, et al. Recurrent aneurysms of the upper arteries of the lower limb: an atypical manifestation of fibromuscular dysplasia: a case report. Angiology 1987;38:411–416.
45. Stinnett DM, Graham JM, Edwards WD. Fibromuscular dysplasia and thrombosed aneurysm of the popliteal artery in a child. J Vasc Surg 1987;5:769–772.
46. Mehigan JT, Stoney RJ. Arterial microemboli and fibromuscular dysplasia of the external iliac arteries. Surgery 1977;81:484–486.
47. Walder J, Mosimann F, Van Melle G, Mosimann R. Iliac endofibrosis in 2 cycling racers. Helv Chir Acta 1985;51:793–795.
48. Paraf F, Petit B, Roux J, Bertin F, Laskar M, Labrousse F. External iliac artery endofibrosis of the cyclist. Ann Pathologie 2000;20:232–234.
49. Abraham P, Bickert S, Vielle B, Chevalier JM, Saumet JL. Pressure measurements at rest and after heavy exercise to detect moderate arterial lesions in athletes. J Vasc Surg 2001;33:721–727.
50. Abraham P, Chevalier JM, Saumet JL. External iliac artery endofibrosis: a 40-year course. J Sports Med Phys Fitness 1997;37:297–300.
51. Abraham P, Saumet JL, Chevalier JM. External iliac artery endofibrosis in athletes. Sports Med 1997; 24:221–226.
52. Wijesinghe LD, Coughlin PA, Robertson I, et al. Cyclist's iliac syndrome: temporary relief by balloon angioplasty. Br J Sports Med 2001; 35:70–71.
53. Rabkin DG, Goldstein DJ, Flores RM, Benvenisty AI. Spontaneous popliteal artery dissection: a case report and review of the literature. J Vasc Surg 1999; 29:737–740.
54. Cook PS, Erdoes LS, Selzer PM, Rivera FJ, Palmaz JC. Dissection of the external iliac artery in highly trained athletes. J Vasc Surg 1995; 22:173–177.
55. Killewich LA, Martin R, Cramer M, Beach KW, Strandness DE, Jr. Pathophysiology of venous claudication. J Vasc Surg 1984; 1:507–511.
56. Brulisauer M, Jager K, Bollinger A. Intermittent venous claudication: a rarely diagnosed walking disability. Schweiz Med Wochen 1987; 117:123–126.
57. Qvarfordt P, Eklof B, Ohlin P, Plate G, Saltin B. Intramuscular pressure, blood flow, and skeletal muscle metabolism in patients with venous claudication. Surgery 1984; 95:191–195.
58. Alimi YS, DiMauro P, Fabre D, Juhan C. Iliac vein reconstructions to treat acute and chronic venous occlusive disease. J Vasc Surg 1997; 25:673–681.
59. Bartram C, Edwards RH, Beynon RJ. McArdle's disease-muscle glycogen phosphorylase deficiency. Biochim Biophy Acta 1995; 1272:1–13.
60. Schimrigk K, Mertens HG, Ricker K, Fuhr J, Eyer P, Pette D. McArdle's syndrome (myopathy in muscle phosphorylase deficiency). Klin Wochen 1967; 45:1–17.
61. Lewis SF, Haller RG. The pathophysiology of McArdle's disease: clues to regulation in exercise and fatigue. J Appl Physiol 1986;61:391–401.
62. Chaussain M, Camus F, Defoligny C, Eymard B, Fardeau M. Exercise intolerance in patients with McArdle's disease or mitochondrial myopathies. Eur J Med 1992;1:457–463.
63. Lewis SF, Haller RG, Cook JD, Nunnally RL. Muscle fatigue in McArdle's disease studied by 31P-NMR: effect of glucose infusion. J Appl Physiol 1985;59:1991–1994.
64. Hertzer NR. The natural history of peripheral vascular disease: implications for its management. Circulation 1991;83:112–119.
65. Jonason T, Bergstrom R. Cessation of smoking in patients with intermittent claudication: effects on the risk of peripheral vascular complications, myocardial infarction and mortality. Acta Med Scand 1987;221:253–260.
66. Jonason T, Ringqvist I. Diabetes mellitus and intermittent claudication: relation between peripheral vascular complications and location of the occlusive atherosclerosis in the legs. Acta Med Scand 1985; 218:217–221.
67. Hedberg B, Angquist KA, Henriksson-Larsen K, Sjostrom M. Fibre loss and distribution in skeletal muscle from patients with severe peripheral arterial insufficiency. Eur J Vasc Surg 1989;3: 315–322.
68. Farinon AM, Marbini A, Gemignani F, et al. Skeletal muscle and peripheral nerve changes caused by chronic arterial insufficiency: significance and clinical correlations: histological, histochemical and ultrastructural study. Clin Neuropathol 1984;3:240–252.

69. Vogt MT, Cauley JA, Kuller LH, Nevitt MC. Functional status and mobility among elderly women with lower extremity arterial disease: the study of osteoporotic fractures. J Am Geriatr Soc 1994;42: 923–929.
70. Coffman JD. Intermittent claudication: not so benign. Am Heart J 1986;112:1127–1128.
71. Criqui MH, Langer RD, Fronek A, et al. Mortality over a period of 10 years in patients with peripheral arterial disease. N Engl J Med 1992;326:381–386.
72. Hertzer NR, Beven EG, Young JR, et al. Coronary artery disease in peripheral vascular patients: a classification of 1000 coronary angiograms and results of surgical management. Ann Surg 1984;199: 223–233.
73. Hiatt WR, Hirsch AT, Regensteiner JG, Brass EP. Clinical trials for claudication: assessment of exercise performance, functional status, and clinical end points. Vascular Clinical Trialists. Circulation 1995;92:614–621.
74. Criqui MH, Denenberg JO, Bird CE, Fronek A, Klauber MR, Langer RD. The correlation between symptoms and non-invasive test results in patients referred for peripheral arterial disease testing. Vasc Med 1996;1:65–71.
75. Regensteiner JG, Steiner JF, Panzer RJ, Hiatt WR: Evaluation of walking impairment by questionnaire in patients with peripheral arterial disease. J Vasc Med Biol 1988;2:142–152.
76. Gardner AW, Womack CJ, Sieminski DJ, Montgomery PS, Killewich LA, Fonong T. Relationship between free-living daily physical activity and ambulatory measures in older claudicants. Angiology 1998;49:327–337.
77. Gardner AW, Killewich LA, Katzel LI, et al. Relationship between free-living daily physical activity and peripheral circulation in patients with intermittent claudication. Angiology 1999;50:289–297.
78. Hiatt WR, Wolfel EE, Regensteiner JG, Brass EP. Skeletal muscle carnitine metabolism in patients with unilateral peripheral arterial disease. J Appl Physiol 1992;73:346–353.
79. Montgomery PS, Gardner AW. The clinical utility of a six-minute walk test in peripheral arterial occlusive disease patients. J Am Geriatr Soc 1998;46:706–711.

4

Hemodynamics and the Vascular Laboratory

D. E. Strandness, Jr., MD, D MED (HON.)

CONTENTS

INTRODUCTION

The arterial system can be divided anatomically into the large, medium, and small sized arteries and the microcirculation. Atherosclerosis is a disease of the large and medium sized arteries. The large arteries are those confined to the body cavities, with the medium sized arteries being the vessels with proper names outside the chest and abdomen. The small arteries such as the digital vessels generally are not affected in atherosclerosis, but, on occasion, may become involved secondarily. The same applies to the microcirculation. Thus, this chapter focuses on the large and medium sized arteries from both a hemodynamic and a vascular laboratory standpoint.

THE NORMAL ARTERIAL SYSTEM

The arteries supply blood to a variety of tissues with entirely different metabolic needs. Under normal circumstances, the vessels are required not only to provide the necessary blood flow, but to do it with minimal loss of energy. In general terms, the organs and tissues of the body can be considered as either low- or high-resistance systems. The low-resistance systems are those with a high demand for blood flow during the entire day.

From: *Contemporary Cardiology: Peripheral Arterial Disease: Diagnosis and Treatment*
Edited by: J. D. Coffman and R. T. Eberhardt © Humana Press Inc., Totowa, NJ

The organs that fulfill this definition include the brain, liver, and kidney. The high-resistance systems are those with relatively low demands under resting or baseline conditions. Here, the intestine and the blood supply of the extremities come into play. Obviously, with an increase in demand such as with exercise or ingestion of a meal, the demands for more blood increase very rapidly. The time course for the demand for more blood flow will depend on the time and extent of the activity that is in place. For example, in the case of the limbs, any period of exercise will be accompanied by the requisite requirements for an immediate increase in flow to maintain function at a normal level. In the case of the intestine during digestion, flow will slowly increase, reach a peak, and then, after many minutes, the flow will slowly decrease back to the baseline levels *(1)*.

The needs of the lower extremities are of great importance physiologically, as atherosclerosis often limits the amount of blood flow that is available. This will alter the normal pressure/flow relationships in a manner that will determine the degree of disability the patient suffers *(2)*. As will be noted, the other major factor that plays an important role in the pressure/flow relationships is the collateral arteries. These are vessels that are already present but can and will respond to the needs of the tissues if given sufficient time. This is an area of obvious interest today with the emergence of the new field of angiogenesis and gene therapy *(see* Chapter 11). Our ideas relative to the development of collateral vessels may have to be modified.

Another factor that must be remembered is that the structure of the artery walls themselves varies depending on location. For example, the media of the large arteries of the thorax and abdomen are dominated by elastin. In contrast, the medium sized arteries of the lower limbs are stiffer and have a higher collagen/elastin ratio. As will be noted, this does affect their function and our interpretation of the hemodynamic data obtained in the course of studying the peripheral arterial system *(3)*. There is also a dramatic increase in the cross-sectional area with each arterial subdivision. It has been estimated that the cross-sectional area at the level of the arterioles is 125 times that of the aorta *(4)*.

The small unnamed arteries and arterioles are not involved with atherosclerosis. Although there have been suggestions that the arterioles of diabetic patients show a specific lesion that may be responsible for the increased limb loss, this remains unproven *(5–7)*.

THE PHYSICS OF ARTERIAL BLOOD FLOW

Poiseuille's Law

Most discussions of blood flow start with a consideration of Poiseuille's law, which describes the relationship between pressure and flow in rigid tubes of constant diameters. For fluids to follow this law, the flow must be steady and laminar. Obviously none of these conditions are satisfied in the arterial system, but the law does serve as a useful starting point *(8)*. In addition, because blood is a non-Newtonian fluid, the energy losses and their effects are also related to shear rates *(9)*. The following is the basic equation that is commonly used to express this law:

$$Q = \frac{KPd_i^4}{L}$$

where:

Q =   volume flow
P =   pressure drop along the tube

d_i = inside tube diameter
L = tube length
K = a constant depending on fluid viscosity

Decreases in the radius of the tube add little to the pressure gradient until the tube becomes very small. This is illustrated by the fact that the mean pressure drop along the entire arterial system from the level of the heart to the arterioles is very small, in the range of 10 mmHg *(10)*. Arteries the size of a normal iliac artery can accommodate large volume flows without a measureable pressure gradient. This becomes important when the hemodynamics of arterial stenosis are considered.

Obviously, the use of the Poiseuille formulation is far removed from reality in terms of the actual situation with arterial blood flow. Flow is pulsatile, the fluid is non-Newtonian, and the tubes are elastic. However, one can use a simplified model as proposed by Womersley in 1955 to begin to approach the situation as it is actually encountered *(11)*. His handling of the problem is based on a cylindrical vessel without tapering and a rigid wall. The flow is assumed to be laminar and without the development of turbulence. The fluid is assumed to be Newtonian. The relationship between the pressure recorded from two points in the femoral artery is shown in Fig. 1. This was adapted from McDonald *(10)*. The pressure waves recorded over one pulse cycle (360°) show that the pressure at point A is slightly greater than that at point B, until a point is reached beyond 90° when there appears to be a reversal of the gradient, as shown in the differential recording. In humans, as shown in the latter part of the pulse cycle, a reversal of the gradient occurs that should lead to a transient reversal of blood flow. This is an important aspect in determining if blood flow patterns at specific points in the arterial system are indeed normal.

Turbulence

A point of considerable interest relates to the issue of turbulent blood flow, as it leads to energy losses that are considerably greater. In a laminar flow system with a Newtonian fluid and steady flow in a rigid pipe, flow will remain laminar until the Reynold's number (a dimensionless quantity) exceeds 2000. However, if the flow conditions are rigidly kept in the flow model, Reynold's numbers as high as 50,000 have been reached without the development of full-blown turbulence *(12)*. However, there is an intermediate state referred to as unsteady flow in which the laminar flow pattern may transiently "break up" but is then restored downstream from the site of the disturbance.

$$Re = \frac{\Delta d_i \rho}{\eta}$$

where:
Re = Reynold's number
Δ = average velocity
ρ = fluid density
η = viscosity
d_i = inside diameter

The importance of these flow patterns is reflected in terms of both their detection by diagnostic methods and their influence on the delivery of blood flow to the limbs.

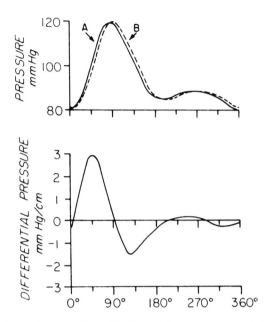

Fig. 1. The *upper tracing* shows the recording of differential pressures recorded simultaneously from two points along the femoral artery only a few centimeters apart. Curve A is proximal; curve B is distal. The *lower curve* is the differential pressure obtained by subtracting curve B from curve A. (Reproduced from Strandness DE Jr, Sumner DS: Hemodynamics for Surgeons. Grune & Stratton, New York, 1975, by permission.)

Laminar Blood Flow—Is it Present in the Human Peripheral Arteries?

If laminar flow requires rigid tubes with a Newtonian fluid in a steady flow system, the answer is obviously no. However, given our current knowledge of the blood flow patterns over a single pulse cycle in the femoral artery of a normal person, the answer may be a qualified yes. For example, when the velocity profiles are plotted over a single pulse cycle, it can be seen that just before the reversal of flow occurs, the picture is much like what is seen with steady flow (Fig. 2) *(10)*. These changes can now be studied to some degree noninvasively and have become important factors in determining the status of the arterial system.

Volume Flow: Normal and with Arterial Obstruction

When an organ or tissue is deprived of its normal arterial input, the total flow to the site during the ischemic episode has to be reduced. Thus, it would appear to be the logical variable to measure. However, this is not the case for both technological and practical reasons. First, there is a wide range for normal values for limb blood flow. Second, many of the flow abnormalities that occur are regional within the limb and may not be reflected when the total flow to the limb is measured. For example, gangrene of the forefoot can occur even with entirely normal calf blood flow. A major compounding factor is our limited ability to measure regional blood flow. Plethysmography measuring blood flow in the calf has been widely applied with great success, but it has found only a limited role in evaluating the hemodynamics of the arterial system affected by disease of the large and medium sized arteries.

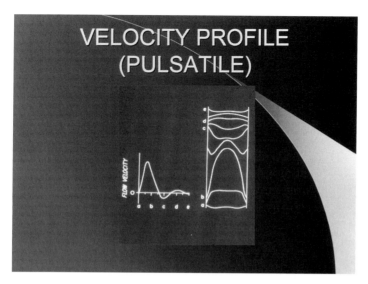

Fig. 2. Velocity distribution over a single pulse cycle. The waveform on the left is what one would expect from a normal peripheral artery. Points *a–e* represent different points in the cycle with *a* representing the onset of systole and *e* the end of diastole. The velocity distribution shown for point *b* has a laminar flow pattern but this is quickly broken up as the reverse flow component appears at *c*.

However, estimates of calf blood flow measured by plethysmography have added insight into the pressure flow relationships that occur in response to exercise *(2)*. This information has enhanced our understanding of the changes that occur when a patient develops claudication. The changes that occur normally and in the presence of an arterial lesion sufficient to produce intermittent claudication include the following:

1. Normally with exercise, calf blood flow will increase very rapidly to reach a level commensurate with the workload. One of the striking facts is the very short time required for the calf blood flow to return to normal, usually within the first few minutes. This is referred to as the period of postexercise hyperemia (Fig. 3).
2. Another very important finding is the change that occurs in the perfusion pressure. Normally, the ankle systolic pressure will remain unchanged or increase slightly postexercise. However, if the workload is heavy, there may be a transient fall in the ankle systolic pressure, but it will return to baseline levels within 3 min. The drop is normally <20% of the baseline level recorded at the ankle.
3. It is also important to remember that arm blood pressure after exercise will increase in relation to the work load *(13)*. Thus, if one were to measure the arm pressure at regular time intervals after exercise, it would increase.
4. When there is arterial inflow obstruction sufficient to produce claudication, the pressure–flow relationships are drastically altered. While the resting calf blood flow will be in the normal range, the ankle systolic pressure will usually be below normal. When the patient walks and develops progressive ischemia of the skeletal muscle, calf blood flow will increase but not to the extent seen in normal individuals, and, most important, will require much longer to return to the baseline levels. Thus, the period of postexercise hyperemia is prolonged. The same will be seen with the ankle systolic pressure; it will fall often to low levels and require a prolonged period of time to recover to preexercise levels (Fig. 4) *(14–17)*.

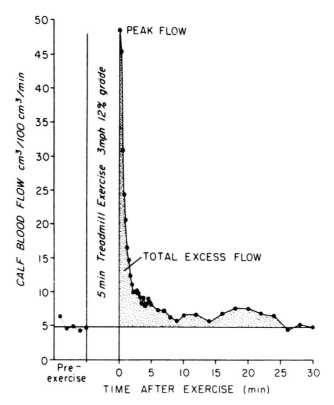

Fig. 3. Postexercise hyperemia in a normal subject who has exercised for 5 min on a treadmill set at 3 mph on a 12% grade. This was done with a plethysmograph on the calf. Please note the very high peak flows and the very short time for recovery to baseline levels. (Reproduced from Strandness DE Jr, Sumner DS: Hemodynamics for Surgeons. Fig. 9.7, Grune & Stratton, New York, 1975, with permission.)

Velocity of Flow and Pressure

Fortunately, we are able to estimate two aspects of vascular function that are diagnostically of great importance for obstructive arterial disease. As noted previously, the viscoelastic properties of the arterial tree change as one progresses down the limb. The arteries become progressively stiffer owing to a change in the elastin/collagen ratio. This stiffness leads to what is referred to as amplification of the systolic pressure levels. Thus, as one proceeds down the limb, the systolic pressure will normally be shown to gradually increase *(10,18)*. However, as is well recognized, there has to be a gradual fall in the mean arterial pressure. As noted in Fig. 5, this change in pressure is also accompanied by a change in the shape of the pulsatile arterial waveform. The dicrotic wave moves further from the systolic peak *(10)*.

On the other hand, when comparing the velocity waveforms recorded from similar sites, there are obvious differences in that there is a gradual decrease in the peak systolic velocity as one approaches the periphery. However, as noted, an important finding relates to the observation of a reverse flow component, which should always be present if there are no pressure and flow reducing lesions proximal to the recording site (Fig. 5) *(1,19)*.

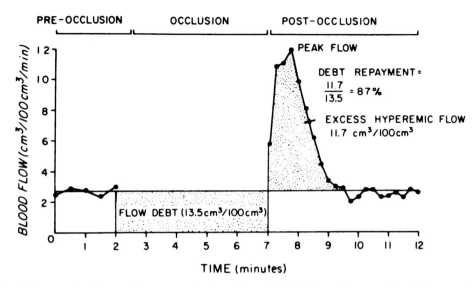

Fig. 4. The reactive hyperemia response in the right calf of a 54-yr-old man with a right superficial femoral artery occlusion. Note the very low peak blood flow response and the very slow recovery time back to baseline levels. Compare this with the flow response in a normal shown in Fig. 3. (Reproduced from Strandness DE Jr, Sumner DS. Hemodynamics for Surgeons, Fig. 9.14, Grune & Stratton, New York, 1975, with permission.)

COLLATERAL ARTERIES IN PERIPHERAL ARTERIAL DISEASE
Hemodynamics

Fortunately, the arterial system has been provided with a set of channels that are referred to as the collateral arteries. As previously noted, these are preexisting vessels that, if given time, can respond to need and keep limb perfusion within normal levels under resting flow conditions with arterial obstructions. A variety of facts are well known and accepted:

1. Collateral arteries consist of three components: the exit, midzone, and reentry vessel *(20)*. An example of an exit collateral would be the profunda femoris with the geniculate arteries representing the reentry channel(s). Normally the midzone connecting the two will not be visible on an arteriogram because of their small size. However, this is the zone that will undergo the greatest change in diameter when ischemia develops. In fact, with acute arterial occlusion, limb survival will often depend on the ability of the midzone collaterals to increase in diameter and carry enough nutritive blood flow to permit limb survival.

2. The problems with collateral arteries is that they present an increase in resistance to flow which limits their capability of providing enough blood flow to reach the levels necessary to prevent claudication from occurring. Thus, they may be sufficient for resting flow needs but cannot respond to the added stress of exercise.

3. Another problem relates to resistance to flow when more than one set of collateral arteries are in series in a limb with multisegmental obstructions. The resistance to flow is additive for each set of collaterals, so this further adds to the problems not only with exercise but in some cases at rest as well. For this reason multisegment arterial disease is

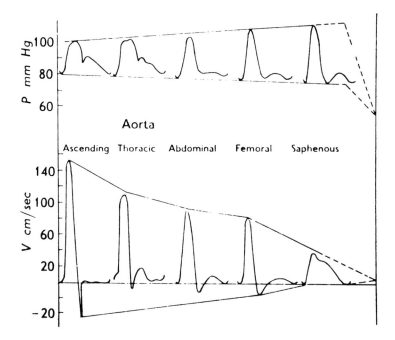

Fig. 5. This is a diagrammatic representation of the changes in pressure and flow velocity recorded from the arteries of a dog proceeding from the central aorta to the saphenous artery. There is a progressive decline in the peak velocity while there is amplification of the amplitude of the systolic pressure. (Reproduced from Strandness DE, Jr, Sumner DS: Hemodynamics for Surgeons. Modified from McDonald DA: Blood Flow in Arteries, Williams & Wilkins, Baltimore, 1960).

nearly always more severe than single-segment occlusion *(2)*. As will be noted, it is the patient with multisegment disease who presents the greatest challenges in management.

Anatomical Considerations of Collateral Arteries

Anatomically, there are profound differences in the collateral capabilities of some areas of the circulation that are important hemodynamically. In the case of the aorta and iliac arteries, the collateral pathways that may be called into action are often not visible by arteriography unless special techniques are used. The collaterals are described as parietal, as they arise and course in the body wall taking their origin from intercostal and subcostal arteries. Visceral collaterals to supply the limb can also come from the inferior mesenteric arteries that connect with the arteries of the pelvis. These are generally considered to be high-resistance collaterals that are rarely, if ever, able to supply enough blood to the ischemic limb to prevent claudication from occurring.

Below the inguinal ligament, as noted, the profunda femoris is the most important. It should also be noted that flow in the profunda may actually be reversed as the collaterals from a higher level perfuse this artery in a reverse direction. This is now easily documented by ultrasonic duplex scanning.

The geniculate pathways across the knees are fairly constant and critical to limb survival with acute arterial occlusions of the popliteal artery.

Below the knee the anatomic arrangement, in terms of potential collateral flow, is so much different. The blood supply to the gastrocnemius muscle is from a single source—the sural artery. Within the muscle, the arteries branch much like those of a tree; however, and most critically, there are relatively few arterial connections with the gastrocnemius muscle from outside sources. In a sense, it almost has an isolated blood supply. In sharp contrast, the soleus muscle is supplied by multiple side branches that freely communicate up and down the limb with other branches that permit inflow in cases of chronic arterial obstruction *(21)*.

These extensive intercommunications are usually able to provide adequate levels of blood flow even in the presence of extensive chronic arterial occlusion in the arteries below the knee. They are particularly important when considering the problem of diabetic arterial disease, in which extensive pathology in this area is very common.

ARTERIAL MEDIAL CALCIFICATION

There is a common misconception that the medial calcification seen in the tibial–peroneal arteries of diabetic individuals may adversely affect blood flow to the limb. This is not true because there is no association between these lesions of the media and those seen with atherosclerosis, which is a disease of the intima plus media. Interestingly, this type of problem is associated with diabetes mellitus, in which there is also a very high incidence of atherosclerosis involving these same vessels. The differences in the pattern of calcium deposition can be seen on radiographs of the limb *(22)*. Hemodynamically, the calcium in the media poses a problem in terms of measuring the ankle systolic pressure, which is discussed in more detail later in this chapter.

THE ROLE OF HEMODYNAMIC MEASUREMENTS IN DIAGNOSIS

It had been a dictum that a good history and a well performed physical examination followed by arteriography was, in some cases, all that was needed. However, it is now appreciated that atherosclerosis not only affects the anatomy of the delivery system but also perturbs it in such a way as to lead to symptoms that can be quantitatively expressed. These have become, or certainly should now become, a part of the evaluation process, not only at the time of first encounter but also for following the progress of the disease with and without therapy. In fact, a whole series of steps can be followed to document in rather precise detail the impact of the arterial disease on function. It is the view of this author that the testing procedures available should be used in a tailored fashion to answer the questions posed.

Because atherosclerosis progressively narrows and ultimately occludes the affected arteries, any form of testing is designed to both make the proper diagnosis and, in the final analysis, localize the sites of involvement. What is a significant lesion from a hemodynamic standpoint? This has been referred to as a "critical" stenosis. It is generally accepted that the plaque must narrow the diameter of the artery by at least 50% to reduce pressure and flow beyond the lesion *(23)*. When a large or medium sized artery is narrowed by this amount, a pressure gradient will develop across the lesion. This can limit the amount of flow available during exercise, leading to flow reduction and the development of intermittent claudication.

However, this is not the complete story as it is recognized that lesser degrees of stenosis, although not hemodynamically significant at resting flow rates, will become so during exercise *(24–26)*. This problem was recognized by DeWeese in 1960, who noted that palpable peripheral pulses in some patients disappeared when the individuals exercised to the point of calf pain *(27)*. The explanation for this finding was discovered at a later time but it is now known that with exercise some stenotic lesions develop turbulent blood flow with an accentuated energy loss, a fall in arterial blood flow, and the development of intermittent claudication. This hemodynamic change can now be documented by appropriate methods to be discussed.

Although coverage of aneurysmal disease is not a part of this text, it is important to remember that when present, it may present complications that affect outcome. However, we do not associate the presence of an aneurysm with a reduction in peripheral blood flow unless accompanied by a stenotic lesion or serves as a source for embolic material. Atheroembolism is considered in some detail, so the detection of the potential sites for embolization is considered (*see* Chapter 17). As will be noted, the modern diagnostic methods used to document hemodynamic problems will also be useful for the detection of the aneurysms at one or more sites.

VASCULAR DIAGNOSTIC TESTING

Fortunately, a whole series of examinations can be used in a cost-effective manner to provide the necessary data for clinical decision making. These can be applied to confirm a clinical impression, document the site(s) of involvement, and propose therapies that are likely to be effective. In addition, it is possible to use these same tests to document long-term outcome with and without therapy.

Ankle–Brachial and Toe–Brachial Systolic Pressure Index

When the patient is first seen and suspected of having peripheral arterial disease, the underlying diagnosis is usually not difficult if a proper history and physical examination is performed. However, it is important to confirm the suspicion with a test that is easily done, reproducible, and useful in the long term as well. For this purpose the ankle–brachial index (ABI) or in the diabetic patient the toe–brachial systolic pressure index (TSPI) can be measured.

TECHNICAL ISSUES

The most commonly used method for measuring the ABI is the continuous wave (CW) Doppler. With this pocket sized device, it is possible to detect flow from all three of the arteries at the level of the ankle/foot. In practice the systolic pressure is measured from the dorsalis pedis and posterior tibial arteries at the level of the ankle, although the pressure in the peroneal artery can be measured as well. It is very important to measure the brachial artery pressure with the CW Doppler as well and not rely on the stethoscope method. In the case of the diabetic patient, medial calcification of the tibial/peroneal arteries may prevent the measurement of a pressure owing to noncompressibility of the arteries. In this case, it is important to measure the systolic pressure in the toe—usually the great toe. To do this, one needs specially designed toe cuffs and a photoplethysmograph to document the pressure at this level. The rules guiding these measurements are as follows *(25,28,29)*:

1. The patient should rest at least 10 min before the measurement is taken to permit stabilization of the pressures.
2. When the cuff is inflated, it must be inflated to well above systolic pressure levels.
3. The point at which the opening or systolic pressure is recorded is during slow cuff deflation and not during cuff inflation, which is a common error.
4. The pressure is expressed both in absolute terms and as a ratio to the arm pressure. The normal ABI should be equal to or higher than 1.0 and the TSPI should be >0.69.
5. It is common practice to express the ratio for each of the tibial arteries and also the peroneal artery if that is measured.
6. The intraobserver variability for the ABI is ±0.15 and for the TSPI it is ±0.17. This is important as any change in these indices that exceeds these boundaries is a reflection of either improvement in the collateral blood flow or progression of the underlying arterial disease.
7. The ABI assessment can be done in the clinic at the time of the patient visit. However, it is necessary to have the toe measurement done in the vascular diagnostic laboratory.

INTERPRETATION OF THE ABI AND TSPI

For clinical purposes, a normal ABI is considered to be ≥0.90. For any value less than that, the patient will be found to have some occlusive disease proximal to the recording site. The same applies for toe–brachial pressure indices of <0.69. For clinical purposes, the indices can be useful as rough guides as to the level and extent of arterial disease.

1. An ABI >0.5 but < 0.9 is consistent with single-segment arterial disease such as an occlusion of the superficial femoral artery.
2. An ABI <0.5 is commonly found with multisegment disease.
3. The absolute systolic pressure levels at the ankle level are also useful in a general sense as they represent one aspect of the perfusion pressure. The systolic pressures can be very useful in the case of acute arterial occlusion. For example, an ankle systolic pressure of 50 mmHg or greater is consistent with adequate collateral blood flow. If the pressure is lower than this, serial measurements combined with clinical observation are helpful in predicting outcome.
4. Although it makes sense to use the ABI as an index of severity of claudication, this has not worked out well. However, very low ABIs are worrisome in terms of the development of critical limb ischemia. If an ABI is <0.40, it is important to follow these patients closely as blood flow typically is very marginal.
5. The TSPI has also been used to estimate the chances of healing of an open lesion that developed on a toe. TSPI >0.30 are indicative of adequate nutritional blood flow unless there is involvement of tendon or bone by an infectious process *(26,30)*.
6. A major advantage of these simple measurements is their use following the progress of disease and after any form of intervention. If an interventional procedure is successful, the ABI will increase by >0.15. If this level is not achieved, the procedure is considered a failure. Likewise, if during follow-up the ABI falls by >0.15, this is consistent with disease progression.

Treadmill Exercise Testing

The diagnosis of PAD is often very clear from the history, physical examination, and ABI but occasionally it is necessary to verify the diagnosis by an exercise test. This becomes very important in the case of an aging population who may also suffer from neurospinal problems giving rise to what is commonly called pseudoclaudication *(31)* (*see* Chapter 3). Verification of the diagnosis can now be done within the setting of the vascular laboratory. As noted above, claudication is produced by the failure of the arterial circulation to provide adequate inflow to the exercising muscle. The treadmill testing can be done in a variety of ways but in general, a standard test at 2 mph on a 12% grade is used. Even the elderly can walk at this speed and elevation *(15,16)*. It is common practice to terminate the exercise if the patient can walk for 5 min. Although some recommend EKG monitoring during the test, we have not done this, but we do, of course, stop the test if the patient complains of chest discomfort. We have not had an adverse cardiac event using these guidelines. The procedure and interpretation of the treadmill exercise test is as follows:

1. The patient must have been resting for at least 10 min to allow the ankle systolic pressure to stabilize.
2. The cuffs used for the ankle and arm are left in place during the testing.
3. The patient is asked to inform the technologist when and where the pain occurs. This is recorded as the initial claudication distance (ICD). When the patient is forced to stop, this is called the maximum walking distance (MWD).
4. When the patient stops, they are returned to the bed quickly and the ankle and brachial systolic pressures are recorded at intervals of approx 1 min. While some laboratories record the postexericse pressures in terms of an ABI, this is not what should be done. The arm pressure will increase in relation to the workload. Thus, it is possible to have a normal ankle blood pressure response postexercise but an abnormal ABI.
5. There are two important elements of the postexercise response: the magnitude of the ankle systolic pressure drop and the time required for it to return to the preexercise level. Normally, the ankle systolic pressure at the ankle should not fall more than 20% of the baseline and require less then 3 min to return to prewalking levels (Fig. 4) *(13)*.
6. The more severe the claudication, the greater the ankle pressure fall and the longer it takes to recover. In some cases, the ankle systolic pressure may be unrecordable after exercise and require > 30 min to recover to baseline. This period is referred to as the postexercise ischemic period.

With pseudoclaudication, there will not be an abnormal postexercise response unless there is coexisting arterial disease. One helpful suggestion with regard to the exercise test is that patients with pseudoclaudication are often forced to stop walking very early due to pain and they do not demonstrate the ankle pressure fall and recovery that is expected for true vascular claudication. This dissociation is useful to distinguish which of the two disorders is causing the patient's symptoms. This same testing procedure can be done after any form of intervention. However, it is not commonly performed because the changes in the ABI are often sufficient to determine the result.

Duplex Scanning

TECHNICAL ISSUES AND DIAGNOSTIC CRITERIA

With the availability of high-resolution imaging, color and power Doppler combined with real-time spectral analysis, it is now possible to accurately assess the location and degree of arterial involvement from the level of the aorta to the ankles. This type of information can be very useful for planning and evaluating the results of any therapeutic intervention.

The critical items that need to be determined relate to site(s) and their hemodynamic significance. The significant technological elements can be summarized as follows *(19,32–34)*:

1. The B-mode image quality has improved greatly so one can visualize areas of plaque formation, calcification, and aneurysmal changes. However, it is not possible to define the degree of diameter reduction based on the B-mode imaging alone.
2. The availability of color Doppler has been an important advance in scanning peripheral arteries. It provides a very useful roadmap for the technologist, who has the following options *(35,36)*:
   a. Setting the color to cover the expected ranges of velocity.
   b. Determining the direction of flow.
   c. Documenting the triphasic flow patterns in normal peripheral arteries.
   d. Visualizing arteries down to the level of the foot.
   e. Using the B-mode/color image for accurate placement of the sample volume of the pulsed Doppler for recording the spectral velocity patterns.
   f. Documenting poststenotic flow and turbulence by the visualization of a "Doppler bruit."
3. A more recent addition to ultrasound technology is Power Doppler. This color display is dependent on the amplitude of the backscattered signal and not the velocity. It has become useful for following the arteries in areas of tortuosity.
4. Real-time spectral analysis is also used. There is no doubt that examining the velocity information has been the most useful for documenting the flow patterns and estimating the degree of narrowing. The proper application of the actual velocity data to estimate the degree of stenosis is to calculate the ratio of the peak systolic velocity at the site of narrowing divided by that found in the prestenotic segment *(32,37,38)*. The reason for using this type of information in contrast to the absolute velocity change at the site of narrowing is that velocities in peripheral arteries vary a great deal in normal subjects. The manner in which one arrives at an estimate of arterial narrowing requires the following:
   a. The scan must be along the artery prior to, in, and after the stenosis. Color makes this much simpler as it provides the "roadmap" for the technologist.
   b. It is mandatory that the angle of the incident sound beam be kept at of 60° to the long axis of the artery. If this simple rule is not followed, the observed velocities will vary so much as to render them useless.
   c. An assumption is made that the lesions of greatest interest are those that narrow the artery by >50% diameter reduction (critical stenosis) *(23)*. This has been tested by more than one group. Our own findings comparing the ultrasound data with arteriography support this approach. While there are differences between investigators, the procedure and outcome are relevant to the problem in general. These considerations are as follows:
      i. For clinical decision making relative to intervention it is important to document the presence of a 50% stenosis or greater. The ratio of the peak systolic velocity at the site of the stenosis divided by that immediately proximal to the stenosis should be > 1.5 *(32)*. Other investigators prefer a higher ratio (2.0–2.5), which is probably more conservative but will also work well. If the ratio is <2.0–2.5 *(39)*, it must be remembered that lesions <50% in terms of diameter reduction can become hemodynamically significant when the velocity increase is enough to lead to the development of turbulence.

    ii. With these kinds of data relative to areas of narrowing/occlusion, it is possible to determine which form of intervention might be feasible.

SITES OF DISEASE AND IMPLICATIONS OF STUDIES

Aortoiliac Disease. Lesions involving the common iliac/external iliac artery can produce disabling intermittent claudication. Because of the proximal location of these arteries, the entire limb is deprived of normal arterial input during exercise. This is also an area where treatment by endovascular means has been successful in properly selected patients. To plan a therapeutic approach, it is necessary to document the site of the disease (stenosis/occlusion) and the artery in which it is found. The best candidates for endovascular therapy are those with common iliac stenoses and an external iliac artery that is free of significant disease. In addition, it is important to know if there is coexisting disease in the superficial femoral artery/popliteal artery. The finding of multilevel disease adds to the hemodynamic problems because, as noted earlier, every additional set of collaterals adds to the resistance to flow. Correction of one proximal level of disease will render the patient's symptoms dependent on the resistance offered by the next set of collaterals.

There is no doubt that duplex ultrasound can be used to make these determinations. The studies that have been done examining the role of ultrasound here have shown this to be the case *(40)*. The studies provide useful information as the patient can be informed of the plan and the endovascular therapist can use this information to determine the site for catheter entry. It is this author's view that the endovascular procedure can be planned without having to resort to arteriography to make this decision.

If there is combined two level disease—aortoiliac/femoropopliteal disease—it may be difficult to determine which of the levels is most important in leading to the exercise-induced pain. However, as is well known, isolated superficial femoral artery occlusive disease does not, in general, produce the severe claudication seen with disease proximal to the inguinal ligament.

Superficial Femoral/Popliteal Artery Disease. This segment of the lower limb arterial supply is a very common site for the development of atherosclerosis and can easily be studied by duplex ultrasound *(41)*. The lesions are most commonly seen in the adductor canal. It is possible to determine the site(s) of involvement and most importantly, their distribution. This becomes critically important for planning surgical therapy. It should be noted that endovascular therapy for the femoral/popliteal area is not as successful as proximal to the inguinal ligament owing to the very difficult problem of myointimal hyperplasia.

The ability to perform surgical revascularization on the basis of ultrasound findings alone is often questioned *(37,39,42)*. This is possible as long as the inflow arteries and those below the knee can also be shown to be free of significant disease. It is certain that with experience, preoperative arteriography will not be needed for isolated disease in this location. It is also likely that more intraoperative arteriograms will be done to verify the plan, resulting in considerable overall cost reduction and avoidance of complications for the patient.

Infrapopliteal Occlusive Disease. This is an interesting area both in terms of hemodynamics and the role of the vascular laboratory in evaluating this problem. It is well known that diabetic patients will have a much higher incidence of involvement at this level *(43,44)*. Another fact that has been poorly appreciated is the infrequency of intermittent claudication when the arterial occlusions are confined to this segment of the circulation. As mentioned earlier, there are differences in the potential collateral input to both the gastrocnemius and soleus muscle, which might explain at least why this is the case. It is assumed that the pain of "calf" claudication is from ischemia of the gastrocnemius and not from the soleus muscle. Because the major blood supply to the gastrocnemius comes from a level above the muscle itself (popliteal artery via the sural arteries), it is not surprising that lesions below the level of this major source of blood do not lead to claudication. Also, the arrangement of the collateral blood supply to the soleus muscle explains why this muscle is rarely the site of ischemic pain with exercise.

The diagnosis of infrapopliteal disease is suspected both from a reduced ABI and from either absence of flow by CW Doppler or abnormal flow patterns (monophasic). This assumes that the flow patterns detected from the popliteal artery and higher are entirely normal. It must always be remembered that there are three arteries below the knee. It is also well known that either the posterior tibial or peroneal artery alone is capable of providing a normal blood supply to both the calf and the foot.

Is the area "hemodynamically silent"? The answer is a qualified no, but it is very rare, in my experience, to have patients note claudication due to disease in this location alone. Thus, it is possible to have occlusions below the popliteal artery level and have a normal response to treadmill exercise. The problems dealing with this area become evident when it is not the sole area of occlusive involvement.

THE DIABETIC PATIENT

It is important to review in some detail how patients with diabetes are evaluated. It is well known that this group has the most virulent form of occlusive disease. The peculiarities of their problems explain why the evaluation may be more difficult (*see* Chapter 15). Some of these differences are as follows:

1. The frequent occurrence of a peripheral neuropathy, which not only leads to a loss of deep pain sensation but also results in an "autosympathectomy." As a consequence the foot will become dry but warm, reflecting the increased skin blood flow that is a part of the process *(6)*.
2. The frequent occurrence of medial calcification, which as noted earlier is not associated with any restriction in blood flow to the leg or foot. It is nearly always confined to the tibial/peroneal arteries.
3. The need for measurement of the TSBI to circumvent the problem of medial calcification of the tibial/peroneal arteries. This needs to be performed by a vascular laboratory using an indirect sensor such as a photoplethysmograph *(45)*.

The vascular laboratory plays a crucial role in localizing the extent of involvement in this population. The most important patients are those with femoropopliteal involvement and occlusive disease below the knee arteries. The evaluation at these levels is critical as these patients may require distal arterial bypass to improve flow in patients with critical ischemia. While some laboratories do not routinely scan these arteries, with the improvement in duplex scan technology these arteries can and should be scanned. The availability of color and power Doppler has made this feasible *(35,36)*.

SELECTING PATIENTS FOR THERAPY

When patients are seen, and after a proper diagnosis has been made, the next obvious step relates to therapy. Interventional therapy has one role only and that is to increase blood flow to the limb. These techniques involve angioplasty with or without stenting vs operative procedures. In the past, these procedures were never done without the benefit of arteriography. This practice is gradually changing and will change more in the future as physicians become more comfortable with alternative forms of imaging combined with flow velocity determinations. One possible avenue will be magnetic resonance arteriography, which can be used without contrast, but more recently, gadolinium is being used to enhance imaging of some areas of the circulation. This workup remains controversial for two reasons: cost and availability. While the cost issue might become moot if it is cheaper than standard contrast methods, it must be remembered that, even if it works, it remains no better than a standard contrast study. In addition, one of the major problems with such procedures is that they are not suitable for long-term follow-up studies, which in the view of this author remain a key issue for patients with vascular disease. The method chosen must be useable on a regular basis, and duplex scanning fits that requirement.

LONG-TERM FOLLOW-UP

Two categories are worthy of comment as the methods of follow-up will be different.

Without Interventional Therapy

As the majority of patients with PAD will not have any direct interventional therapy, how should these patients be followed? Hemodynamically, there are two changes that can occur—the disease may remain stable with or without improvement in the collateral circulation or the disease may progress either at the same site or at others. The simplest method of documenting these changes is by simply measuring the ABI. As collateral circulation improves, the resistance to flow in the mid-zone collaterals will decrease and the ABI will increase. Conversely, if the disease progresses at the same site or new ones, new collaterals may be called into play. When this occurs, the resistance to flow increases and the ABI decreases. It is accepted that an increase or decrease of 0.15 or more in the ABI is sufficient to note progression of disease or improvement in the collateral circulation.

With Interventional Therapy

Any procedure designed to improve blood flow to the leg must lead to an increase in the ABI of at least 0.15 (as noted earlier). This is now considered the standard and simplest method of documenting an improvement following intervention. However, with the availability of duplex scanning this can now be used for documenting outcome changes in patients who have infrainguinal saphenous vein grafts placed. The saphenous vein grafts rapidly acquire the compliance characteristics of the host artery. However, there is a high incidence of myointimal hyperplasia, which threatens the long-term function of the graft. It appears that this process may begin very quickly after placement of the graft. Therefore, it is important that the surveillance program begin soon after placement *(46–49)*. The hemodynamic criteria used for follow-up are as follows:

1. When functioning properly, a femoropopliteal/distal graft should not show any discrete areas of narrowing within the graft itself. The velocities should be uniform along the length of the graft. If the graft were an *in situ* vein graft, the peak systolic velocity should increase near its distal end owing to the tapering of the vein graft. The opposite will be seen with the reverse saphenous vein graft.
2. Uniformly low velocities along the graft (<45 cm/s) may be seen in large grafts or in those with an outflow stenosis.
3. When a focal stenosis is found within the graft, it is important to express that change as a ratio of the peak systolic velocity at the site of narrowing to that immediately proximal to that point. The magnitude of this ratio will, in part, determine the need for intervention. For example, if that ratio exceeds 3.5, there is good evidence that an intervention may be needed to promote long-term graft patency. It is thought that a ratio of this magnitude is associated with a reduction of the cross-sectional area of 75% or greater.
4. Because myointimal hyperplasia can occur at either anastomosis, these areas need to be studied as well. The geometry of these areas is more complex, making the use of ratios unrealistic. For this reason, the findings at any visit should be compared with that found previously.
5. Progressive disease in the inflow and outflow arteries is detected and assessed in the manner outlined previously.

SUMMARY

It is clear from our past experience that a better understanding of hemodynamics of the arterial system along with modern study methods will provide us with the type of objective information that we need. It is no longer acceptable to use only the history and physical examination as the sole method of documenting the presence of disease and its location. As noted in this chapter, we now have the tools to move ahead. It is also becoming obvious that as a result of such an approach, we will be able to reduce the number of invasive diagnostic procedures that have for so many years been the mainstay of our approach.

REFERENCES

1. Strandness DE, Jr. Hemodynamics of the normal arterial and venous system. In: Strandness DE, Jr., ed. Duplex Scanning in Vascular Disorders, 2nd edit. New York: Raven Press, 1993; pp.45–79.
2. Sumner DS, Strandness DE, Jr. The relationship between calf blood flow and ankle pressure in patients with intermittent claudication. Surgery 1969;65:763–771.
3. Mozersky DJ, Sumner DS, Hokanson DE, et al. Transcutaneous measurement of the elastic properties of the human femoral artery. Circulation 1972;46:948
4. Burton AC. Arrangement of the many vessels. In: Physiology and Biophysics of the Circulation, 1st edit. Chicago: Year Book, 1965; pp.61–71.
5. Goldenberg S, Alex M, Joshi RA, et al. Non-atheromatous peripheral vascular disease of the lower extremity in diabetes mellitus. Diabetes 1959;8:261–273.
6. Strandness DE, Jr, Priest RR, Gibbons GE. A combined clinical and pathological study of nondiabetic and diabetic vascular disease. Diabetes 1964;13:366–372.
7. Conrad MC. Large and small artery occlusion in diabetics and nondiabetics. Circulation 1967;36: 83–91.
8. Burton AC. Transmural pressures, pressure gradients and resistance to flow in the vascular bed. In: Physiology and Biophysics of the Circulation, 1st edit. Chicago: Year Book, 1965; pp. 84–92.
9. Strandness DE, Jr, Sumner DS. Hemodynamics for Surgeons, 1st edit. New York: Grune & Stratton, 1975.

10. McDonald DA. The pulsatile flow pattern in arteries. In: McDonald DA, ed. Blood Flow in Arteries. Baltimore: Williams & Wilkins, 1960; pp.129–145.

11. Womersley JR. Method for calculation of velocity rate of flow and viscous drag in arteries where the pressure gradient is known. J Physiol 1955;127:553–563.

12. Forrester JH, Young DF. Flow through a converging-diverging tube and its implications in occlusive vascular disease. J Biomech 1970;3:297–307.

13. Stahler C, Strandness DE, Jr. Ankle blood pressure response to graded treadmill exercise. Angiology 1967;18:237–241.

14. Carter SA. Response of ankle systolic pressure to leg exercise in mild or questionable arterial disease. N Engl J Med 1972;287:578–582.

15. Skinner JS, Strandness DE, Jr. Exercise and intermittent claudication: I. Effect of repetition and intensity of exercise. Circulation 1967;36:15–22.

16. Strandness DE, Jr. Exercise testing in the evaluation of patients undergoing direct arterial surgery. J Cardiovasc Surg 1970;11:192–200.

17. Clement DL, Shepherd JT. Regulation of peripheral circulation during muscular exercise. Prog Cardiovasc Dis 1976;19:23–31.

18. Taylor MG. Wave travel in arteries and design of the cardiovascular system. In: Attinger EO, ed. Pulsatile Blood Flow, 1st edit. New York: McGraw-Hill, 1964.

19. Jager KA, Ricketts HJ, Strandness DE, Jr. Duplex scanning for the evaluation of lower limb arterial disease. In: Bernstein EF, ed. Vascular Diagnosis, 4th edit. St. Louis: CV Mosby, 1985; p.619

20. Longland CJ. The collateral circulation to the limb. Ann Roy Coll Surg (Engl) 1953;13:161–176.

21. de Saunders CH, Lawrence J, Maciver DA, et al. The anatomic basis of the peripheral circulation in man. In: Redisch WT, ed. Peipheral Circulation in Health and Disease, 1st edit. New York: Grune & Stratton, 1957; pp.113–145.

22. Lindbom A. Arteriosclerosis and arterial thrombosis in the lower limb: a roentgenological study. Acta Radiol Scand 1950;80(Suppl):38–48.

23. May AG, Vandeberg L, DeWeese JA, Rob DG. Critical arterial stenosis. Surgery 1963;54:250–259.

24. Carter SA. Arterial auscultation in peripheral vascular disease. JAMA 1981;246:1682–1686.

25. Carter SA. Clinical measurement of systolic pressures in limbs with arterial occlusive disease. JAMA 1969;207:1869–1874.

26. Carter SA. The relationship of distal systolic blood pressures to healing of skin lesions in limbs with arterial occlusive disease, with special reference to diabetes mellitus. Scand J Clin Lab Invest 1973; 31(Suppl 128):239–243.

27. DeWeese JA. Pedal pulses disappearing with exercise: a test for intermittent claudication. N Engl J Med 1960;262:1214–17

28. Strandness DE, Jr, Bell JW. Peripheral vascular disease: diagnosis and objective evaluation using a mercury strain gauge. Ann Surg 1965;161(Suppl):1–35.

29. Carter SA, Tate RB. The effect of body heating and cooling on the ankle and toe systolic pressures in arterial disease. J Vasc Surg 1992;16:148–153.

30. Ramsey DE, Mankey DA, Sumner DS. Toe blood pressure: a valuable adjunct to ankle pressure measurement for assessing peripheral arterial disease. J Cardiovasc Surg 1983;24:43–48.

31. Goodreau JJ, Greasy JK, Flanigan DP, et al. Rational approach to the differentiation of vascular and neurogenic claudication. Surgery 1978;84:749–757.

32. Jager KA, Phillips DJ, Martin RL, et al. Noninvasive mapping of lower limb arterial lesions. Ultrasound Med Biol 1985;11:515–521.

33. Kohler TR, Nance DR, Cramer MM, Vandenburgh N, Strtandness DE. Duplex scanning for diagnosis of aortoiliac and femoropopliteal disease: a prospective study. Circulation 1987;76:1074–1080.

34. Kohler TR, Andros G, Porter JM, Clowes A, Goldstone J, Johansen K. Can duplex scanning replace arteriography for lower extremity arterial disease? Ann Vasc Surg 1990;4:280–287.

35. Hatsukami TS, Primozich J, Zierler RE, Strandness DE. Color Doppler characteristics in normal lower extremity arteries. Ultrasound Med Biol 1992;16:167–171.

36. Hatsukami TS, Primozich JP, Zierler RE, et al. Color Doppler imaging of infrainguinal arterial occlusive disease. J Vasc Surg 1992;16:527–533.

37. Elsman BH, Legemate DA, van-der-Heijden FH, de Vos HJ, Mali WP, Eikelboom BC. Impact of ultrasonographic duplex scanning on therapeutic decision making in lower-limb arterial disease. Br J Surg 1995;82:630–633.

38. Legemate DA, Teeuwen C, Hoeneveld H, Eikelboom BC. How can the assessment of the hemodynamic significance of aortoiliac arterial stenosis by duplex scanning be improved? A comparative study with intraarterial pressure measurement. J Vasc Surg 1993;17:676–684.
39. Elsman BH, Legemate DA, van-der-Heyden FW, de Vos H, Mali WP, Eikenbloom BC. The use of color-coded duplex scanning in the selection of patients with lower extremity arterial disease for percutaneous transluminal angioplasty: a prospective study. Cardiovasc Intervent Radiol 1996;19: 313–316.
40. Edwards JM, Coldwell DM, Goldman ML, Srandness DE. The role of duplex scanning in the selection of patients for transluminal angioplasty. J Vasc Surg 1991;13:69–74.
41. Cossman DV, Ellison JE, Wagner WH, et al. Comparison of contrast arteriography to arterial mapping with color-flow imaging in the lower extremities. J Vasc Surg 1989;10:522–529.
42. Legemate DA, Teeuwen C, Hoeneveld H, Ackerstaff RG, Eikelboom. The potential for duplex scanning to replace aortoiliac and femoropopliteal angiography. Eur J Vasc Surg 1989;3:49–54.
43. Gensler SW, Haimovici H, Hoffert P, Steinman C, Beneventano TC. Study of vascular lesions in diabetic, non-diabetic patients. Arch Surg 1965;91:617–622.
44. Wheelock FC, Jr. Transmetatarsal amputation and arterial surgery in diabetic patients. N Engl J Med 1961;264:316–320.
45. Orchard TJ, Strandness DE, Jr. Assessment of peripheral vascular disease in diabetes. Circulation 1993;88:819–828.
46. Caps MT, Cantwell-Gab K, Bergelin RO, Strandness DE. Vein graft lesions: time of onset and rate of progression. J Vasc Surg 1995;22:466–474.
47. Bandyk DF, Schmitt DD, Seabrook GR, Adams MB, Towne JB. Monitoring functional patency of in situ saphenous vein bypasses: the impact of a surveillance protocol and elective revision. J Vasc Surg 1989;9:286–296.
48. Idu MM, Buth J, Hop WCJ, Cuypers P, van de Pavoordt ED, Tordoir JM. Vein graft surveillance: is graft revision without angiography justified and what criteria should be used? J Vasc Surg 1998;27: 399–411.
49. Mills JL, Bandyk DF, Gahtan V, Esses GE. The origin of infrainguinal vein graft stenosis: a prospective study based on duplex surveillance. J Vasc Surg 1995;21:16–22.

5

Vascular Imaging with X-Ray, Magnetic Resonance, and Computed Tomography Angiography

John A. Kaufman, MD

CONTENTS

INTRODUCTION

The peripheral arteries can now be imaged with a variety of modalities *(1)*. Selection of the appropriate technique for an individual requires consideration of the type of information that is needed, the risks to the patient, and the availability of the imaging technology. This chapter reviews the basic principles of catheter angiography, magnetic resonance angiography (MRA), and CT angiography (CTA) as applied to the peripheral arteries.

CATHETER ANGIOGRAPHY

The basis of modern angiography is the Seldinger technique, the percutaneous introduction of a plastic catheter into an artery *(2)*. Utilizing sophisticated guidewires and catheters, catheters as small as 3 French (1 mm in outer diameter) can be used, although more usual sizes are 4- and 5-French *(3)*. The most frequent site of catheter introduction is the common femoral artery, but a variety of options exist including axillary artery, radial artery, subclavian artery, and direct translumbar aortic puncture *(4)*. With rare exceptions diagnostic procedures can be performed utilizing local anesthetic and intravenous sedation. The need for surgical cutdown to obtain arterial access for catheter introduction is almost nonexistent. Following femoral artery catheter removal

From: *Contemporary Cardiology: Peripheral Arterial Disease: Diagnosis and Treatment*
Edited by: J. D. Coffman and R. T. Eberhardt © Humana Press Inc., Totowa, NJ

with manual compression patients remain at bedrest for 4–6 h, but can be discharged directly home *(5)*. Diagnostic angiography is an outpatient procedure unless dictated otherwise by clinical circumstances.

Contrast Agents

The development of safe contrast agents has been a major advance in peripheral arterial angiography *(6)*. There are two major classes of tri-iodinated contrast agents, ionic and nonionic. Ionic contrast agents are bound to a nonradiopaque cation, usually sodium and meglumine (*N*-methylglucamine). The result is a highly osmolar (two particles per iodinated ring) solution. High osmolarity is believed to be a major contributing factor to adverse reactions. Nonionic contrast agents have no electrical charge, so that binding to a cation is unnecessary. This greatly lowers the osmolality of the contrast agent (one particle per iodinated ring), but increases viscosity. Thromboembolic complications may be more common with nonionic agents *(7)*.

Adverse reactions to iodinated contrast agents are distressingly common, but the majority are minor (Table 1). The overall incidence is lower with nonionic contrast agents *(8)*. Complications such as nausea and vomiting are related to a central nervous system mechanism, and seem more frequent with venous rather than arterial injections. The incidence of life-threatening anaphylaxis is approx 1 per 40,000–170,000, with mild reactions such as urticaria and nasal stuffiness occurring more commonly (especially with ionic contrast).

There are two alternative contrast agents that can be used for peripheral arteriography in patients with contraindications to iodinated contrast. Carbon dioxide gas (CO_2) is highly soluble, completely nonallergenic, and nonnephrotoxic *(9)*. Injected intraarterially, CO_2 briefly displaces blood and acts as a negative contrast agent (the vessel lumen is less radioopaque than surrounding tissues). The gas is totally absorbed within seconds, and ultimately exhaled by the patient. This agent can be safely used even in patients with severe CO_2 retention due to chronic lung disease. However, use is limited to the infradiaphragmatic arteries owing to reports of seizures and loss of consciousness if CO_2 reaches the cerebral arteries *(10)*.

Gadolinium chelates were developed as contrast agents for magnetic resonance imaging (MRI), but are sufficiently radioopaque to be used in conventional angiography *(11)*. The safety profile of these contrast agents is superior to that of iodinated contrast, and there appears to be lower nephrotoxicity *(12)*. Volumes of contrast in the range of 40–60 mL have been used for many years without complications. Gadolinium-based contrast agents have been used safely in every vascular application, including the carotid arteries. The main limitations are the expense, the small total volume that can be used, and the relatively low radioopacity.

Film-Screen and Digital Angiography

A key element of angiography is the record of the contrast injection. There are two basic modes, film-screen and digital subtraction angiography (DSA). Film-screen imaging currently provides the highest resolution, and is the traditional "gold standard" against which digital imaging is compared. However, this modality is rapidly disappearing, as all new angiographic equipment have been only digital for almost a decade.

DSA is the most widely used angiographic technique. DSA has lower resolution than film-screen, but provides extremely rapid acquisition of images and processing and the

Table 1
Contrast Reactions

Reaction	Incidence with ionic contrast	Incidence with nonionic contrast
Nausea	4.6%	1%
Vomiting	1.8%	0.4%
Itching	3.0%	0.5%
Urticaria	3.2%	0.5%
Sneezing	1.7%	0.2%
Dyspnea	0.2%	0.04%
Hypotension	0.1%	0.01%
Death	1:40,000	1:170,000

ability to manipulate the image appearance on-line to compensate for poor opacification. Images can be viewed in either subtracted or unsubtracted (raw) format. Filming can be as rapid as 30 frames per second with some units, with continuous acquisition while moving the angiographic table (bolus chasing) or the tube (rotational angiography). Lower contrast concentrations can be used (30–50% less iodine than for film-screen angiography), without altering the injection rates. The exquisite sensitivity of this technique allows the use of alternative negative contrast agents such as CO_2 for angiography. Limitations of DSA in addition to lower resolution include subtraction artifacts from involuntary motion such as bowel peristalsis, respiration, and cardiac pulsation.

Suprainguinal Angiography

Angiographic evaluation of the lower extremities includes, in most patients, the diaphragm to the ankle (Fig. 1). An abdominal aortogram is of particular importance when renovascular or visceral artery occlusive disease is suspected. Pelvic arteriography is performed with a pigtail catheter just proximal to the aortic bifurcation. Anterior–posterior and bilateral oblique views are obtained whenever iliac artery pathology is suspected. Typical parameters are 8–10 mL/s of contrast injected for 2–3 s, and an exposure rate of two to four frames per second for DSA. Pressure gradients should be measured across any stenosis.

Infrainguinal Angiogram

Bilateral lower extremity runoffs are obtained with the catheter at the aortic bifurcation. Full-strength low-osmolar contrast should be injected at 6–10 mL/s for 12 s. Runoffs with DSA can be obtained with two basic strategies. The simplest and most reliable is stationary overlapping DSA down the legs. The volume of contrast necessary is dependent on the severity of disease; as the length and number of occlusions increase, more contrast is needed to opacify distal reconstituted vessels. Typical injections range from 10 to 30 mL. The second basic approach is termed "bolus chase," in which the physician activates the position change based on real-time assessment of vascular opacification. Images can be acquired as either digital angiograms or DSA. A standard contrast injection can be used. Although less overall contrast is typically used compared to stationary runs, the likelihood of underfilling a segment of vessel is greater.

Single-limb angiography usually produces more visually appealing images than bilateral run-offs. After the necessary views of the pelvis are obtained, a catheter is positioned in the external iliac artery. Stationary DSA runs with injections of 4 mL/s

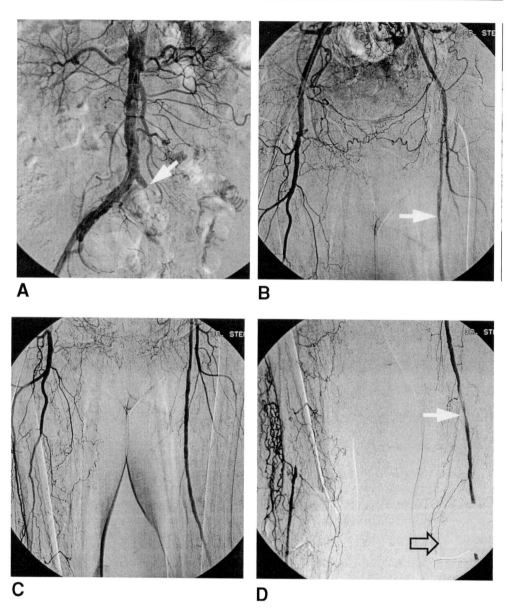

Fig. 1. Digital subtraction angiogram (DSA) performed with the bolus chase technique.
(A) Aortic injection with a pigtail catheter at the level of the visceral artery segment. There is a left common iliac artery occlusion (*arrow*). **(B)** The left lower extremity runoff is reconstituted via hypogastric collaterals, resulting in less intense opacification of the left superficial femoral artery (SFA) (*arrow*). The right SFA is occluded. **(C)** Image at the level of the thighs. **(D)** Image at the level of the adductor canal and above-knee popliteal artery. The contrast column in the left SFA appears attenuated as it crosses the bony cortex owing to subtraction artifact (*solid arrow*). The patient has a metallic knee prosthesis on the left that completely obscures the popliteal artery (*open arrow*). **(E)** Image at the level of the popliteal arteries. Note the metallic prosthesis on the left (*arrow*). A repeat angiogram with the knee turned in profile confirmed a normal popliteal artery. **(F)** Image at the level of the tibial arteries. **(G)** Image at the level of the ankles. The pedal vessels are not well visualized from this aortic injection.

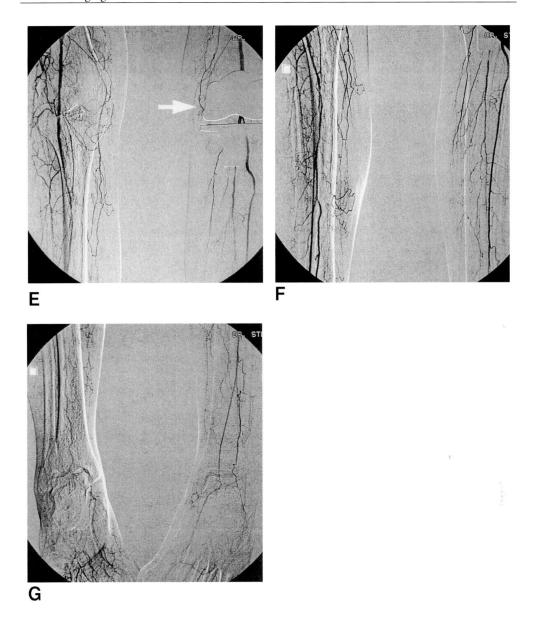

E

F

G

for 2 s each is a quick technique that produces excellent images. On some occasions it may be advantageous to image the right and left legs individually in the same procedure rather than to film both legs from an aortic injection.

The origins of the superficial femoral artery (SFA) and profound femoris artery (PFA) are usually viewed best from an ipsilateral anterior oblique projection (Fig. 2). These views should be obtained when the vessel origins are not clearly seen in anterior–posterior projections. Additional oblique and even lateral views of specific abnormalities are not usually obtained, but can be important to grade stenoses accurately, particularly in the tibial arteries where overlying bone can obscure vessels or create subtraction artifacts.

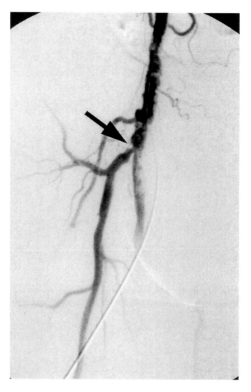

Fig. 2. Anterior oblique DSA of the right groin in a patient with SFA occlusion and severe claudication. The stenosis of the profunda femoris origin (*arrow*) was visible only in this projection.

Foot Angiography

Whenever pathology is present in the foot, dedicated views are necessary. A single lateral view that includes the malleolus to the toes is usually sufficient, although an anterior–posterior projection may be necessary for specific indications (Fig. 3). Positioning the catheter tip in the external iliac artery or SFA maximizes the delivery of contrast to the foot. The foot should be carefully taped in position (with special attention to delicate skin and pressure points). In the presence of extensive proximal occlusive disease, it is important to use reactive hyperemia and prolonged image acquisition.

Evaluation of Stenoses

The angiographic detection of hemodynamically significant stenoses is considered to be highly accurate. However, in an interesting study by Wikstrom and colleagues, pressure measurements were obtained across all iliac lesions with 50% reduction in luminal diameter *(13)*. When a peak systolic gradient of 20 mmHg was used as the threshold for hemodynamic significance, the sensitivity of DSA was 86% and specificity 88%. The severity of a lesion cannot be judged solely by angiographic appearance, a fact that has been lost in the recent excitement over expanded application of percutaneous interventions.

Complications of Angiography

The complications of conventional angiography are related primarily to the arterial puncture and the contrast agent *(14–16)* (Table 2). Bleeding complications can be

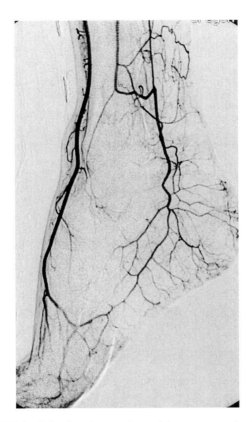

Fig. 3. Dedicated lateral DSA of the foot in a patient with severe proximal occlusive disease and a foot ulcer. Contrast was injected into the ipsilateral external iliac artery. Visualization of the pedal vessels is excellent.

Table 2
Complications of Angiography

Complication	Acceptable incidence
Hematoma (requiring transfusion, surgery, or delayed discharge)	<3%
Access artery occlusion	<0.5%
Pseudoaneurysm	<0.5%
Arteriovenous fistula	<0.1%
Distal emboli	<0.5%
Arterial dissection/subintimal passage	<2.0%
Subintimal injection of contrast	<1.0%

minimized using small catheters, careful compression, and arterial closure devices. The latter technology permits percutaneous arterial procedures in patients with severely deranged coagulation parameters. However, complications due to the closure device itself can occur in up to 5% of patients *(17)*. The use of renal protective strategies such as hydration, acetylcysteine, or fenoldapam can reduce the incidence of contrast-induced nephropathy *(18–20)* (Table 3). Cholesterol embolization is a rare (<1%) but potentially

Table 3
Measures to Prevent Contrast-Induced Acute Renal Failure

Agent	Protocol
Hydration	1 mL/kg D_5W for 12 h prior to procedure; 0.5 mL/kg D_5W for 12 h post-procedure
Fenoldopam	Begin infusion 2 h before procedure at 0.1 g/kg/min; increase 0.1 μg/kg/min every 20 min to maximum 0.5 g/kg/min or decrease in systolic blood pressure (BP) 20 mmHg (maintain systolic BP $\geq$ 100 mmHg). Infuse throughout procedure and for 4 h post-procedure. This may be stopped abruptly as the half-life is 5 min.
Acetylcysteine	600 mg orally every 12 h beginning 24 h before the procedure, including one dose the morning of the angiogram, and one dose the night after the procedure. Total of four doses

catastrophic event *(14,15)* (*see* Chapter 17). Patients with Erhlos–Danlos syndrome are at risk of puncture-site pseudoaneurysms and catheter-induced dissections.

INTRAVASCULAR ULTRASOUND

Intravascular ultrasound (IVUS) combines features of angiography and ultrasound imaging. A probe on the end of a catheter (usually 3–9 French in diameter) is inserted into the vascular lumen over a guidewire *(21)*. With IVUS the artery is seen from inside out. This technique can be an important adjunct to conventional angiography when evaluating processes such as dissections, stenoses, extent of plaque, or the results of an intervention. One limitation of the technique is the expense of the equipment, as probes can cost $500 or more.

MAGNETIC RESONANCE ANGIOGRAPHY

MR imaging is based on the detection of radiofrequency signals emitted by protons within a powerful static magnetic field *(22)*. Protons in the tissue being imaged align their axes with the strong magnetic field in the MR scanner (longitudinal magnetization). Application of an additional radiofrequency pulse to the protons tips the spins out of alignment with the magnetic field, in a plane perpendicular to the magnetic field (transverse magnetization). The natural tendency of the protons is to realign themselves with the magnetic field (relaxation), which creates a detectable signal (echo). Images are created from the signals emitted during longitudinal (T1) or transverse (T2) relaxation of the spins. In general, images based on short echo times are T1 weighted (longitudinal magnetization), while those based on long echo times are T2 weighted (transverse magnetization).

Advantages and Techniques

One of the most powerful features of MR imaging is the ability to create images in any plane, with large fields of view. The images are acquired directly in the plane of interest, rather than recreated after the fact utilizing post-processing techniques. This

Table 4
MRI Techniques

Technique	Basic principle	Blood/background signal
Black blood	No signal from rapidly flowing blood, normal signal from surrounding tissues	Dark/bright
Time of flight (TOF)	Signal from fresh protons in flowing blood; suppression of signal from background tissues and slowly moving blood by saturation pulses; venous/arterial selection by saturation of opposite inflow	Bright/dark
Phase contrast (PC)	Measurement of phase shift of spinning proton at two time points as it moves through magnetic field; directional and velocity information; stationary protons have no phase shift	Bright/dark
Gadolinium enhanced	Signal from intravascular contrast agent; timing critical, especially to separate arteries and veins; background signal present but minimal	Bright/dark

characteristic can be extremely useful when imaging blood vessels, as these structures can assume a serpentine course through the truncal cavities.

The first clinical MRA was described in 1985 *(23)*. There are now numerous MRA techniques, each reliant upon a different aspect of MR imaging to visualize blood flow (Table 4). Time-of-flight (TOF) and phase-contrast (PC) MRA image flowing protons, and are susceptible to signal loss due to turbulence, slow flow, and rapid changes in velocity. These conditions frequently exist in diseased blood vessels. These techniques acquire images either slice by slice (two-dimensional [2-D]) or volume (three-dimensional [3-D]) acquisitions. In general, 2-D imaging provides excellent vascular signal at the expense of image resolution, whereas 3-D imaging provides superior resolution but is susceptible to signal loss as volumes increase in size. Of the techniques described above, 2-D TOF imaging was initially most widely applied to the peripheral arteries (Fig. 4). Scan times were long, and signal loss due to slow, in-plane, or turbulent flow, particularly in the pelvis, decreased the accuracy of the technique *(24)*. TOF and PC imaging decreased in importance following the introduction of gadolinium enhanced 3-D MRA by Prince in 1993 *(25)*.

Gadolinium-Enhanced MRA

Gadolinium-enhanced MRA images the contrast agent, with only a slight flow-related enhancement. There is very little signal degradation by abnormal flow patterns. The gadolinium contrast agent is injected rapidly through a peripheral vein, with a 3-D acquisition timed to occur as the contrast enters the arterial circulation in the region of interest. Large fields of view can be imaged with this technique in a single breathhold. Although 3-D volumes are routinely used, there is no loss of signal due to saturation

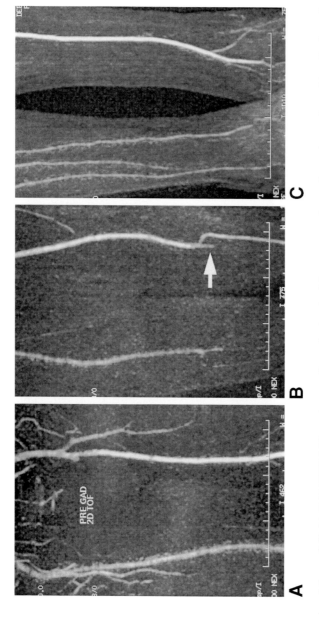

Fig. 4. Two-dimensional time-of-flight (2-D TOF) MR angiogram from the level of the common femoral arteries to the ankles. Each station was acquired separately, requiring a total of 1 h of scan time. (**A**) There is decreased signal and pulsatility artifact on the normal right side. This is common with 2-D TOF MR angiography. (**B**) There is proximal occlusion of the tibioperoneal trunk on the left (*arrow*). The right popliteal artery is poorly visualized but normal. (**C**) There is single-vessel runoff on the left and three-vessel runoff on the right

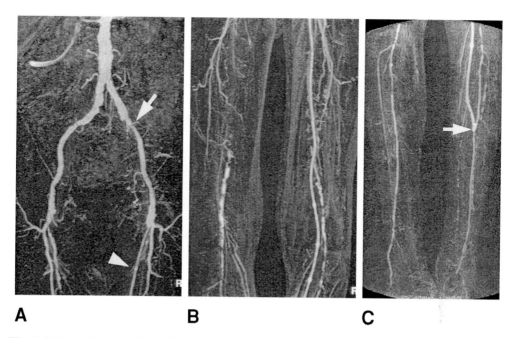

A   **B**   **C**

Fig. 5. 3-D gadolinium-enhanced bolus chase runoff. The study was completed in 15 min. **(A)** Image from the renal arteries to the proximal thighs. There is a left common iliac artery stenosis (*arrow*). A femoral to tibial bypass graft is also present on the left (*arrowhead*). **(B)** Image at the level of the thighs and knees. **(C)** Image at the level of the tibial arteries. The distal anastomosis of the bypass graft is widely patent (*arrow*).

effects as seen with noncontrast techniques. With fast scanners and moving tables, stepping studies can be obtained from the renal arteries to the ankle *(26)* (Fig. 5).

Contrast-enhanced MRA studies are highly specific and sensitive for occlusions and normal vessels *(27,28)*. Reid and colleagues found a 100% sensitivity and 92% positive predictive value for identification of lesions requiring intervention *(29)*. The precise degree of stenosis is typically still overestimated by MRA owing to the limited spatial resolution. However, stenotic lesions that reduce the diameter of the lumen by 50% are accurately detected *(13)*. In addition, visualization of distal runoff vessels in the presence of multilevel inflow occlusions (i.e., aorta to tibial artery) is frequently superior when compared to conventional angiography *(30)*. The major limitation in this setting is the inability to visualize intimal calcification, which is sometimes an important factor when selecting a distal bypass target.

Disadvantages of MRA

MR imaging techniques are subject to a number of limitations. Spatial resolution remains less than that of DSA, and calcium in the vessel wall cannot be visualized. Patients with cardiac pacemakers, defibrillators, intraocular or intra-aural metallic foreign bodies, and claustrophobia cannot be imaged. Specialized MR-compatible equipment is required for hemodynamic monitoring of unstable patients during scanning. Uncooperative or demented patients who are not able to hold still during image acquisition can render a study useless.

CT ANGIOGRAPHY

The development of helical CT scanners revitalized the vascular applications of this imaging modality. Conventional scanners image one slice at a time, with the table in a stationary position. Although conventional CT is recognized as an excellent modality for visualizing blood vessel morphology, the imaging is too slow to be used for angiographic studies. Helical (or spiral) CT scanners image continuously as the patient is moved rapidly through the gantry (31,32). Slip-ring technology in the CT scan gantry allows continuous rotation of the X-ray tube, without the need to stop and "rewind" between slices. Data are acquired in a volume, much like 3-D MRA, rather than as individual slices. The scan time is dramatically reduced compared to conventional CT, so that a bolus of contrast can be imaged as it opacifies a vascular bed. Large anatomic areas can be scanned in 20–30 s, usually during a single breath-hold. Multidetector row helical scanners with multiple row detectors further decrease scan times, so that imaging of the entire body in < 30 s is a reality. Unstable patients, such as those with suspected aortic transection or rupture, can be scanned expeditiously and without special monitoring equipment. The helical data are reconstructed in the axial plane, as in conventional CT.

Important information can be obtained about the vascular system without the use of intravenous contrast. All CT scans for vascular pathology should begin with a noncontrast scan. The size of the blood vessel and the degree of vascular calcification can be easily assessed on noncontrast CT. Acute extravascular blood appears dense on noncontrast CT, so that the diagnosis of acute hemorrhage from vascular injury or rupture does not require intravenous contrast.

Contrast Agents

The basic principle of CT angiography (CTA) is a carefully timed helical acquisition during the rapid peripheral infusion of iodinated contrast. Information from background tissues is not suppressed, as in MRA. Three factors are important in choosing a contrast agent for CTA: injection rate, total volume, and concentration of iodine. Visualization of small vessels improves as the concentration of iodine in the blood increases. Most CTA studies utilize injection rates of 3–5 mL/s for a total volume of 100–150 mL. Contrast agents containing at least 60% iodine provide the best results in most instances (Fig. 6).

Advantages of CTA

One of the major advantages of CTA is that the source images are simply axial slices with intense vascular opacification. All of the information that one would normally expect regarding the vascular wall and perivascular structures on a CT scan is still present. This allows more comprehensive evaluation of the vascular structures than with MRA. CTA of the lower extremity arteries is just entering clinical practice (33). The sensitivity and specificity for hemodynamically significant occlusive disease are unknown at this time.

Limitations of CTA

CTA has certain important limitations. Spatial resolution is less than that of DSA. Opacification of small peripheral vessels is suboptimal owing to overlap of enhancing veins. Patients with contrast allergies or renal failure may not be candidates for elective studies, as well as those with contraindications to ionizing radiation (such as patients in the first trimester of pregnancy). Heavily calcified vessels are difficult to evaluate, as

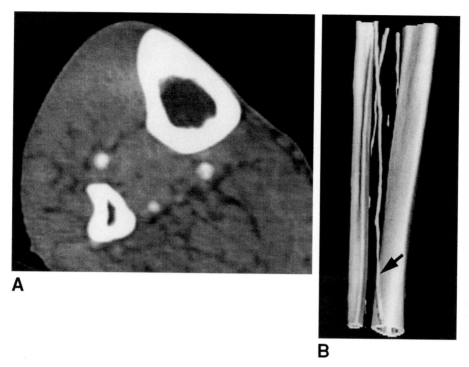

Fig. 6. CT angiography of the lower extremties. **(A)** Axial source image from the mid-calf showing enhancement of the three runoff vessels. **(B)** Anterior view of 3-D reconstruction showing the anterior tibial artery (arrow).

bulky intimal calcium can be indistinguishable from the opacified vessel lumen. Uncooperative patients introduce motion or respiratory artifacts that seriously degrade the final images.

Image Post-Processing

To view the data from MRA and CTA studies as angiograms, post-processing of source data on an independent workstation is necessary (Figs. 6 and 7). This crucial step occurs after the study has been completed, and frequently after the patient has been removed from the scanner *(34)*. A number of post-processing options are available, ranging from simple reformating of data into different planes (i.e., coronal slices from axial data) to three-dimensional renderings that permit an endoscopic view of the vascular lumen (Table 5). The accuracy of the final output requires a thorough knowledge of vascular pathology and the imaging technique. Excellent post-processed images can be created only from excellent original data. Review of source data is important whenever post-processed images do not correlate with the clinical picture.

CHOICE OF TECHNIQUE FOR IMAGING PAD

What is the best approach to imaging a patient with peripheral arterial disease? The answer to this deceptively simple question is complex. The clinical presentation, presence of comorbid diseases, past experience of the clinician treating the patient, and the availability of specific imaging modalities are all factors that must be considered.

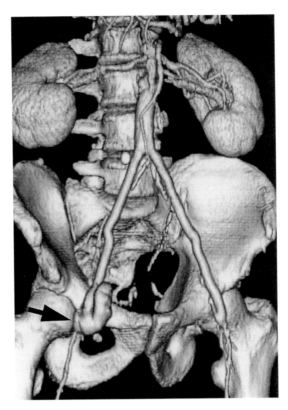

Fig. 7. 3-D shaded surface display of an aortopelvic CTA in a patient with an aortobifemoral graft. There is a distal anastomotic pseudoaneurysm on the right (*arrow*). Image post-processing allows display of the vascular data within a model of the bones. The remainder of the soft tissue data has been removed.

Acute Limb Ischemia

Patients with acute, limb-threatening ischemia require immediate imaging to determine the precise level and extent of the occlusion, the status of the inflow vessels, and identification of distal target vessels. The clinical features and radiographic appearance of the occlusion often are suggestive of the etiology (Table 6). Furthermore, the ideal imaging modality allows rapid conversion to potential therapeutic catheter-based intervention. Based on these criteria, conventional angiography remains the optimal imaging modality for patients presenting with acute ischemia.

Chronic Limb Ischemia

Patients with chronic ischemia are most effectively imaged with either MRA or conventional angiography. Few imaging departments have the expertise to perform peripheral arterial CTA, although this may well change within a few years. Where available and appropriate (based on patient factors), MRA is less expensive, less invasive, and more comfortable than conventional angiography *(30,35)*. An important added benefit of MRA is that patients with lesions amenable to percutaneous intervention can be referred for a focused angiographic procedure, rather than undergoing a preliminary complete peripheral arterial angiogram *(36)*. This improves patient outcomes in that pro-

Table 5
Post-Processing Techniques

Technique	Basic principle	Strength/weakness
Maximum intensity projection (MIP)	Displays brightest voxels in user defined 2-D planes, discards background information.	Quick; bright vessels with no background/ threshold for display may result in loss of critical information, 2-D display only.
Reformat	Allows display of all data in volume in user defined (2-D) planes, including curved.	Quick; no loss of data; can display complex anatomy/overlap of structures can be confusing, 2-D display only.
Shaded surface display (SSD)	Displays brightest voxels as a virtual surface (i.e., empty cup) shaded to have 3-D appearance.	3-D-like rendition of complex structures/ threshold for model may result in loss of critical information.
Volume Rendering	Displays brightest voxels as a virtual volume (i.e., full cup) shaded to have 3-D appearance.	3-D-like rendition of complex objects with ability to evaluate internal structures/ threshold for model may result in loss of critical information.
Endoscopic	Displays tubular structures without intraluminal contents with 3-D appearance.	Allows viewer to enter and travel through lumen of blood vessel/intraluminal perspective only.

Table 6
Distinguishing Features of Acute Arterial Occlusion

	Embolic	*Thrombotic*
Identifiable source of emboli	Frequent	Rare
Preexisting claudication	Rare	Frequent
Physical examination	Normal proximal and contralateral pulses	Evidence of peripheral vascular disease in ipilateral and contra-lateral limb
Degree of ischemia	Frequently profound	Frequently threatened but viable
Imaging findings	Normal vessels with abrupt occlusion (sometimes multiple), frequently at major bifurcation of vessel, no collaterals, meniscus sign	Diffuse atherosclerotic disease, well developed collaterals, usually midvessel occlusion

cedures are shorter and require less contrast, and promotes efficient utilization of imaging resources. Nevertheless, conventional angiography remains the primary pre- intervention imaging modality for patients with chronic ischemia in many centers.

Aortoiliac Disease

When aortoiliac occlusive disease is suspected on the basis of pulse examination and clinical symptoms, and imaging of the distal runoff is required, MRA should be considered as the initial imaging modality. Femoral arterial access for conventional angiography may not be possible in these patients. Axillary arterial catheterization has 0.5% risk of stroke (related to the catheter crossing the origins of one or more great vessels) and peripheral upper extremity nerve injury (owing to nerve compression by a hematoma in the medial brachial fascial compartment) *(14)*. Although angiographers have become less familiar with translumbar aortography, this is actually the safest access in patients with infrarenal aortic occlusion, yet opacification of distal vessels in patients with multilevel occlusions is difficult.

Vasculitis and Small Vessel Disease

The relatively low spatial resolution of MRA and CTA limit the applicability of these modalities to patients with small vessel disease such as vasculitis or digital artery emboli. Conventional angiography is necessary in these patients to obtain detailed views of the affected vessels. However, the finding of wall thickening and enhancement of large vessels on MRA and CTA is a very useful in the workup of a patient with aortic vasculitis *(37,38)* (*see* Chapter 19).

CONCLUSION

Imaging modalities for angiographic evaluation of the lower extremities include conventional angiography, MRA, and CTA. Conventional angiography remains the reference standard, and has improved greatly in safety and accuracy with newer contrast agents and imaging equipment. However, for purely diagnostic procedures, it is likely that conventional angiography will be equaled or replaced by both MRA and CTA in the future. In turn, combined modality procedures, such as DSA and MRA, will someday replace the current paradigm in which the choice is "either/or."

REFERENCES

1. Reimer P, Landwehr P. Non-invasive vascular imaging of peripheral vessels. Eur Radiol 1998;8: 858–872.
2. Seldinger, SI. Catheter replacement of the needle in percutaneous arteriography. Acta Radiol 1953;39: 368–376.
3. Fitzgerald J, Andrew H, Conway B, Hackett S, Chalmers N. Outpatient angiography: a prospective study of 3 French catheters in unselected patients. Br J Radiol 1998;71:484–486.
4. Cowling MG, Buckenham TM, Belli AM. The role of transradial diagnostic angiography. Cardiovasc Intervent Radiol 1997;20:103–106.
5. Cragg AH, Nakagawa N, Smith TP, Berbaum KS. Hematoma formation after diagnostic angiography: effect of catheter size. J Vasc Interv 1991;2:231–233
6. Bettmann MA. Safety and efficacy of iodinated contrast agents. Invest Radiol 1994; 29:S33–36.
7. Hoffmeister HM, Heller W. Radiographic contrast media and the coagulation and complement systems. Invest Radiol 1996;31:591–595.
8. Cochran ST, Bomyea K, Sayre JW. Trends in adverse events after IV administration of contrast media. Am J Roentgenol 2001;176:1385–1388.
9. Back MR, Caridi JG, Hawkins IF, Seeger JM. Angiography with carbon dioxide (CO2). Surg Clin North Am 1998;78:575–591.
10. Caridi J, Hawkins IJ. CO2 digital subtraction angiography: potential complications and their prevention. J Vasc Interv Radiol 1997;8:383–391.
11. Kaufman JA, Geller SC, Waltman AC. Renal insufficiency: gadopentetate dimeglumine as a radiographic contrast agent during peripheral vascular interventional procedures. Radiology 1996;198: 579–581.
12. Spinosa D, Angle J, Hagspiel K, Kern J, Hartwell G, Matsumoto A. Lower extremity arteriography with use of iodinated contrast material or gadodiamide to supplement CO2 angiography in patients with renal insufficiency. J Vasc Interv Radiol 2000;11:35–43.
13. Wikstrom J, Holmberg A, Johansson L, et al. Gadolinium-enhanced magnetic resonance angiography, digital subtraction angiography and duplex of the iliac arteries compared with intra-arterial pressure gradient measurements. Eur J Vasc Endovasc Surg 2000;19:516–523.
14. Abu Rahma AF, Robinson PA, Boland JP, et al. Complications of arteriography in a recent series of 707 cases: factors affecting outcome. Ann Vasc Surg 1993;7:122–129.
15. Egglin TK, O'Moore PV, Feinstein AR, Waltman AC. Complications of peripheral arteriography: a new system to identify patients at increased risk. J Vasc Surg 1995;22:787–794.
16. Spies JB, Bakal CR, Burke DR, et al. Standard for diagnostic arteriography in adults. J Vasc Interven Radiol 1993;4:385–395.
17. Sprouse LR, Botta DM, Hamilton IN. The management of peripheral vascular complications associated with the use of percutaneous suture-mediated closure devices. J Vasc Surg 2001;33:688–693.
18. Barrett BJ. Contrast nephrotoxicity. J Am Soc Nephrol 1994;5:125–137.
19. Solomon R, Werner C, Mann D, D'Elia J, Silva P. Effects of saline, mannitol, and furosemide to prevent acute decreases in renal function induced by radiocontrast agents. N Engl J Med 1994;331: 1416–1420.
20. Tepel M, van der Giet M, Schwarzfeld C, Laufer U, Liermann D, Zidek W. Prevention of radiographic-contrast-agent-induced reductions in renal function by acetylcysteine. N Engl J Med. 2000;343: 180–184.
21. Nissen SE, Yock P. Intravascular ultrasound: novel pathophysiological insights and current clinical application. Circulation 2001;103:604–616.
22. Mistretta CA. Relative characteristics of MR angiography and competing vascular imaging modalities. J Magn Reson Imaging 1993;3:685–698.

23. Wedeen VJ, Meuli RA, Edelman RR, et al. Projective imaging of pulsatile flow with magnetic resonance. Science 1985;230:946–948.
24. Kaufman JA, McCarter D, Geller SC, Waltman AC. Two-dimensional time-of-flight MR angiography of the lower extremities: artifacts and pitfalls. Am J Roentgenol 1998;171:129–135.
25. Prince MR, Yucel EK, Kaufman JA, Harrison DC, Geller SC. Dynamic gadolinium-enhanced three-dimensional abdominal MR arteriography. J Magn Reson Imaging 1993;3:877–881.
26. Stein B, Leary CJ, Ohki SK. Magnetic resonance angiography: the nuts and bolts. Tech Vasc Intervent Radiol 2001;4:27–44.
27. Ho KY, de Haan MW, Kessels AG, Kitslaar PJ, van Engelshoven JM. Peripheral vascular tree stenoses: detection with subtracted and nonsubtracted MR angiography. Radiology 1998;206:673–681.
28. Rofsky NM. MR angiography of the aortoiliac and femoropopliteal vessels. Magn Reson Imaging Clin N Am 1998; 6:371–384.
29. Reid SK, Pagan-Marin HR, Menzoian JO, Woodson J, Yucel EK. Contrast-enhanced moving-table MR angiography: prospective comparison to catheter arteriography for treatment planning in peripheral arterial occlusive disease. J Vasc Interv Radiol 2001;12:45–53.
30. Koelemay MJ, Lijmer JG, Stoker J, Legemate DA, Bossuyt PM. Magnetic resonance angiography for the evaluation of lower extremity arterial disease: a meta-analysis. JAMA 2001;285:1338–1345.
31. Rubin GD, Shiau MC, Schmidt AJ, et al. CT angiography: historical perspective and new state-of-the-art using multi detector-row helical CT. JCAT 1999;23:S83–89.
32. Rubin GD. Techniques for performing multidetector-row computed tomographic angiography. Tech Vasc Interven Rad 2001;4:2–14.
33. Rubin GD, Schmidt AJ, Logan LJ, Sofilos MC. Multi-detector row CT angiography of lower extremity arterial inflow and runoff: initial experience Radiology 2001;221:146–158.
34. Hany TF, Schmidt M, Davis CP, Gohde SC, Debatin JF. Diagnostic impact of four postprocessing techniques in evaluating contrast-enhanced three-dimensional MR angiography. Am J Roentgenol 1998; 170:907–912.
35. Swan JS, Langlotz CP. Patient preference for magnetic resonance versus conventional angiography: assessment methods and implications for cost-effectiveness analysis: an overview. Invest Radiol 1998; 33:553–559.
36. Sharafuddin MJ, Wroblicka JT, Sun S, Essig M, Schoenberg SO, Yuh WT. Percutaneous vascular intervention based on gadolinium-enhanced MR angiography. J Vasc Interv Radiol 2000;11:739–746.
37. Choe YH, Kim DK, Koh EM, Do YS, Lee WR. Takayasu arteritis: diagnosis with MR imaging and MR angiography in acute and chronic active stages. J Magn Reson Imaging 1999;10:751–757.
38. Yamada I, Nakagawa T, Himeno Y, Numano F, Shibuya H. Takayasu arteritis: evaluation of the thoracic aorta with CT angiography. Radiology 1998;209:103–109.

6

Chronic Critical Limb Ischemia

Diagnosis and Treatment

Frank A. Schmieder, MD and
Anthony J. Comerota, MD, FACS

CONTENTS

INTRODUCTION

Chronic critical limb ischemia (CLI) represents the most advanced form of athero-sclerotic lower extremity vascular disease. By definition, the term characterizes patients with distal extremity perfusion so limited as to produce rest pain and/or tissue necrosis in the form of ischemic ulcers and gangrene. Clinically, patients with CLI differ from those with intermittent claudication (IC) by symptoms of ischemia present at rest as well as evidence of tissue breakdown or loss due to hypoperfusion. Acute limb ischemia (ALI), on the other hand, describes the patient in whom blood supply is suddenly inter-rupted, leading to sensory–motor symptoms and potential tissue destruction in short order if perfusion is not restored (*see* Chapter 7). ALI may occur in conjunction with CLI when a vessel with high-grade stenosis undergoes thrombosis or an embolus is superimposed on preexisting disease.

Although comparatively smaller in numbers than other groups with vascular disease, patients with CLI represent a disproportionately larger workload for the medical system and individual vascular practices. Diagnostic efforts, hospitalization rates, treatment modalities, and general medical care are usually significantly more intensive than in patients with IC. At the same time, risks and benefits are often close, rendering deci-sion-making for both patients and physicians more difficult. With advances in various treatment strategies including novel techniques of lower extremity revascularization as well as overall patient care, specific data about cost and effectiveness are not generally available but much needed. Wahlenberg and colleagues illustrated an interesting paradox

From: *Contemporary Cardiology: Peripheral Arterial Disease: Diagnosis and Treatment*
Edited by: J. D. Coffman and R. T. Eberhardt © Humana Press Inc., Totowa, NJ

when they reported that one third of all amputees in one major hospital had not been assessed by a vascular surgeon *(1)*.

Rutherford's classification (Table 1) is the currently recommended standard for describing the clinical assessment of patients with peripheral arterial disease (PAD) *(2,3)*. Accordingly, patients with CLI fall into categories 4–6, designated by ischemic rest pain, and minor and major tissue loss, respectively. Foot pain at rest—generally referred to as ischemic rest pain—is considered a milder form, whereas any tissue loss represents a more advanced state of CLI. Categories 0–3 are assigned to asymptomatic patients and those with mild, moderate, and severe IC.

CLI is most commonly the result of progressive multisegmental atherosclerosis. Ultimately, blood flow rates are so impaired that basal metabolic needs of the peripheral tissue are no longer met. Collateral circulation and local physiologic mechanisms may compensate to some degree for the occlusions, whereas decreased cardiac output and chronic venous disease may further compromise distal perfusion. In contrast to intermittent claudication in which predominately skeletal muscle is affected during exercise, CLI pathophysiology prominently involves the skin microcirculation. Rest pain and trophic changes are thought to be mediated by an interruption of the microvascular flow regulating system as well as an inappropriate activation of normal defense mechanisms *(4)*. Obliteration of precapillary arteriolar function by vasospasm and capillary collapse through interstitial edema has been experimentally observed along with abnormalities in nitric oxide and prostacyclin release *(5)*. Also, platelet and leukocyte activation sets the inflammatory cascade into motion, eventually leading to microthrombosis and endothelial damage further impairing flow *(6,7)*. To date, the precise steps leading from macrovascular atherosclerosis to rest pain and tissue necrosis remain unknown. Figure 1 is a summary of the suggested pathogenesis in CLI *(8)*.

BACKGROUND

Risk Factors

The basic risk factors of CLI are those of atherosclerosis and indisputably include age, gender, smoking, diabetes, and the more recently recognized role of hyperhomocysteinemia (*see* Chapter 2). These factors are considered independent of each other and additive. The relative risk of developing PAD as well as CLI increases about two- to threefold for each additional decade of life and male gender *(9)*. Similarly, smokers carry at least a three times higher risk of PAD and progress at a more rapid rate to rest pain and tissue loss *(10)*. In fact, a Swedish survey demonstrates that the group of male patients smoking more than 10 cigarettes a day incurred a major limb amputation an average of 13 yr earlier when compared to their matched nonsmoking counterparts *(11)*. The Framingham study shows that smokers are twice as likely to develop PAD as coronary artery disease (CAD) *(12)*. Abnormal endothelium (nitric oxide)-dependent vasodilatation has been implicated for the smoking-induced development and progression of atherosclerosis *(13)*.

Diabetes predisposes the patient to PAD with an odds ratio between 2 and 3, and the risk of progression to CLI is even stronger. Population-based surveys estimate that diabetics require amputations about 10 times more frequently as nondiabetic PAD patients and at a younger age *(14)*. Diabetic neuropathy associated with loss of sensation and functional foot changes as well as impaired immune function with increased

Table 1
Classification of Peripheral Arterial Disease—Rutherford's Categories

Grade	Category	Clinical description
0	0	Asymptomatic
I	1	Mild claudication
I	2	Moderate claudication
I	3	Severe claudication
II	4	Ischemic rest pain
III	5	Minor tissue loss
III	6	Major tissue loss

From ref. 2.

susceptibility to infection are likely explanatory mechanisms. Although there is strong evidence that tight control of blood sugar delays the onset of microvascular diabetic retinopathy and nephropathy, the effect of such control on progression of macrovascular disease remains in dispute (9).

Hyperhomocysteinemia has recently been recognized as an important risk factor with an odds ratio of >6 for developing PAD (15). It remains to be determined why hyperhomocysteinemia is related to premature atherosclerosis and preferentially associated with PAD compared with CAD. It is, however, known that homocysteinemia and hypercoagulability are linked through downregulation of thrombomodulin and inhibition of tissue plasminogen activator as well as endothelial protein C activation.

The association between PAD and hyperlipidemia as well as hypertension remains a subject of debate. The association of hyperlipidemia and the progression of coronary and carotid atherosclerosis is well established but research has both supported and refuted a similar link of total cholesterol to PAD (16,17). However, the ratio of total to high-density lipoprotein has been recognized as an accurate predictor of arterial disease. Furthermore, Cheng and colleagues found lipoprotein(a) to be an independent PAD risk factor (18). Similarly, data are divergent about the role of hypertension, which may have both a cause and effect relationship to PAD. Also, aggressive blood pressure control in newly diagnosed hypertensive patients may decrease perfusion sufficiently to unmask an unrecognized but now hemodynamically significant lesion.

Comorbidities: Risk to Limb and Life

Because atherosclerosis represents a systemic process, PAD—particularly in the more advanced form of CLI—should be expected to coexist with both coronary and cerebrovascular disease. An often-cited study from the Cleveland Clinic evaluated 1000 consecutive patients scheduled for elective peripheral vascular surgery with coronary arteriography without regard to their cardiac symptoms. Ninety-one percent of PAD patients had documented CAD and 25% presented with severe, correctible and 6% with inoperable coronary atherosclerosis (19). The relationship between PAD and cerebrovascular disease (CVD) appears to be less prominent. Asymptomatic carotid stenosis >60% was present in 15% of patients with severe limb ischemia admitted for infrainguinal bypass procedures in a study by Gentile and colleagues from the University of Oregon (20). Alexandrova and colleagues observed that about 20% of all PAD patients studied had carotid stenosis >50% and 15% had stenosis >75% (21). Aronow and Ahn studied 1886 patients age 62 and above and found that 73% of the group had

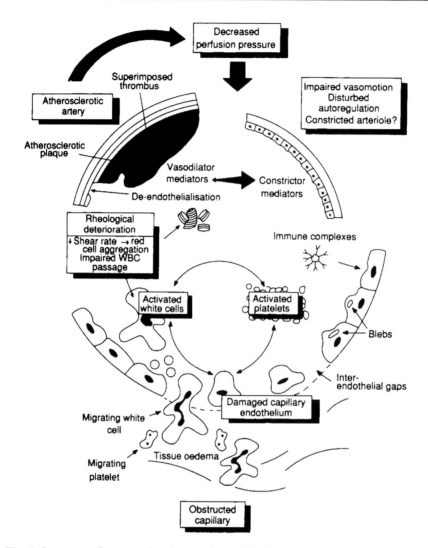

Fig. 1. Summary of suggested pathogenesis in CLI *(8)*.

clinical evidence of either PAD, CAD, or CVD; thus, only 37% were devoid of these diseases (Fig. 2) *(22)*. The specific overlap of disease in various vascular territories certainly depends on the sensitivity of the diagnostic test and the population under observation. Summarizing evidence from available studies, the Transatlantic Inter-Society Consensus (TASC) working group concluded that about 60% of PAD patients have significant CAD, CVD, or both whereas approx 40% of those with CAD and CVD will also have PAD *(3)*.

Fate of the Patient with CLI

Information on the natural history of CLI in contrast to IC is sparse since the majority of patients with CLI are evaluated for and offered a revascularization procedure. However, placebo group pharmacological trial data, from patients without an option for revascularization because of a high risk for serious morbidity and mortality, showed that

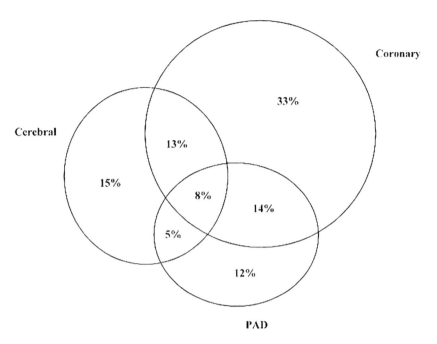

Coronary

33%

Cerebral

13%

15%

8%

14%

5%

12%

PAD

Fig. 2. Overlap between PAD, CAD and CVD in 1,886 patients above age 62 *(22)*.

at 6 mo about 80% were alive of which 35% required amputation, while 20% died *(23)*. Dormandy and colleagues summarized information from several surgical trials conducted between 1978 and 1997 of newly presenting CLI patients. Accordingly, about half of all patients underwent a revascularization procedure, while the other half of the group was evenly divided among those with primary amputation and medical treatment only. At 1 yr, about a quarter of the entire group had died, required amputation, or continued to suffer from or had been cured of CLI (Fig. 3) *(23)*. Five-year survival of patients with limb-threatening ischemia treated by an operation has been documented between 50% and 60% while only 12% of the subset requiring reoperative surgery in one study were still alive at that time *(24–26)*. In comparison, about 75% of all patients with IC will improve or remain stable without operative intervention within 5 yr of their initial diagnosis. Only about 5% will ultimately require amputation and 70% are alive at 5 yr *(3,27)*. Clearly, the diagnosis of CLI portends a particularly high risk to life and limb. Aggressive risk factor modification and management strategies for systemic atherosclerosis must be adopted concurrent with efficient patient evaluation for a timely revascularization procedure.

Epidemiology

Epidemiological information about CLI is sparse and often indirectly derived. Catalano in Northern Italy assessed the incidence of CLI in patients with and without IC in a prospective 7-yr survey and obtained regional data on CLI hospital admissions and amputation rates *(28)*. British and Irish vascular societies surveyed their members about practice experience with CLI *(29)*. Data also have been extrapolated from IC studies and the proportion of IC patients developing CLI. Interestingly, despite varied approaches and assumptions the overall incidence of CLI in these studies is similar ranging from

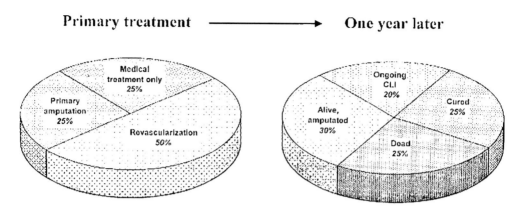

Fig. 3. Initial treatment and one-year status of patients with CLI *(23)*.

0.4 to 1 per 1000 patients per year. In comparison, CLI occurs annually about 5–10 times less frequently than IC but 3–6 times as often as ALI *(30,31)*.

The overall incidence and prevalence of PAD and CLI is likely to increase significantly with the aging of the population. One current estimate expects that the number of individuals aged >65 in the United States will grow by 70% between 2010 and 2030 *(32)*. Despite progress in risk factor modification, early detection and intervention, and improved general medical care, this demographic trend is likely to significantly increase the overall vascular disease workload. Associated costs for diagnostic procedures, intervention, and follow-up care will furthermore directly affect individual patients and the public's allocation for health care services.

CLINICAL PRESENTATION AND EVALUATION

History

A complete medical history and physical examination is a *sine qua non* for proper patient evaluation and management. Detailed information on the signs and symptoms of coronary and cerebrovascular disease should be elicited and existing risk factors listed to plan for their subsequent modification as well as systemic therapy. Furthermore, a patient may suffer from a disease aggravating, though not causing, chronic CLI. Identifying and managing diabetes, congestive heart failure, chronic pulmonary disease, or anemia may significantly alleviate lower extremity symptoms.

Ischemic rest pain is typically described as a constant severe pain with intermittent sharp exacerbation affecting the dorsum of the forefoot and the toes. Initially, these symptoms occur in a supine position yet they can also significantly impair a patient's ambulation. Patients obtain relief by placing the limb into a dependent position, by application of warmth, or from ambulation. Some patients can no longer sleep in bed and find rest only in a recliner. Unfortunately, the dependent limb position and repeated cycles of ischemia and reperfusion may ultimately lead to foot and ankle edema, further exacerbating ischemia and pain. Ischemic peripheral neuropathy often contributes to rest pain in the form of a sharp, shooting pain, disturbed temperature sensation, and heightened sensitivity to compression or pressure.

The more severe form of CLI presents with various degrees of tissue loss manifested by gangrene or ulceration. Often a history of antecedent trauma can be elicited that may be as minor as new shoes producing pressure points on marginally perfused tissue or the cutting of toenails with adjacent soft tissue trauma. Trauma plays a significant role in the diabetic patient who may not perceive the initial insult due to sensory impairment. The ischemic, uninfected, gangrenous toe may desiccate, mummify, and autoamputate with or without healing of the amputation site. In the presence of cellulitis or wet gangrene, the local infectious process may quickly spread in an ascending fashion and progress to sepsis and shock. A subgroup of (mostly sedentary) patients with severely impaired circulation may not have suffered from symptoms of impaired circulation prior to presenting with severe and progressive lower extremity tissue breakdown and infection.

Physical Examination

The physical examination centers on but is not limited to the circulatory system. The general examination may reveal hyper- or hypotension, arrhythmias, a cardiac murmur, generalized edema, anemia, or bony deformities. Blood pressure is measured in both upper extremities and any gradient between the arms is noted. Evaluation of the lower extremity commonly starts with an inspection for trophic changes such as hair loss, dry and shiny skin, loss of subcutaneous fat, and thickened nails. Depending on the severity of the underlying disease, calf and foot muscle atrophy, either uni- or bilateral, may be present. The frequently "skeletonized" appearing limb, however, may be obscured by the presence of edema resulting from the constant dependent position in order to minimize discomfort. Skin color may range from pale and mottled cyanotic to the rubor of dependency due to persistent dilatation of pre- and postcapillary sphincters/vessels secondary to increased local tissue lactic acidosis. Elevating the leg above the heart quickly changes rubor to pallor.

Ulcers resulting from decreased arterial perfusion are most commonly found at the most distal point in the vascular distribution, that is, the tip of the toes and the heel as well as pressure points. They may also appear as "kissing ulcers" on the inner digital surfaces. The ulcer margins are usually sharp and the ulcer base may be pale or in the case of concomitant inflammation or infection contain exudate and pus. Gangrene is frequently localized to the digits but in more advanced cases may affect the forefoot. Uninfected or "dry" gangrene may lead to tissue desiccation, mummification, and ultimately autoamputation. Infected or "wet" it may be associated with local or more extensive soft tissue, fascial plane, or deep space infection. The extremity examination must therefore identify any associated cellulitis, lymphangitis, and lymphadenopathy. Occasionally this local process will develop into a systemic process especially in the diabetic patient.

A careful pulse examination at the base of the neck and in both upper and lower extremities follows. It is most practical to grade pulses according to whether they are absent (0), questionable (1), diminished (2), normal (3), or prominent (4). While the majority of patients with CLI will exhibit diminished or absent pulses, severe ischemia may occasionally be present with a palpable distal pulse such as in diabetic patients or those with distal atheromatous emboli. Auscultation for cervical bruits is an integral part of the circulatory exam. The neurological exam focuses on extremity motor and sensory function and reflexes.

Bedside Doppler evaluation and calculation of the ankle–brachial index (ABI) is part of the complete physical examination (Table 2). The brachial, posterior tibial, and

Table 2
Ankle brachial index (ABI) values and clinical classification—Temple University Hospital

Clinical presentation	ABI
Normal	≥ 0.96
Claudication	0.50–0.95
Rest pain	0.21–0.49
Tissue loss	≤ 0.20
Significant *change* in consecutive studies	≥ 0.15

dorsalis pedis pressures are measured using an appropriately sized blood pressure cuff placed on the arms and above the ankles. On gradual cuff deflation, resumption of a Doppler signal and thus systolic pressure in each artery is determined with a continuous wave hand-held Doppler probe. The ABI is calculated by dividing the highest pressure obtained at the ankle by the highest brachial pressure. Values > 0.95 are considered normal, those between 0.50 and 0.95 fall into the claudication range, measurements between 0.21 and 0.49 are in the ischemic rest pain range, and those < 0.21 are consistent with tissue necrosis. Values < 0.90 are thought to represent vessel stenosis greater than 50% and, independent of presence or absence of symptoms, serve as marker for systemic atherosclerosis (33–35). ABI values above 1.25 are considered falsely elevated, most commonly from vessel wall rigidity due to medial calcinosis frequently associated with diabetes. This rigidity may be so severe that meaningful pressures cannot be obtained, in which case the result is recorded as noncompressible.

Differential Diagnosis

Causes other than severe peripheral ischemia may cause rest pain and ulceration. Diabetic sensory neuropathy usually leads to decreased sensation and function but in some patients may cause a sharp, shooting foot pain. The symmetrical distribution, associated cutaneous hypersensitivity, lack of relief from placing the limb in a dependent position, and evidence of adequate arterial perfusion help to exclude this etiology. Causalgia or reflex sympathetic dystrophy may be mistaken for ischemic rest pain. However, burning pain, vasomotor symptoms commonly in the form of mottling cyanosis, as well as hyperhidrosis and the hypersensitivity in a dermatomal or peripheral nerve distribution characteristic for causalgia will establish the diagnosis. Nerve root compression may also produce persistent foot pain in a dermatomal distribution but is usually associated with back pain. Other causes of foot pain come from peripheral sensory neuropathy due to alcohol abuse, vitamin B_{12} deficiency, and toxins, as well as inflammatory etiologies such as arthritis.

The differential diagnosis of ulceration includes venous ulcers secondary to chronic venous insufficiency. Venous ulcers are distinguished by their preceding hyperpigmentation, less severe pain, and distribution in the so-called gaiter area above the medial and lateral malleolus. About 10–15% of venous ulcers may occur together with arterial ulcers posing both a diagnostic and therapeutic challenge. Ulcers in diabetic patients may also arise due to sensory, sympathetic, and motor neuropathy in the absence of or in addition to ischemia. A normal pulse can identify the diabetic patient with a predominantly neuropathic etiology. The important judgment, which follows the diagnosis of diabetic neuropathic ulceration, is whether the patient has adequate perfusion to heal the ulcer once proper local care is instituted. Other etiologies causing leg and foot ulceration include vasculitis (*see* Chapter 19) and collagen vascular disease, those associated with hematological disease (sickle-cell anemia, chronic leukemia, polycythemia), inflammatory bowel disease (pyoderma gangrenosum), and malignancy (skin primary, metastatic, Kaposi's sarcoma, lymphoma, degeneration from chronic venous ulceration). Atheromatous emboli from a proximal source such as an abdominal aortic aneurysm may also lead to tissue loss in the form of toe ulcers and gangrene (*see* Chapter 17).

DIAGNOSTIC STUDIES

Doppler-derived segmental pressures and pulse volume recordings represent powerful noninvasive diagnostic modalities beyond the bedside ABI measurement (*see* Chapter 4). Through analysis of segmental pressure gradients and pulse waveform contours, a more objective assessment of the presence and location of PAD can be made. Rutherford and colleagues used these modalities with an accuracy of 97% in predicting level and extent of arteriocclusive disease *(36)*. Segmental pressures are obtained in much the same way as the ABI but at the level of the high thigh, low thigh, the calf, ankle, and foot. The high thigh pressure should be greater than the reference arm pressure and subsequent segments should exhibit no pressure drop >20 mmHg or they are considered hemodynamically significant. In addition, a photoplethysmographic probe may be used to measure toe pressures. The digital arteries are usually spared from medial calcinosis, which makes toe pressures particularly useful in patients with falsely elevated limb pressures or if there is disease of the digital arch or pedal arteries. A toe pressure index below 0.6 is considered abnormal. An absolute toe pressure < 30 mmHg supports the diagnosis of ischemic rest pain and indicates a poor prognosis for healing of a foot ulcer or foot incision *(37)*. Pulse volume recordings (PVR) are particularly helpful when pressures are falsely elevated or vessels are noncompressible. They represent the volume change of the leg segment studied with each heartbeat and are independent of vessel wall calcification. PVR values are obtained by plethysmography with a cuff placed at the arm, the thigh, the calf, and foot. The cuff is inflated to a preset pressure and the change in volume of the compartment under the cuff with each heartbeat is recorded. Analysis of the pulse waveform helps determine the presence, location, and the severity of disease (Fig. 4).

A number of tests are available to assess the status of the microcirculation and the likelihood of ulcer healing. Perhaps the best known method is transcutaneous oxygen tension measurement (TCPO$_2$) via modified Clark polarographic electrodes. The values obtained depend on a complex interplay between cutaneous blood flow, oxyhemoglobin dissociation, metabolic activity, and tissue oxygen diffusion. Limitations arise since the measurements are indirect with a wide range of normal values. An oxygen tension value <30 mmHg suggests severe ischemia. Values <20 mmHg are considered to predict nonhealing of an existing ulcer, whereas those >40 mmHg suggest the possibility of ulcer or skin incision healing without need for a revascularization procedure *(3)*.

In contrast to patients with IC in whom noninterventional treatment is most frequently indicated, endovascular therapy and/or surgery is usually considered in CLI. Arteriography is obtained in CLI patients considered surgical candidates to plan the appropriate revascularization procedure (*see* Chapter 5). The imaging modality of choice for most patients remains digital subtraction angiography with nonionic contrast

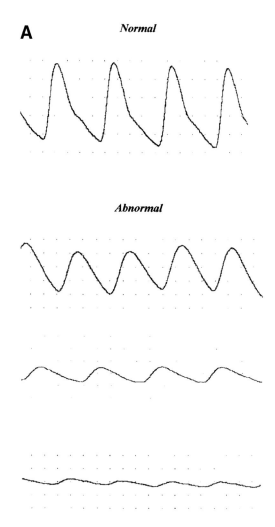

Fig. 4. PVR and Doppler derived segmental pressures: **(A)** Normal and abnormal waveforms. *Normal*—with characteristic sharp upstroke and peak, and dicrotic notch. *Abnormal*—with various degrees of dampening including loss of dicrotic notch (first sign of stenosis), gradual upstrokes, and rounded peaks. **(B)** Tibioperoneal disease, typically seen in patients with diabetes **(C)** Aorto-iliac occlusive disease.

B

Vascular Laboratory
Department of Surgery
Temple University Hospital
Philadelphia, PA.

Lower Arterial

Name: R		Patient ID:
Date: 02/03/2001Time:		Date of Birth: 08/13/1925
Sex: F		Age: 75
Room ID: 614		Examined by: BO
Ref. Dr.: V		Read by Dr.:

History

Hypertensive:	Yes	Diabetic:	Yes	M.I.:		No
CVA:	Yes	Smoke:	No	Vasc. Surgery:		No
Claudication:	Yes	Rest Pain:	Right			

Pulse Volume Recording

Right	Amplitude	Left	Amplitude
Arm:	29 MM	Arm:	22 MM
Thigh:	19 MM	Thigh:	16 MM
Calf:	17 MM	Calf:	22 MM
Metatarsal:	5 MM	Metatarsal:	5 MM
Great Toe:	2 MM	Great Toe:	5 MM

Segmental Limb Pressures

Right			Left		
Brachial:	134		Brachial:	147	
High Thigh:	175-	1.19	High Thigh:	179-	1.22
Low Thigh:	163-	1.11	Low Thigh:	160-	1.09
Calf (DP):	150-	1.02	Calf (DP):	162-	1.10
Calf (PT):	150-	1.02	Calf (PT):	159-	1.08
Ankle (DP):	89-	0.61	Ankle (DP):	100-	0.68
Ankle (PT):	120-	0.82	Ankle (PT):	103-	0.70
Gr. Toe:	35-	0.24	Gr. Toe:	42-	0.29

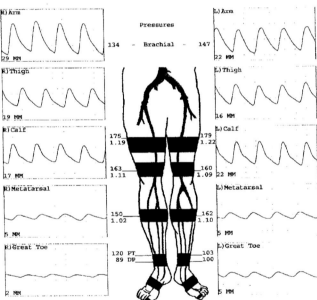

Pulse Volume Recording

0.82 -Ankle/Brachial- 0.70
Index

Fig. 4. *Continued*

C

Vascular Laboratory
Department of Surgery
Temple University Hospital
Philadelphia, PA.

Lower Arterial

Name: M   Patient ID:
Date: 01/20/2001Time: Date of Birth: 08/27/1958
Sex: F   Age: 42
Room ID: 505A   Examined by: EO
Ref. Dr.: R   Read by Dr.:

History
  Hypertensive: Yes   Diabetic: No   M.I.:   Yes
  CVA: Yes   Smoke: Yes   Smoke # Yrs: 30
  Vasc. Surgery: No   Claudication: Yes   Rest Pain: Left

    CLAUDICATION X 1 BLOCK B/L
    SMOKES 1/2 PPD X 30 YRS

Pulse Volume Recording
Right	Amplitude	Left	Amplitude
Arm:	16 MM	Arm:	15 MM
Thigh:	6 MM	Thigh:	8 MM
Calf:	11 MM	Calf:	17 MM
Metatarsal:	2 MM	Metatarsal:	2 MM
Great Toe:	1 MM	Great Toe:	4 MM

Segmental Limb Pressures
Right			Left		
Brachial:	108		Brachial:	134	
High Thigh:	75-	0.56	High Thigh:	79-	0.59
Low Thigh:	70-	0.52	Low Thigh:	77-	0.57
Calf (DP):	68-	0.51	Calf (DP):	77-	0.57
Calf (PT):	67-	0.50	Calf (PT):	74-	0.55
Ankle (DP):	67-	0.50	Ankle (DP):	68-	0.51
Ankle (PT):	65-	0.49	Ankle (PT):	70-	0.52
Gr. Toe:	44-	0.33	Gr. Toe:	85-	0.63

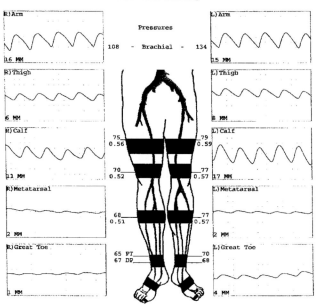

Pulse Volume Recording

Fig. 4. *Continued*

to visualize the vascular tree from the perirenal aorta to the pedal arteries. Intraarterial pressure measurements are obtained across any suspicious aortic, iliac, and femoropopliteal stenosis, which should be corrected if a gradient >10 mmHg is detected. Alternative contrast agents including gadolinium and carbon dioxide are used in patients with renal insufficiency. Magnetic resonance arteriography with gadolinium enhancement has been proposed as an alternative to conventional arteriography, particularly in patients with renal dysfunction or difficult vascular access *(38)*. However, current magnetic resonance angiography (MRA) techniques occasionally cannot distinguish between a tight stenosis and occlusion *(3,38,39)*. Color duplex ultrasound also has been used for preoperative evaluation, avoiding the need for arteriography altogether (*see* Chapter 4) *(40)*. Nevertheless, owing to the expertise and time required for proper examination and the inability to print complete images of the arterial system, duplex examination is unlikely to fully replace arteriography as a "surgical roadmap."

Beyond studies directed specifically at the evaluation of CLI, a number of general laboratory tests are recommended for all patients on initial presentation including the CBC, BUN, creatinine, electrolytes, glucose, and hemoglobin A1C and a lipid profile. An EKG is routinely obtained unless already available from a previous, recent workup. All patients presenting with concomitant symptomatic coronary or cerebrovascular disease require specific workup and management. Whether patients without signs or symptoms or family history of coronary disease should be screened routinely for CAD remains controversial. Liberal use of the carotid duplex examination is recommended based on the NASCET and ACAS data showing significant benefit of carotid endarterectomy in both symptomatic and asymptomatic patients *(41,42)*.

THERAPY
General Measures

Patients with CLI who present with ischemic rest pain should have their bed placed in reverse Trendelenburg position to allow gravity to assist with distal perfusion. An automatic bed may be adjustable to such a position or alternatively the head of the bed should be elevated at least 25 cm with blocks. The urge by some staff to elevate the chronically ischemic, edematous extremity must be resisted as perfusion will be diminished and pain increased (Fig 5). Foot protection plays an important role in general therapy of the CLI patient, whether diabetic or not. This includes proper footwear to minimize pressure points, soft gauze pads to prevent enlarging sores and protection of the feet from the bed by "egg crates" or special boots to avoid decubitus ulcers. Lambs wool or gauze can be placed between toes to prevent "kissing ulcers" that may develop from pressure exerted by adjacent toes or toenails. Gauze roll (instead of tape) to secure dressings and lanolin-base skin lotions may help avoid skin breakdown and cracking. Extremes of cold or heat must be avoided.

Aggressive risk factor modification is part of routine patient care (*see* Chapter 9) *(43)*. First among those is smoking cessation. A concerted effort through medical staff encouragement, pharmacological aids, and support groups appears to have the best success. Patients with CLI and diabetes should be managed with aggressive blood sugar control. Current recommendations include a fasting glucose range between 80 and 120 mg/dL, a postprandial target of 180 mg/dL and hemoglobin A1c values at <7% *(44)*. An LDL cholesterol level of <100 mg/dL is targeted through diet control and lipid-

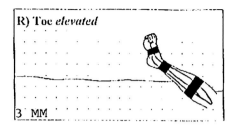

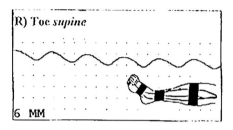

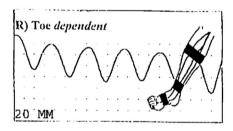

Fig. 5. PVRs and segmental pressures of the ischemic limb in elevated, supine and dependent position.

lowering agents *(45)*. Patients with an underlying hypercoagulable state and a history of venous or arterial thrombosis should be anticoagulated. Based on limited available information, hyperhomocysteinemia is currently treated with vitamin supplementation only if the symptomatic patient has concurrent folic acid or vitamin B_{12} deficiency *(2)*. The treatment of hypertension follows well established guidelines *(46)*.

Based on evidence from numerous well performed studies, platelet inhibition is recommended for both symptomatic and asymptomatic PAD patients *(47)*. Aspirin therapy is most commonly prescribed and has demonstrated benefit in the form of lowering the risk of ischemic stroke, myocardial infarcion, and vascular death. New platelet inhibitors such as clopidogrel appear to further reduce these risks when compared with aspirin alone *(48)*.

The general therapeutic strategy in CLI takes the vascular patient's risk to both life and limb into account. Cardiac and cerebrovascular management takes priority following established clinical guidelines for medical and surgical intervention (*see* Chapter 14). Also, cardiac and cerebrovascular risk assessment plays an important role when deciding on the safety of an intervention and which form it should take.

Endovascular or surgical intervention is generally considered in patients with CLI, in contrast to those with IC who are most commonly managed nonoperatively. The procedure chosen for a particular patient depends on several factors including general health, mobility status, life expectancy, the surgical risk, and the extent and location of the PAD. Open surgical procedures such as bypass grafting are generally considered more durable but entail higher risks when compared to endovascular intervention. Familiarity with each approach and considerable judgment are required to determine which approach offers the least risk and highest durability in the individual patient. Availability of local expertise must also be taken into account.

Aortoiliac Disease

Aortobifemoral bypass grafting using prosthetic conduits has been established as one of the most durable revascularization procedures. Five- and 10-yr patency rates are reported at 86% and 80%, respectively, with operative mortality between 2% and 3% *(49,50)*. Systemic morbidity in the form of myocardial infarct or renal failure has decreased with advances in perioperative care. Graft infection, aortoenteric fistula, and intestinal ischemia are rare. Rates of wound infection and false aneurysm formation have been reported at 3–5% *(3)*. Altered sexual function is a common complication occurring in as many as 20% *(51)*. We routinely perform an end-to-end proximal anastomosis for its beneficial flow characteristics, superior graft patency, and minimization of severe adverse effects such as graft enteric fistula. If the underlying disease precludes proper pelvic perfusion with an end-to-end proximal anastomosis, pelvic blood flow can be restored through internal iliac to graft anastomosis. The distal anastomosis is customized depending on the existing anatomy. In case of external iliac artery occlusion, an end-to-end common femoral anastomosis should be considered. If the superficial femoral artery is occluded or shows significant disease, the graft limb can be extended to the proximal deep femoral artery. A profundaplasty may be needed for disease of the profunda femoris orifice. More than 80% of patients with aortoiliac disease are satisfactorily treated with aortofemoral bypass grafting alone. A smaller subset with significant infrainguinal disease will require further procedures to restore adequate distal blood flow and maintain graft patency.

Percutaneous transluminal angioplasty (PTA) and stenting procedures, first described in the late 1960s by Gruentzig from the University of Aachen, Germany, and Dotter of Oregon, significantly expanded therapeutic options for the patient with CLI (*see* Chapter 12). The most durable application of percutaneous therapy has been in the circumstance of focal, segmental stenosis of the common iliac arteries. Patency rates of about 80%, 75%, and 65% at 1, 3, and 5 yr are well documented *(3,52)*. PTA and stenting have also been successfully applied in arterial occlusions in the iliac system. Vascular stents have proven particularly useful when PTA leads to significant arterial wall dissection, when recoil is present after PTA, and in the case of ulcerated plaques *(53)*.

The TASC working group has summarized current evidence for specific treatment protocols and provides a therapeutic guideline by anatomic classification (Fig. 6). Accordingly, lesions classified as (A) including short segment iliac artery lesions are best treated by endovascular therapy, whereas class (D) lesions describing long segment aortoiliac obstruction and multisegment occlusive disease are best approached with surgical therapy. Longer segment iliac artery lesions classified as (B), or lesions of 5–10 cm length in category (C) are most commonly treated with endovascular or surgical therapy respectively. However, clear evidence of superiority for the most commonly performed treatment strategies of class (B) and (C) lesions is not currently available.

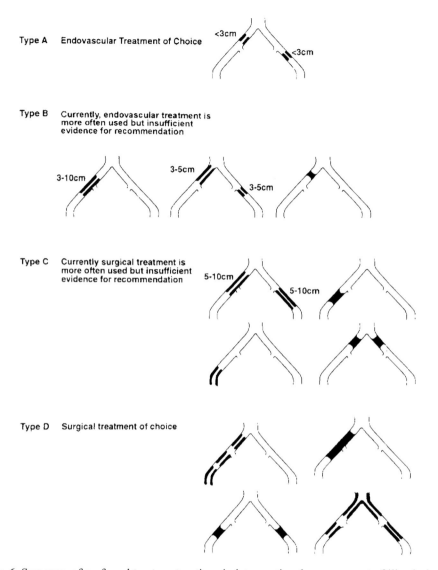

Fig. 6. Summary of preferred treatment options in interventional management of iliac lesions *(3)*.

On occasion, patients will present with disease not amenable to endovascular therapy and comorbidities such as severe pulmonary or cardiac disease or a hostile abdomen prevent aortobifemoral bypass grafting at reasonable risk. Extraanatomic approaches in the form of femoral–femoral or axillofemoral revascularization may offer the best treatment options in this circumstance. These procedures are technically less demanding and can be performed with shorter operative times, yet do not have the same durability. Primary patency rates between 30% and 75% at 5 yr are documented *(2)*.

Infrainguinal Disease

Multisegmental infrainguinal disease is common in patients with CLI and may be isolated or coexist with aortoiliac disease. For reasons incompletely understood, diabetics frequently present with arterial stenosis or occlusion limited to an infrainguinal or infrageniculate distribution. Owing to the diffuse nature of infrainguinal disease and technical limitations, less invasive percutaneous revascularization applies only to a relatively small, carefully selected group of patients at the present time. The TASC working group has categorized femoropopliteal lesions and their preferred treatment based on anatomic characterization (Fig. 7). Accordingly, type A lesions designated as stenosis < 3 cm are preferentially treated by endovascular therapy. Tandem stenosis/occlusion < 3 cm or a single lesion < 5 cm in length (type B) are most commonly treated with percutaneous approaches. Conversely, longer stenosis and occlusions (types C and D) are more frequently and best managed with bypass procedures.

In general, the most effective and durable revascularization procedure is a bypass graft to the best available outflow vessel regardless of (distal) location using autogenous vein. Adequate inflow to the bypass graft must be ensured and is most commonly obtained at the level of the common femoral artery (CFA) although the superficial femoral artery (SFA), profunda (PFA), or popliteal arteries are appropriate sources provided there is no significant proximal stenosis. A more distal inflow site is important if the length of suitable autogenous vein is limited. The quality of the distal artery and its runoff to the foot determines outflow resistance and is critical for graft patency. All distal arteries, including those of the foot, may be acceptable outflow targets *(54,55)*. Patency of femoroinfrapopliteal and femorodistal vein bypass grafts is similar, demonstrating that length alone is not a significant factor *(3)*. Also, there is no difference in outcome of autogenous femorodistal grafts in diabetic and nondiabetic patients *(56)*. When a satisfactory distal target vessel and adequate autogenous vein is not available, and no direct communication except through collaterals exists between the popliteal artery and the distal vessels, a more proximal bypass graft to an isolated popliteal artery may be indicated. Success for such a procedure is higher when the segment of popliteal artery is at least 7 cm and at least one major, large collateral vessel drains the popliteal segment *(57)*.

Several large, well conducted clinical trials have demonstrated the superiority of autogenous conduit most commonly in the form of greater saphenous vein (GSV) for surgical revascularization *(3,58,59)*. This holds both for above knee and below knee bypass grafting. Sources for venous conduits other than the GSV include the lesser saphenous system and arm veins *(60)*. The ideal venous conduit demonstrates no vessel wall thickening, and has an intact endothelium and a diameter of >4 mm. Ultrasound can help determine the quality of the veins preoperatively. When a suitable autogenous conduit is not available, synthetic bypass grafts are the next option. Prosthetic material in form of polytetrafluoroethylene (PTFE) or Dacron is available. Proponents of prosthetic bypass surgery have argued for preservation of vein for potential future cardiac or tibial revascularization. However, < 5 % of patients ever require vein for cardiac use. Also, prosthetic graft failure often leads to occlusion of additional segments of the arterial tree, something rarely observed in failed autogenous bypass grafts. Cryopreserved veins or arteries have shown disappointing patency results *(61)*. However, their relative resistance to infection confers an advantage when revascularization is needed in a contaminated environment.

Whether venous conduits should be used *in situ*, requiring valve lysis, or in excised, reversed form remains a matter of preference. Early and late patency rates are comparable, emphasizing the importance of other factors such as anastomotic technique and vein preparation *(3)*. Adjunctive surgical techniques intended to improve patency

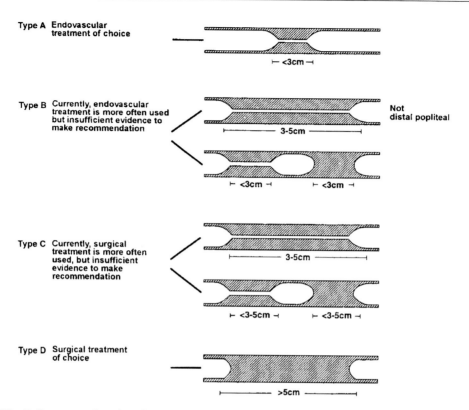

Fig. 7. Summary of preferred options for interventional treatment of femoral–popliteal lesions *(3)*.

include vein patch angioplasty at the proximal anastomosis (Linton patch), an interposition vein cuff at the distal anastomosis in infrageniculate prosthetic revascularization (Miller cuff), and distal arteriovenous fistulas *(62–64)*. Fig. 8 shows average results for surgical treatment.

Occlusive atherosclerotic disease of the CFA, profunda femoris orifice, and the proximal SFA may be treated with more limited surgical procedures including endarterectomy and profundaplasty. Autogenous vein patch profundaplasty has proven initial and long-term success in patients with (1) occlusion of the SFA and stenosis of the PFA orifice; (2) a normal distal profunda with good collaterals to the popliteal and/or tibial arteries; (3) a profunda popliteal collateral index (i.e., above knee pressures – below knee pressures divided by above knee pressures) < 0.3 *(65,66)*.

While the benefit of endovascular therapy is well established for iliac lesions, comparable supportive data for femoropopliteal and infrapopliteal lesions are lacking *(see* Chapter 12}. Lesion length, distribution, and character as well as runoff status and the presence of diabetes and end-stage renal disease affect initial technical success, long-term patency, and limb salvage. Many published studies regarding endovascular therapy are difficult to assess and compare because these factors are incompletely defined. In addition, whether patients were treated for IC or CLI is frequently not specified.

For femoropopliteal PTA, between 50% and 77% of patients with favorable anatomy show clinical benefit at 2 yr (Table 3). Infrapopliteal angioplasty is limited to short segment stenosis. It has been shown to yield an 80% limb salvage rate at 2 yr in carefully selected patients with subsequent "straight line flow" in one tibial vessel to the foot *(67)*.

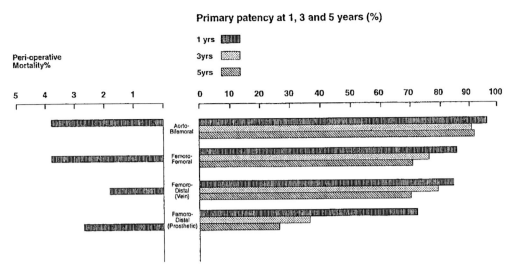

Fig. 8. Average results for surgical treatment *(3)*.

Table 3
Morphologic Stratification of Infrapopliteal Lesions

TASC type A infrapopliteal lesions:
1. Single stenoses shorter than 1 cm in the tibial or peroneal vessels

TASC type B infrapopliteal lesion:
2. Multiple focal stenoses of the tibial or peroneal vessel, each < 1 cm in length
3. One or two focal stenoses, each <1 cm long, at the tibial trifurcation
4. Short tibial or peroneal stenosis in conjunction with femoropopliteal PTA

TASC type C infrapopliteal lesions:
5. Stenoses 1–4 cm in length
6. Occlusions 1–2 cm in length of the tibial or peroneal vessels
7. Extensive stenoses of the tibial trifurcation

TASC type D infrapopliteal lesions:
8. Tibial or peroneal occlusions >2 cm
9. Diffusely diseased tibial or peroneal vessels

From ref. *3*.

Less favorable anatomy has led to primary patency rates of < 15% and frequent early failures *(3,68)*. Technical advances in terms of smaller hardware size, more versatility and instrument maneuverability, and improved imaging will likely increase applicability.

Adjuvant Treatment Following Revascularization

Antiplatelet therapy in the form of aspirin (ASA) has been shown to reduce events of acute and subacute thrombosis in lower extremity revascularization *(69)*. Unless contraindicated, ASA is begun preoperatively, then continued indefinitely in patients undergoing endovascular and surgical therapy. Ticlopidine and more recently clopidrogel, which has the same mechanism of action but causes fewer adverse effects than ticlopidine, have been given together with ASA in coronary angioplasty and stenting. This combination therapy has improved outcome when compared to ASA alone or ASA with full anticoagulation (70,71). Combined platelet inhibition with ASA and clopidrogel is also administered frequently in peripheral angioplasty and stenting. While reasonable based on the coronary interventional experience, randomized studies will need to help clarify the benefit for peripheral percutaneous intervention.

Controversy exists regarding long-term anticoagulation for all patients following peripheral surgical revascularization balancing possible beneficial effects on patency with increase of bleeding risks. We consider full anticoagulation in all patients with below knee prosthetic grafts as well as those considered "disadvantaged" primarily due to their poor runoff status whether prosthetic or autogenous conduits were used. Dextran reduces platelet deposition on graft surfaces and red cell aggregation, increases microcirculation and fibrin clot lysis, and serves as volume expander. Dextran significantly improves early graft patency in infrainguinal revascularization as well as longer-term patency in infrageniculate bypass grafting with vein (72,73). Dextran is particularly useful in patients undergoing the "difficult" lower extremity bypass.

Other Therapeutic Modalities

Other forms of therapy are occasionally employed when surgical or percutaneous interventions are contraindicated or unlikely to succeed. Lumbar sympathectomy has been advocated for a highly selected group of patients, with better response observed in treating rest pain than tissue loss (74). The TASC working group suggests that specific sympathectomy selection criteria should include an ABI of >0.3, tissue necrosis limited to the digits, absence of diabetic neuropathy, and symptomatic relief after test lumbar sympathetic blockade (2). Intermittent pneumatic compression of the foot and calf also has been used in end-stage CLI without reasonable options for revascularization. Elegant physiologic studies have shown significantly increased blood flow at the level of the popliteal artery and increased skin perfusion (75,76). Case reports suggest benefit for ulcer healing and rest pain alleviation (77). Directed pharmacotherapy for CLI (other than commonly administered platelet inhibition and selected anticoagulation) has played only a minor role owing in part to the still evolving understanding of the underlying pathophysiology (Fig. 9). Prostanoids represent the most widely studied drug group in recent years. Potential beneficial effects include down-regulation of platelet and leukocyte activation and modulating the thrombosis potentiating effect of the damaged endothelium. Based on available evidence, the TASC working group recommends prostanoid treatment for the end-stage CLI patient with a viable limb but no revascularization options (2). However, prostanoids are not approved for this indication in the United States. Vasoactive drugs or defibrinogenating agents are not recommended. Growth factors remain investigational agents but offer the hope of improved limb perfusion by stimulating the growth of blood vessels in a process known as *therapeutic angiogenesis* (see Chapter 11).

Surveillance and Follow-Up

Ongoing surveillance after revascularization is important especially following autogenous vein bypass grafting and percutaneous interventions to identify and correct lesions before they progress to occlusion. Surveillance protocols include scheduled follow-up visits with interval history and physical examination, ABI assessment at rest and if feasible postexercise, and color flow duplex examination. Angiography is not useful

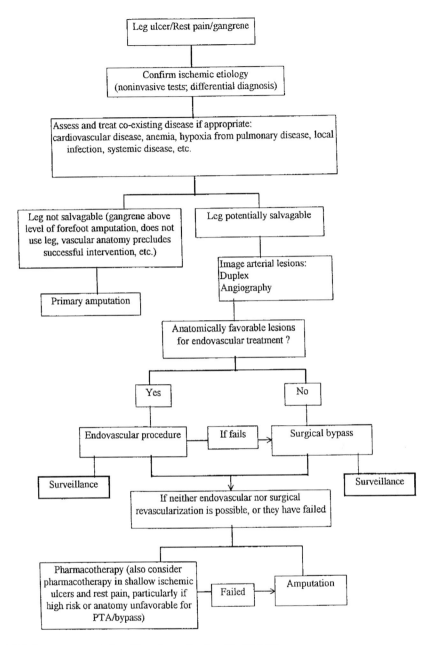

Fig. 9. TASC management algorithm for patients with CLI *(3)*.

for routine surveillance but may be helpful to confirm findings of the duplex examination, to reassess for the feasibility of a percutaneous intervention, or to better evaluate
a failing graft. Once a stenosis of 50–75% is detected, plans for intervention in the form
of PTA, patch angioplasty, segmental resection, and vein interposition grafting are considered. In failing saphenous vein grafts, timely revision results in assisted primary
patency rates that are essentially equivalent to primary patency rates *(78,79)*. Similar
observations have been reported following surveillance of patients after angioplasty.

Significantly lower technical success, higher complication rates, and less durable long-term results are noted when revision follows thrombosis *(80,81)*. Follow-up examination includes also the contralateral extremity. Dawson and colleagues point out that disease progression leads to contralateral amputation annually in about 10% of all patients *(82)*.

Amputation

Primary amputation is considered for selected patients with advanced distal ischemia and uncontrollable pain, infection, or tissue necrosis. Most commonly, the existing arterial anatomy precludes any other option. First-line treatment by amputation may also be required when a patient presents with necrosis of the majority of the weight-bearing area of the foot. Increasing numbers of nonambulatory patients from long-term care facilities are presenting with CLI and major joint contracture. Because these patients are not candidates for rehabilitation, an above knee amputation is the most appropriate procedure. Finally, primary amputation may also be indicated in cases of terminally ill patients or those with a short life expectancy who would otherwise require complex but low-yield revascularization interventions.

Secondary amputation is performed when all revascularization options have been exhausted following prior intervention and the extremity continues to deteriorate. Persistent infection and deterioration despite a functioning bypass graft may also justify amputation. Preservation of the knee joint is a top priority to maximize mobility, minimize ambulatory energy requirements, and facilitate the use of a prosthesis. A check for pulses, capillary refill, muscle mass, warmth and integrity of the skin, and absence of infection are key elements of the evaluation for the most distal possible amputation site. Additional information can be obtained from segmental Doppler-derived pressure measurements, pulse volume recordings, and transcutaneous oxygen assessment.

Dormandy and colleagues reviewed the outcome of 713 patients requiring below knee amputations in European medical centers and found that at 3 mo about 60% of stumps had healed, 20% required an amputation at a higher level, and 10% remained unhealed *(83)*. The perioperative death rate was 10%. Perioperative mortality rates near 20% are reported in several series of above knee amputations *(3)*. This increase is likely related to more advanced systemic atherosclerosis and more significant comorbidities rather than the higher level of amputation. At 2 yr, mortality rates of 25–35% for below knee and of 45% for above knee amputees are well documented *(3)*. Of those patients with well-healed stump sites, the chance for independent ambulation has been reported with a range of 66–81% for below knee and <50% for above knee amputees *(84,85)*. Rehabilitation time commonly exceeds 9 mo *(83)*. Poor general health status and cardiac and pulmonary comorbidities most frequently limit return to full mobility.

SUMMARY

Significant advances have been achieved in the prevention, diagnosis, and therapy of CLI in the past three decades. Ongoing efforts in primary care target earlier detection, improved prevention in form of risk factor modification, and timely referral for definitive treatment *(43)*. New technology is rapidly emerging for diagnosis, including MRA and contrast ultrasound, as well as therapy such as increasingly versatile endovascular instrumentation facilitating more sophisticated interventional and surgical techniques.

Basic science research continues to elucidate the pathophysiologic mechanisms underlying CLI *(5,6)*. Applications of this knowledge can be found in the use of markers of inflammation for the study of CLI or development of in vitro growth models for autogenous conduits used in revascularization. In gene therapy, compounds such as vascular endothelial growth factor (VGEF) are now past safety assessment and have entered the clinical study phase *(86)*. Regarding clinical research, the TASC working group has recommended strategies for CLI study design and defined several critical areas including outcome and quality of life assessment *(2)*. Expectations appear justified that these ongoing efforts will contribute many novel strategies to improve the status of our patients suffering from CLI, the most advanced manifestation of atherosclerotic PAD.

REFERENCES

1. Wahlenberg E, Lepner U, Olofsson P. Limb loss in association with vascular surgery: a five year series of major lower limb amputation. Eur J Vasc Surg 1994;160:561–567.
2. Rutherford RB, Baker JD, Ernst C, et al. Recommended standards for reports dealing with lower extremity ischemia: revised version. J Vasc Surg 1997;26:517–538.
3. Transatlantic Inter-Society Consensus (TASC) Working Group. Management of peripheral arterial disease (PAD). J Vasc Surg 2000;31:S5–S34, S54–S56, S176–188, S192–274, S281–288.
4. Kempczinski RF. The chronically ischemic leg: An overview. In: Rutherford RB, ed. Vascular Surgery, 5th edit. Philadelphia: WB Saunders, 2000; pp.917–927.
5. Lowe GD. Pathophysiology of critical limb ischemia. In: Dormandy J, Stock G, eds. Critical Limb Ischemia: Its Pathophysiology and Management. Berlin: Springer-Verlag, 1990; pp.17–38.
6. Berliner JA, Navab M, Fogelman AM et al. Atherosclerosis: basic mechanisms. Oxidation, inflammation and genetics. Circulation 1995;91:2488–2496.
7. Ross R. Cellular and molecular studies of atherosclerosis. Atherosclerosis 1997;131: S3–4.
8. Dormandy J, Verstraete M, Andreani D, et al. Second European consensus document on chronic critical leg ischemia. Circulation 1991;84(Suppl 4):1.
9. Dormandy J, Heeck L, Vig S. Predictors of early disease in the lower limbs. J Vasc Surg 1999;12: 109–117.
10. Powel JT. Vascular damage from smoking: disease mechanisms at the arterial wall. Vasc Med 1998;3: 21–28.
11. Liedberg E, Perrson BM. Age, diabetes and smoking in lower limb amputation for arterial occlusive disease. Acta Orthop Scand 1983;54:383–388.
12. Murabito JM, D'Agostino RB, Silbershatz H, et al. Intermittent claudication: a risk profile from the Framingham heart study. Circulation 1997;96:44–49.
13. Celermajer DS, Sorenson KE, Georgakopoulos D, et al. Cigarette smoking is associated with dose-related and potentially reversible impairment of endothelium-dependent dilation in healthy young adults. Circulation 1993;88:2149–2155.
14. DaSilva A, Widmer LK, Ziegler HW et al. The Basle longitudinal study; report on the relation of initial glucose level to baseline ECG abnormalities, peripheral artery disease, and subsequent mortality. J Chron Dis 1979;32:797–803.
15. Boushey CJ, Beresford SA, Omenn GS, et al. A quantitative assessment of plasma homocysteine as a risk factor for vascular disease. JAMA 1995;274:1049–1057.
16. Martin MJ, Hulley SB, Browner WS, et al. Serum cholesterol, blood pressure, and mortality: implications from a cohort of 361,662 men. Lancet 1986;2:933–936.
17. Blauw GJ, Lagaay AM, Smelt AH, et al. Stroke, statins and cholesterol: a meta-analysis of randomized, placebo-controlled, double blind trials with HMG-CoA reductase inhibitors. Stroke 1997;28: 946–950.
18. Cheng SWK, Ting ACW, Wong J. Lipoprotein (a) and its relationship to risk factors and severity of atherosclerotic peripheral vascular disease. Eur J Vasc Endovasc Surg 1997;14:17–23.
19. Hertzer NR, Beven EG, Young JR, et al. Coronary artery disease in peripheral vascular patients: a classification of 1000 coronary angiograms and results of surgical management. Ann Surg 1984;199: 223–233.

20. Gentile AT, Taylor LM, Moneta GL, Porter JM. Prevalence of asymptomatic carotid artery stenosis in patients undergoing infrainguinal bypass surgery. Arch Surg 1995;130:900–904.
21. Alexandrova NA, Gibson WC, Norris JW et al. Carotid artery stenosis in peripheral vascular disease. J Vasc Surg 1996;23:645–649.
22. Aronow WS, Ahn C. Prevalence of coexistence of coronary artery disease, peripheral arterial disease, and atherothrombotic brain infarction in men and women less than 62 years of age. Am J Cardiology 1994;74:64–65.
23. Dormandy J, Heeck L, Vig S. The fate of patients with critical leg ischemia. J Vasc Surg 1999;12: 142–147
24. Veith FJ, Gupta SK, Samson RH, et al. Progress in limb salvage by reconstructive arterial surgery combined with new or improved adjunctive procedures. Ann Surg 1981;194:386–401.
25. Hickey NC, Thompson IA, Shearman CP, et al. Aggressive arterial reconstruction for critical lower limb ischaemia. Br J Surg 1991;78:1476–1478.
26. Edwards JM, Taylor LM, Porter JM. Treatment of failed lower extremity bypass grafts with new autogenous vein bypass. J Vasc Surg 1990;11:132-
27. Coffman JD. Intermittent claudication: not so benign. Am Heart J 1986;112:1127-1128.
28. Catalano M. Epidemiology of critical limb ischemia. North Italian data. Eur J Med 1993;2:1–4.
29. The Vascular Surgical Society of Great Britain and Ireland: critical limb ischaemia: management and outcome. Report of a national survey. Eur J Vasc Endovasc Surg 1995;10:108–113.
30. Dormandy J, Heeck L, Vig S. Intermittent claudication: underrated risks. J Vasc Surg 1999;12: 96–108.
31. Dormandy J, Heeck L, Vig S. Acute limb ischemia. J Vasc Surg 1999;12:148–53.
32. Stanley JC, Barnes RW, Ernst CB, et al. Work Force Issues Report of the Society for Vascular Surgery and the International Society for Cardiovascular Surgery, North American Chapter, Committee on Workforce Issues. J Vasc Surg 1996;23:172–181.
33. McDermott MM, Feinglass J, Slavensky R, Pierce WH. The ankle–brachial index as predictor of survival in patients with peripheral vascular disease. J Gen Intern Med 1994;9:445–449.
34. Newman AB, Shemanski L, Manolio T, et al. Ankle-arm index as predictor of cardiovascular disease and mortality in the cardiovascular health study. Arterioscler Thromb Vasc Biol 1999;19:538–545.
35. Hiatt WR, Hoag S, Hammen RF. Effect of diagnostic criteria on the prevalence of peripheral arterial artery disease. Circulation 1995;92:1472–1479.
36. Rutherford RB, Lowenstein DH, Klein, MF. Combining segmental arterial pressures and plethysmography to diagnose arterial disease in the legs. Am J Surg 1979;38:211–218.
37. Katz ML, Comerota AJ. Noninvasive evaluation of lower extremity arterial disease. In: Kerstein MD, White JV eds. Alternatives to Open Vascular Surgery. Philadelphia: JB Lippincott, 1995; pp.215–224.
38. Cambria R, Kaufman JA, L'Italien, et al. Magnetic resonance angiography in the management of lower extremity arterial occlusive disease: a prospective study. J Vasc Surg 1997;25:380–389.
39. Baum RA, Rutter CM, Sunshine JH, et al. Multicenter trial to evaluate vascular magnetic resonance angiography of the lower extremity. American College of Radiology Rapid Technology Assessment Group. JAMA 1995;274:875–880.
40. Elsman BH. Impact of ultrasonographic duplex scanning on therapeutic decision making in lower limb arterial disease. Br J Surg 1995;82:630–633.
41. North American Symptomatic Carotid Endarterectomy Trial Collaborators. Beneficial effect of carotid endarterectomy in symptomatic patients with high-grade carotid stenosis. N Engl J Med 1991;325:445–453.
42. Executive Committee for the Asymptomatic Carotid Atherosclerosis Study. Endarterectomy for asymptomatic carotid artery stenosis. JAMA 1995;273:1421–1428.
43. Hiatt WR. Medical treatment of peripheral arterial disease and claudication. N Engl J Med 2001;344: 1608–1621.
44. UK Prospective Diabetes Study (UKPDS) Group. Intensive blood-glucose control with sulphonylureas or insulin compared with conventional treatment and risk of complications in patients with type 2 diabetes. Lancet 1998;352:837–853.
45. Gould AL, Rossouw JE, Santanello NC, et al. Cholesterol reduction yields clinical benefit: impact of statin trials. Circulation 1998;97:946–952.
46. The sixth report of the joint National Committee on prevention, detection, evaluation and treatment of high blood pressure. Arch Intern Med 1997; 157:2413–2446.

47. Antiplatelet Trialists Collaboration. Secondary prevention of vascular disease by prolonged antiplatelet treatment. BMJ (Clin Res Ed) 1988;296:320–331.
48. CAPRIE Steering Committee. A randomized, blinded trial of clopidogrel versus aspirin in patients at risk of ischaemic events (CAPRIE). Lancet 1996;348:1329–1339.
49. deVries SO, Hunink MGM. Results of aortic bifurcation grafts for aortoiliac occlusive disease: a meta-analysis. J Vasc Surg 1997;26:558–569.
50. Brewster DC. Current controversies in the management of aortoiliac occlusive disease. J Vasc Surg 1997;25:365–379.
51. Nevelsteen A, Beyens G, Duchateau J, Suy R. Aorto–femoral reconstruction and sexual function: a prospective study. Eur J Vasc Surg 1990;4:247–251.
52. Bosch Jl, Hunink MGM. Meta-analysis of the results of percutaneous transluminal angioplasty and stent placement for aortoiliac occlusive disease. Radiology 1997;204:87–96.
53. Tettero E, Haaring C, van der Graf Y, van Schaik JP, Van Engelen AD, Mali WP. Intraarterial pressure gradients after randomized angioplasty and stenting of iliac artery lesions. Dutch Iliac Stent Trial Group. Cardiovasc Intervent Radiol 1996;19:411–417.
54. Pomposelli FB, Marcaccio EJ, Gibbons GW, et al. Dorsalis pedis arterial bypass: durable limb salvage for foot ischemia in patients with diabetes mellitus. J Vasc Surg 1995;21:375–384.
55. Darling RC, Chang BB, Shah DM, Leather RP. Choice of peroneal or dorsalis pedis artery bypass for limb salvage. Semin Vasc Surg 1997;10:17–22.
56. Akbari CM, LoGerfo FW. Diabetes and peripheral vascular disease. J Vasc Surg 1999;30:373–384.
57. Kram HB, Gupta SK, Veith FJ, Wengerter KR, Panetta TF, Nwosis C. Late results of two hundred seventeen femoropopliteal bypasses to isolated popliteal artery segments. J Vasc Surg 1991;14:386–390.
58. Rutherford RB, Jones DN, Bergentz SE, et al. Factors affecting the patency of infrainguinal bypass. J Vasc Surg 1988;8:236–246.
59. Johnson WC, Lee KK and members of the Department of Veteran Affairs COOP Study 141. A comparative evaluation of polytetrafluoroethylene, umbilical vein and saphenous vein bypass grafts for femoral-popliteal above knee revascularization: a prospective, randomized Department of Veteran Affairs cooperative study. J Vasc Surg 2000;32:268–277.
60. Gentile AT, Lee RW, Moneta GL, Taylor LM, Edwards JM, Porter JM. Results of bypass to the popliteal and tibial arteries with alternate sources of autogenous vein. J Vasc Surg 1996;23:272-280.
61. Harris L, O'Brian-Irr M, Ricotta JJ. Long-term assessment of cryopreserved vein bypass grafting success. J Vasc Surg 2001;33:528-532.
62. Pappas PJ, Hobson RW, Meyers MG, et al. Patency of infrainguinal polytetrafluoroethylene bypass grafts with distal interposition vein cuffs. Cardiovasc Surg 1998;6:19-26.
63. Kreienberg PB, Darling RC III, Chang BB, et al. Adjunctive techniques to improve patency of distal prosthetic bypass grafts: polytetrafluoroethylene with remote arteriovenous fistulae versus vein cuffs. J Vasc Surg 2000;31:696–701.
64. Dardik H, Silvestri F, Alasio T, et al. Improved method to create the common ostium variant of the distal arteriovenous fistula for enhancing crural prosthetic bypass graft patency. J Vasc Surg 1996;24:240–248.
65. Kalman PG, Johnston KW, Walker PM. The current role of isolated profundaplasty. J Cardiovasc Surg 1990;31:107–110.
66. Tovar-Pardo AE, Bernhard VM. Where the profunda femoris fits in the spectrum of lower limb revascularization. Semin Vasc Surg 1995;8:225–235.
67. Bakal CW, Cynamon J, Sprayregen S. Infrapopliteal percutaneous transluminal angioplasty: what we know. Radiology 1996;200;36–43.
68. Parsons RE, Suggs WD, Lee JL, Sanchez LA, Lyon RT, Veith FJ. Percutaneous transluminal angioplasty for treatment of limb-threatening ischemia. J Vasc Surg 1998;28:1066–1071.
69. Antiplatelet Trialists' Collaboration. Collaborative overview of randomized trials of antiplatelet therapy II: maintenance of vascular graft or arterial patency by antiplatelet therapy. Br Med J 1994;308:159–168.
70. Schomig A, Naumann FJ, Kastrati A, et al. A randomized comparison of antiplatelet and anticoagulant therapy after the placement of coronary artery stents. N Engl J Med 1996;334:1084–1089.
71. Bertrand ME, Legrand V, Boland J, et al. Randomized multicenter comparison of conventional anticoagulation versus antiplatelet therapy in unplanned and elective coronoray stenting: the Full Anticoagulation versus Aspirin and Ticlopidine (FANTASTIC) study. Circulation 1998;98:1597–1603.

72. Rutherford RB, Jones DN, Bergentz SE, et al. The efficacy of dextran 40 in preventing early postoperative thrombosis following difficult lower extremity bypass. J Vasc Surg 1984;1:765–773.

73. Katz SG, Kohl RD. Does dextran 40 improve the patency of autogenous infrainguinal bypass grafts? J Vasc Surg 1998;28:23–26.

74. Persson AV, Anderson LA, Padberg FT. Selection of patients for lumbar sympathectomy. Surg Clin N Am 1985;65:393–403.

75. van Bemmelen PS, Mattos MA, Faught WE, et al. Augmentation of blood flow in limbs with occlusive arterial disease by intermittent calf compression. J Vasc Surg 1994;19:1052–1058.

76. Eze AR, Comerota AJ, Cisek PL, et al. Intermittent calf and foot compression increases lower extremity blood flow. Am J Surg 1996;172:130–134.

77. van Bemmelen PS, Weiss-Olmanni J, Ricotta JJ. Rapid intermittent compression increases skin circulation in chronically ischemic legs with infra-popliteal arterial obstruction. Vasa 2000;29:47–52.

78. Lundell A, Lindblad B, Berqvist D, Hansen F. Femoropopliteal–crural graft patency is improved by an intensive surveillance program: a prospective randomized study. J Vasc Surg 1995;21:26–33.

79. Nehler MR, Moneta GL, Yeager RA, Edwards JM, Taylor LM, Porter JM. Surgical treatment of threatened reversed infrainguinal vein grafts. J Vasc Surg 1994;20:558–563.

80. Kinney EV, Bandyk DF, Mewisson MW, et al. Monitoring functional patency of percutaneous transluminal angioplasty. Arch Surg 1991;126:743–747.

81. Vroegindewij D, Tielbeck AV, Buth S, van Kints MJ, Landman GH, Mali WP. Recanalization of femoropopliteal occlusive lesions: a comparison of long term clinical, color duplex US, and arteriographic follow-up. JVIR 1995;6:331–337.

82. Dawson I, Hajo van Brockel J, Pesch-Batenburg J, et al. Late outcomes of limb loss after failed infrainguinal bypass. J Vasc Surg 1995;21:613–622.

83. Dormandy J, Belcher G, Broos P, et al. A prospective study of 713 below knee amputations for ischaemia and the effect of a prostacyclin analogue on healing. Br J Surg 1994;81:33–37.

84. Moore TJ, Barron J, Hutchinson F, Golden C, Ellis C, Humphries D. Prosthetic usage following major lower extremity amputation. Clin Orthop 1989;238:219–224.

85. Campbell WB, St. Johnston JA, Kernick VF, Rutter EA. Lower limb amputation: striking the balance. Ann R Coll Surg Engl 1994;76:205–209.

86. Comerota AJ, Throm RC, Miller KA, et al. Naked plasmid DNA encoding fibroblast growth factor type 1 (NV1FGF) for the treatment of end-stage unreconstructible lower extremity ischemia: preliminary results from a phase-1 trial. J Vasc Surg (accepted, 2002).

7

Acute Limb Ischemia

Jonathan L. Halperin, MD

INTRODUCTION

Acute limb ischemia arises when a rapid or sudden decrease in limb perfusion threatens tissue viability. This form of critical limb ischemia may be the first manifestation of vascular disease in a previously asymptomatic patient or occur as an acute event causing symptomatic deterioration in a patient with antecedent intermittent claudication. Although the progression of peripheral arterial disease (PAD) from intermittent claudication (IC) to critical limb ischemia (CLI) may occur gradually, it may reflect the cumulative effect of multiple acute events that progressively increase the intensity of ischemia.

The severity of acute limb ischemia depends mainly on the location and extent of arterial obstruction and the capacity of the collateral channels to deliver blood around an obstruction. Severity may be influenced by the status of systemic perfusion (cardiac output and peripheral resistance). In patients with PAD, acute obstruction may occur as a result of embolism, thrombosis, or a combination of both. When embolic occlusion affects a vascular bed not previously conditioned by collaterals, the resulting ischemic syndrome is typically severe. Collateral development in relation to the severity and chronicity of preexisting ischemia due to atheromatous obstructive arterial disease lessens the severity of ischemia when acute thrombotic arterial occlusion develops.

From: *Contemporary Cardiology: Peripheral Arterial Disease: Diagnosis and Treatment*
Edited by: J. D. Coffman and R. T. Eberhardt © Humana Press Inc., Totowa, NJ

Arterial embolism is thus more likely than arterial thrombosis to cause sudden, severe, limb-threatening ischemia. In certain clinical settings, however, arterial embolism can occur without symptoms, while thrombosis can produce sudden, severe limb ischemia.

ARTERIAL EMBOLISM

The clinical diagnosis of arterial embolism is suggested by (1) the sudden onset of symptoms, (2) a known embolic source, (3) the absence of antecedent claudication or other manifestations of obstructive arterial disease, or (4) the presence of normal arterial pulses and Doppler systolic blood pressures in the contralateral limb.

Etiology

Arterial embolism of cardiac origin derives from a diversity of cardiac disorders (Fig. 1). There is a history of nonvalvular atrial fibrillation in about half the cases, valvular heart disease in a quarter, and left ventricular mural thrombus in almost a third *(1)*. Less commonly, the source involves an intracardiac tumor such as an atrial myxoma. In the absence of antithrombotic therapy, the risk of embolism associated with atrial fibrillation is five to six events per 100 patient-years, at least five times the rate among comparably aged patients without this cardiac rhythm disturbance, accumulating to a 35% lifetime risk. The risk is directly related to age, such that over half the embolic events occur in patients over 75 yr old *(2–4)*. As for emboli of left ventricular origin, 60% are associated with acute myocardial infarction *(5)*. Intracavitary thrombus occurs in about one-third of patients in the first 2 wk following anterior myocardial infarction, and in an even greater proportion of those with large infarcts involving the left ventricular apex *(1–4)*. Clinically evident cerebral infarction occurs in approximately 10% of patients with left ventricular thrombus following myocardial infarction in the absence of anticoagulant therapy but the incidence of acute limb ischemia is not known *(6)*. Trials of thrombolytic therapy suggest a lower incidence of left ventricular thrombus formation *(7–9)*, but this is controversial *(10)*. Patients with chronic ventricular dysfunction resulting from coronary artery disease, hypertension, or other forms of dilated cardiomyopathy also face a persistent risk of stroke and systemic embolism.

VENTRICULAR THROMBI

The pathogenesis of intracavitary mural thrombosis follows the triad of precipitating factors established over a century ago by Virchow: endothelial injury, a zone of circulatory stasis, and a hypercoagulable state *(11)*. Shortly after the onset of acute myocardial infarction, leukocyte infiltration separates endothelial cells from their basal lamina *(12)*, exposing subendothelial tissue to intracavitary blood and creating a nidus for thrombus development. Endocardial abnormalities have been identified histologically in specimens from patients with left ventricular aneurysm *(13)*, and in patients with idiopathic dilated cardiomyopathy *(14)*. Experimental and clinical studies have emphasized the importance of wall motion abnormalities in the development of left ventricular mural thrombus, and stasis of blood in regions of akinesia or dyskinesia seems the essential factor *(15–17)*. Stasis is similarly important in the development of atrial thrombus when effective mechanical atrial activity is impaired, as occurs in atrial fibrillation, atrial enlargement, mitral stenosis, and cardiac failure *(18)*. Stasis brings about conditions of low shear rate, and deposition of fibrin plays the predominant pathogenic role in the development of intracavitary thrombus. In patients with acute myocardial

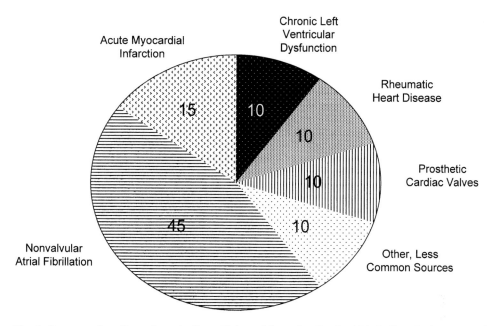

Fig. 1. Sources of cardiogenic embolism. (Adapted from the Cerebral Embolism Task Force, ref. 1.)

infarction, the incidence of thromboembolism is related to plasma fibrinogen level, suggesting a hypercoagulable tendency in this condition. The surface of fresh thrombus is highly thrombogenic, and a local hypercoagulable state may be heightened in the milieu of endocardial injury *(19)*.

PATENT FORAMEN OVALE AND MISCELLANEOUS CAUSES

Transesophageal echocardiography and autopsy studies have identified patent foramen ovale, the most common postnatal residuum of the fetal circulation, occurring in up to 27% of otherwise normal hearts in one series involving cerebral ischemia *(20)*. The prevalence of this anatomical finding is significantly greater, however, in individuals younger than age 55 yr and among those without other identified etiology for ischemia *(21)*. The mechanism in these cases is thought to involve paradoxical embolism of thrombus formed in the peripheral venous system rather than in the cardiac chambers. Aneurysmal deformity of the interatrial septum has been recognized with increased frequency since the advent of transesophageal echocardiography, and may be associated with an increased risk of thromboembolism. However, the mechanism of this association is not clear and may involve coexisting conditions such as patent foramen ovale or atrial fibrillation, rather than thrombus formation on the surface of the aneurysm itself *(22)*. Other sources of embolism include cardiac tumors such as left atrial myxoma, atheromatous plaque in the aorta or proximal limb arteries, or mural thrombus lining the wall of an aortic or arterial aneurysm.

ATRIAL FIBRILLATION

Previously unrecognized atrial fibrillation (AF) is disclosed during cardiac rhythm monitoring in some 20–25% of such cases. Patients with AF associated with rheumatic valvular heart disease or prosthetic heart valves face a particular danger of stroke and systemic embolism—thromboembolic event rates of at least 8–10% per year, 17 times that of patients in normal sinus rhythm in the Framingham Heart Study (23). This is high enough to justify in the minds of most clinicians the hemorrhagic risks associated with maintenance oral anticoagulant therapy with coumarin drugs, even in the absence of randomized trials (24). Among patients with nonvalvular AF, the risk is greatest when stroke or systemic embolism has occurred within the previous 2 yr—in such cases the risk of recurrent ischemic events exceeds 10% per year (25).

During the past decade, randomized clinical trials assessed the efficacy of antithrombotic therapies for stroke prevention in patients with nonvalvular AF. Fifteen randomized trials involving nearly 10,000 participants with atrial fibrillation have compared anticoagulants and antiplatelet platelet agents, alone and in combination, to placebo and to each other (26). Adjusted-dose warfarin is highly efficacious for prevention of thromboembolism in atrial fibrillation patients, with a risk reduction of 61% (95% CI 47, 71) by adjusted-dose warfarin vs placebo (27). By on-treatment analysis (excluding those not taking warfarin), the prophylactic efficacy of warfarin exceeded 80%. Thus, adjusted-dose warfarin has the remarkable potential to reverse almost entirely the increased risk of cardiogenic embolism accompanying AF. The benefit of anticoagulation was not substantially offset by major hemorrhage in the randomized trials, in which participants with a mean age of 69 yr were carefully selected and managed according to strict clinical protocols. It is unclear whether the relatively low observed rates of major hemorrhage apply generally to atrial fibrillation patients in clinical practice (whose mean age is about 75 yr) when anticoagulation administration is less closely regulated (28,29). The target intensity of anticoagulation involves a tenuous balance between prevention of ischemic stroke and accentuation of major bleeding. Targeting the lowest adequate intensity of anticoagulation to minimize the risk of bleeding is particularly important for elderly atrial fibrillation patients, because they have higher risks of bleeding. Maximum protection against ischemic stroke in atrial fibrillation is probably achieved with International Normalized Ratios (INR) between 2.0 and 3.0 (30). Aspirin offers only modest protection against stroke for patients with AF: meta-analysis of five randomized trials showed a stroke reduction of 19% (95% CI 2, 34) (27). The effect of aspirin on stroke in these trials was less consistent than that of warfarin (31). Thus, warfarin may be most beneficial for atrial fibrillation patients at higher intrinsic thromboembolic risk, but offers only modest reductions over aspirin in both the relative risk and absolute rates of stroke for atrial fibrillation patients at low risk (30).

Sites of Embolism

Over 90% of clinically recognized cardioembolic events involve the brain, reflecting both the high relative sensitivity of cerebral tissue to ischemia and the biophysics of the arterial circulation. The limbs and abdominal viscera share the risk, and acute arterial occlusive events may involve virtually any arterial bed. Among the patients with arterial embolism complicating myocardial infarction, multiple sites are involved in approximately one fifth of cases, and a similar proportion is likely in patients with other conditions predisposing to thromboembolism derived from the cardiac chambers.

Arterial emboli typically lodge at branch points in the arterial circulation where the caliber of the arterial lumen diminishes, but relative frequencies are difficult to obtain from the literature. In a series of 89 cases of lower limb ischemia attributed to embolism accumulated between 1959 and 1968 at the Mayo Clinic, 46% lodged in the femoral arteries, 21% in the iliac arteries, 18% in the aorta, 10% in the popliteal arteries, and 5% in the tibial arteries *(32)*. Embolism to the aortoiliac bifurcation ("saddle embolus") may produce bilateral lower limb ischemia variably associated with reversible paraplegia and a high mortality rate *(33,34)* and has been described as a complication of systemic thrombolytic therapy in patients with left ventricular mural thrombus *(35)*. Embolic occlusions at sites of arterial bifurcation may cause more severe ischemia when accessory routes of perfusion are interrupted, as occurs when the profunda femoris artery is compromised by embolism to the common femoral artery.

ARTERIAL THROMBOSIS

The other major cause of acute limb ischemia is acute arterial thrombosis superimposed on a stenotic atherosclerotic plaque. A common site of thrombosis is the superficial femoral artery, although occlusion may occur anywhere from the aorta to the digital arteries. Arterial thrombosis may be precipitated by a decrease in blood flow velocity because of low cardiac output, as may occur in congestive cardiac failure or after myocardial infarction. Rarely, an extrinsic local factor such as popliteal entrapment or cystic adventitial disease may be the precursor of arterial thrombosis. Embolism from cardiac valves and chambers or from other sources may affect atherosclerotic arteries, producing a confusing clinical picture. The location of the obstruction in relation to other axial arteries in the region of the obstructed vessel and the collateral flow they provide also affect the severity of ischemia. The longer the obstructive lesion, the more collateral pathways are interrupted. Thrombosis tends to extend to the next large collateral, but the low-flow state below the obstructing thrombus encourages propagation of thrombus. This is the rationale for the early administration of heparin.

CLINICAL EVALUATION

History and Symptoms

The clinical history should be directed toward detection of symptoms relative to the onset and course of ischemia and background information pertaining to etiology, differential diagnosis, and concurrent disease. Symptoms in acute limb ischemia relate primarily to pain and dysfunction. The pattern of onset may have etiological implications (i.e., embolism tends to present more abruptly than thrombosis), whereas the character and distribution of pain may aid the differential diagnosis. The limb pain associated with severe acute ischemia may share the same acute intensity as the rest pain of chronic severe ischemia; it is less often localized to the forefoot, less influenced by dependency, and usually more diffuse, extending above the ankle in severe cases. In cases of lesser severity, pain may be absent, while in more severe cases it may diminish, either because of improving collateral perfusion or because sensory loss interferes with perception. Weakness and numbness are commonly associated with persistent severe acute limb ischemia, and it is important to determine whether dysfunction is worsening or improving over time. It is also crucial to determine whether the patient had previous claudication or arterial interventions, arterial or aortic aneurysm, and whether there is an established diagnosis of heart disease with particular reference to atrial fibrillation or ventricular dysfunction. The patient should also be asked about concurrent diseases and risk factors for atherosclerosis.

Physical Examination

Pulselessness, pallor, paresthesia, and paralysis characterize acute limb ischemia; assessing these features is aided by comparing the suspect limb with the opposite extremity. It may be difficult to determine whether pulse deficits are new or old in patients with PAD without a history of previous symptoms, a recorded examination, or the finding of similar pulse deficits in the contralateral leg. Pedal pulses may be normal in cases of microembolism due to proximal disruption of atheromatous plaque. Skin pallor may be observed early after the onset of ischemia, but over time cyanosis becomes more common. Coolness, particularly when the opposite extremity is not cool, is a typical finding and an abrupt line of transition in temperature or color is generally one limb segment below the level of arterial obstruction. These levels should be correlated with pulse palpation and should be marked or recorded during the initial examination as a baseline for subsequent comparison. Evaluation of "capillary" return, which reflects the emptying and refilling of subpapillary venules, is subject to considerable environmental and interobserver variation but is usually slow or absent in acute limb ischemia.

Some, but not all, patients with sensory loss describe numbness or paresthesias, but preexisting sensory deficits in diabetics can lead to confusion. Sensory deficits may be subtle in the early phase of acute limb ischemia; appreciation of light touch, two-point discrimination, vibratory perception, and proprioception are usually lost before perception of deep pain and pressure. Motor deficits indicate advanced, limb-threatening ischemia, partly because foot movement is produced mainly by more proximal muscles. Dorsiflexion or plantar flexion of the great toe is produced by muscles originating just below the knee and innervated by the peroneal nerve that passes through the anterior tibial compartment. Ischemia may be less profound in these proximal locations than distally, so detection of early motor weakness requires testing the intrinsic muscles of the foot in comparison with the contralateral foot. Persistent pain, sensory loss, and muscle weakness are among the most important findings that distinguish threatened from viable extremities. Muscle rigor, tenderness, or pain on passive movement are late signs of advanced ischemia predictive of tissue loss.

DIFFERENTIAL DIAGNOSIS

The differential diagnosis in acute limb ischemia involves exclusion of conditions mimicking arterial occlusion, identification of nonatherosclerotic causes of arterial occlusion, and distinguishing ischemia caused by an arterial thrombosis from embolism (Table 1).

Vasospasm may produce the same symptoms as acute limb ischemia. Other conditions that may mimic arterial occlusion are *low cardiac output*, especially when superimposed on chronic lower extremity occlusive disease; acute *deep venous thrombosis,* especially when associated with features of *phlegmasia cerulea dolens* and acute *compressive peripheral neuropathy*. The latter conditions should be distinguishable by palpable pulses unless chronic arterial occlusive disease or an intense vasoconstrictor response coexists. In acute compressive neuropathy, color and temperature are usually normal or above normal, which is quite unusual for ischemia causing similar pain. In cases of venous thrombosis, cyanosis and coolness may be present, and pulses may be difficult to palpate in the

Table 1
Differential Diagnosis of Acute Limb Ischemia

Nonarterial disorders
  Congestive heart failure
  Proximal deep venous thrombosis
  Acute compressive neuropathy

Nonatherosclerotic arterial disorders
  Trauma
  Arteritis
  Hypercoagulable syndromes
  Adventitial cysts and tumors
  Popliteal artery entrapment
  Vasospasm

Atherosclerotic syndromes
  Thrombosis superimposed upon atherosclerotic stenosis
  Thrombosis of an arterial stent
  Thrombosis of an arterial bypass graft
  Cardiogenic embolism
  Embolism from proximal aortic or arterial aneurysm or complex atheromatous plaque
  Embolism complicating endovascular procedure
  Thrombosis of peripheral arterial aneurysm

presence of edema, but edema does not occur with acute arterial occlusion unless diagnosis is delayed long enough to allow dependent swelling to develop.

Vasospasm

Difficulties in palpating arterial pulses may be resolved by detection of unobstructed arterial Doppler signals over distal arteries. This is helpful in cases of vasospasm when distal pulses may be difficult to feel; the velocity signals may sound blunted but remain biphasic. When vasospasm is severe enough to cause acute limb ischemia, a cause such as ergotism *(36,37)* can usually be found (primary, idiopathic vasospasm seldom produces deep tissue ischemia). Patients in advanced congestive heart failure may develop acute limb ischemia, particularly when chronic arterial insufficiency is present.

Atheroembolism

Microembolism from proximal atherosclerotic lesions can cause cool, painful, cyanotic toes or skin mottling akin to livedo reticularis (*see* Chapter 17). The source is usually complex atherosclerotic plaque in the aorta that is thick, irregular, or ulcerated or, typically in the iliac or femoral arteries, narrowed sufficiently to produce flow turbulence prior to the onset of occlusive thrombus. Commonly mistaken for vasculitis or collagen vascular disease, the importance of cholesterol emboli is not so much as a cause of distal gangrene, because most of the initial lesions resolve, than as harbingers of recurrent ischemic events. The source should be sought by ultrasound or magnetic resonance imaging or by arteriography, although the latter carries the risk of dislodgement and recurrent embolic phenomena. Intervention may prove necessary when anticoagulation is not sufficient to prevent recurrent episodes.

Popliteal Artery Aneurysm Thrombosis

Thrombosis of popliteal arterial aneurysms accounts for about 10% of acute arterial occlusions in elderly men. Commonly mistaken for arterial embolic events, the diagnosis is often made intraoperatively *(38,39)*. Severe ischemia usually results because thrombosis occurs in the absence of collateral enhancement, and because the popliteal artery is the sole axial artery traversing the knee. Because popliteal aneurysms are bilateral in approx 50% of cases, detecting a prominent popliteal pulse in the opposite leg may be a valuable clue. These patients also tend to have dilated femoral arteries or an abdominal aortic aneurysm. Once suspected, duplex imaging is the most rapid means of confirming the diagnosis.

Popliteal Arterial Cysts and Entrapment

Popliteal cysts *(40,41)* and popliteal entrapment *(42,43)* may be discovered before they induce thrombosis if the patient develops claudication, but thrombosis is often the first presenting syndrome (*see* Chapter 3). Like popliteal aneurysm, ischemia is often severe. Young age betrays popliteal entrapment, but popliteal cysts present at an older age and may be indistinguishable from atherosclerotic PAD. The absence of atherosclerotic risk factors and the location of the obstruction, best identified by duplex imaging, may suggest the etiology.

Vasculitis

Segmental arterial thrombosis can occur with giant cell arteritis *(44)* but this is more likely to occur in the axillobrachial than the femoral arterial segment (*see* Chapter 19). The erythrocyte sedimentation is usually accelerated. Takayasu's aortitis rarely affects lower extremity circulation and has a gradual onset. Thrombosis with thromboangiitis obliterans (Buerger's disease) *(45)* usually occurs in crural or pedal arteries in smokers younger than age 45 yr, characteristically presenting with ischemic ulcers or focal gangrene. It should rarely be confused with acute arterial thrombosis caused by PAD but can be similar to cases of severe chronic ischemia secondary to peripheral atherosclerosis (*see* Chapter 18).

Arterial Trauma or Dissection

Overt arterial trauma is not difficult to recognize, but iatrogenic trauma, which typically occurs as a result of arterial catheterization, is readily overlooked. This should be considered in patients presenting with femoral artery occlusion following cardiovascular instrumentation. Such trauma also can produce arterial dissections, and the most commonly missed are thoracic aortic dissections that extend to involve the abdominal aorta or into an iliac artery. Tearing interscapular back pain associated with hypertension points to such a thoracic aortic dissection, but this may be obscured by other events or by impairment of the patient's mental status. Another common complication of transfemoral catheterization is perforation of the common iliac artery that produces retroperitoneal hemorrhage associated with compressive arterial insufficiency causing acute limb ischemia. This may be suggested by signs of blood loss, flank ecchymoses, and roentgenographic evidence of compression of the contrast-enhanced urinary bladder by an expanding hematoma.

Arterial Thrombosis Associated with Hypercoagulable Syndromes

Arterial thrombosis secondary to an underlying hypercoagulable state is character-ized by unusual location, lack of atherosclerotic risk factors or other obvious precipi-tating causes, young age, and a past or family history of thrombotic events including deep vein thrombosis (46). Such patients warrant comprehensive evaluation of the coag-ulation system. Acquired or hereditary hyperhomocysteinemia can also lead to acute arterial thrombosis.

ANCILLARY INVESTIGATIONS

Techniques of vascular testing for patients with acute limb ischemia are similar to those used in patients with chronic symptoms. The most important objectives are to eval-uate the arterial circulation in the legs objectively and to evaluate the systemic circula-tion in terms of cardiac disease and possible sources of embolism. Detection of concurrent atherosclerotic involvement of other vascular regions should be investigated as the foundation for assessment of operative risk.

Doppler Velocimetry

Measurement of segmental limb pressures is of little value in patients with acute arte-rial occlusion, and the pressure gradient criteria developed for chronic ischemia do not apply. The ankle–brachial systolic pressure index (ABI) is less useful in the setting of acute ischemia than in situations of chronic critical limb ischemia. In fact, it is often not possible to detect systolic arterial signals in an acutely ischemic limb, and detection of arterial Doppler signals over pedal arteries has been used to assess the severity of ischemia. The presence of audible Doppler arterial signals suggests a less immediate limb threat, but the absence of Doppler arterial signals does not necessarily mean the opposite. Similarly, venous Doppler sounds may be misinterpreted as arterial signals. The risk of misinterpretation of Doppler signals makes it important to emphasize that arterial Doppler analysis cannot substitute for clinical examination in cases of acute limb ischemia. The presence or absence of neurological deficits is an overriding con-sideration (47).

Vascular Imaging

Duplex scanning may help to detect and localize arterial obstruction (48–51), but this technique has been properly evaluated for this purpose only in the setting of trauma. Magnetic resonance angiography (MRA) is an emerging technology, but further studies are needed to determine to what extent MRA may replace angiography (52–59). Angiog-raphy yields greater anatomical detail on which to base therapeutic decisions and is a prerequisite for catheter-directed thrombolytic therapy (see Chapter 12). With this tech-nique, the obstructive lesion can be visualized, although it may be difficult to image the distal arterial tree in patients with acute arterial occlusion. Angiography often facilitates the distinction between embolism and thrombosis, because the former may be associ-ated with either an abrupt cutoff of contrast flow, a convex meniscus, or a clot silhouet-ted by contrast medium, and may help identify patients more likely to benefit from percutaneous treatment than from catheter embolectomy or open surgical revascular-ization.

Contrast-induced injury to the ischemic limb or kidneys may be difficult to dissociate from the effects of ischemia and reperfusion. Digital subtraction enhancement angiography reduces the risks associated with administration of ionic contrast media. Another consideration is the delay imposed by performing formal angiography in the face of limb-threatening ischemia. In patients with acutely threatened limbs, intraoperative angiography can be combined with embolectomy.

Echocardiography

Aside from the identification of mitral stenosis, the main echocardiographic correlate of thromboembolic risk is impairment of left ventricular systolic function *(50,60)*, which may promote stasis of blood within the left atrium in the presence of AF. Enlargement of the left atrium, seemingly a correlate of stasis within the atrial appendage, has some predictive value as a marker of embolic risk *(61–63)*, but left ventricular dysfunction is a more powerful predictor in patients not given antithrombotic medication *(64)*.

Transesophageal echocardiography (TEE) places high-frequency ultrasound transducers in closer proximity to the heart to provide high-quality images of cardiac structure *(65)* and function *(66)*. TEE more frequently identifies potential sources of embolism than transthoracic echocardiography *(67)*, particularly thrombus in the left atrial appendage of patients with AF, found in 5–15% of cases undergoing cardioversion (68). Detection of thrombus in the setting of systemic embolism is convincing evidence of a cardiogenic mechanism *(69)*. When standards for acquisition and interpretation are carefully applied, this technique provides a unique diagnostic window for evaluating the left atrium, left atrial appendage, and thoracic aorta, and also appears more sensitive for detection of spontaneous echo-contrast, which is associated with circulatory stasis and thrombus formation *(70)*. In a study of patients with atrial fibrillation at high risk of thromboembolism (based on age, gender, prior thromboembolism, and/or left ventricular dysfunction), TEE features associated with subsequent ischemic events were abnormalities of the left atrial appendage (reduced emptying velocity, dense spontaneous echo-contrast, or manifest thrombus) or complex atherosclerotic lesions of the proximal aorta *(71)*. These TEE findings support the view that multiple mechanisms may be responsible for thromboembolism even in patients with atrial fibrillation, involving thrombus formation in the cardiac chambers, as well as extracardiac vascular disease.

Other Laboratory Studies

Basic blood tests should be obtained to assess anesthetic risk, and tests of the coagulation system should be obtained before heparin is administered. An electrocardiogram and echocardiogram should be obtained in those with possible embolism, but these need not delay initiation of anticoagulant medication.

CLASSIFICATION OF SEVERITY

The Transatlantic Inter-Society Consensus (TASC) on Management of Peripheral Arterial Disease classified the severity of acute limb ischemia (Table 2) *(72)*. Level I severity refers to a viable limb that is not immediately threatened by ischemia. Continuous pain or neurological deficits are absent, cutaneous capillary perfusion is adequate, and Doppler arterial flow signals are detectable over a pedal artery. Level II severity refers to a threatened but salvageable limb and implies reversible ischemia in which

Table 2
Clinical Categories of Acute Limb Ischemia

| Level | Severity | Description prognosis | Clinical findings | | | Doppler signals | |
			Sensory loss	Muscle weakness	Arterial	Venous
I	Viable	Not immediately threatened	None	None	Audible	Audible
IIa	Marginally threatened	Salvageable with prompt intervention	Minimal and limited to toes	None	Variable	Audible
IIb	Immediately threatened	Salvageable with immediate revascularization	Often extends beyond toes; rest pain	Mild to moderate	Usually inaudible	Audible
III	Probably irreversible[a]	Amputation or permanent damage anticipated	Profound numbness, paralysis or rigor	Extensive	Absent	Absent

Adapted from the Transatlantic Inter-Society Consensus (TASC), ref. 62.
[a]Early in the course after onset, it may be difficult to distinguish level III from level IIb ischemia.

major amputation can be avoided if arterial obstruction is promptly relieved. Doppler signals are not audible over pedal arteries. The subcategory of level IIa ischemia refers to a *marginally* threatened limb, and level IIb to an immediately threatened limb. Patients with marginally threatened extremities (IIa) may experience numbness and have transient or minimal sensory loss, limited to the toes, but not continuous pain. In contrast, *immediately threatened* (IIb) limbs have persistent ischemic pain, loss of sensation, or motor weakness. In level III ischemia, major, irreversible ischemic changes usually result in permanent neuromuscular damage, regardless of therapy, and major amputation is usually required. Profound sensory loss and muscle paralysis extend above the foot, distal capillary skin flow is absent, or there is evidence of more advanced ischemia, such as muscle rigor or skin marbling. Neither arterial nor venous flow signals are audible over pedal vessels. In a small proportion of patients with level III ischemia, particularly those presenting early, the limb may be salvaged by prompt treatment.

More definitive tests of tissue viability are still needed, because even physicians with considerable clinical experience cannot always accurately predict reversibility of ischemia or the potential for limb salvage. However, the grouping of patients into "viable," "threatened," and "irreversible" categories facilitates comparison of the results of different treatment strategies. At one extreme are patients with clearly viable limbs, where time is available for deliberate, detailed evaluation and interventional procedures might not ultimately prove necessary. At the other extreme are patients facing inevitable major tissue loss (amputation) or permanent ischemic neuromuscular damage. In such cases, a painless, functional limb cannot be restored regardless of the rapidity or extent of revascularization. The absence of venous signals in this latter category indicates complete circulatory stagnation. Between these extremes lies an intermediate group in which the limb is threatened and prompt revascularization is necessary for limb salvage. In these cases, operative intervention is undertaken without preliminary diagnostic angiography. There is a subgroup of patients without audible pedal artery Doppler signals but only mild or evanescent sensory loss in which high-dose catheter-directed thrombolytic therapy protocols can rapidly improve perfusion to achieve limb salvage.

TREATMENT

The therapeutic challenge presented by acute limb ischemia is compounded by inadequate opportunities to treat important comorbidities and by the problem of reperfusion injury that follows revascularization. Despite progress in many areas of vascular reconstruction, acute limb ischemia is still associated with substantial limb loss and mortality (10–20%), usually attributable to coexistent cardiac disease *(73–76)*.

The arterial occlusion should be removed without delay, because the risk of limb loss increases with the duration of ischemia. In one study, amputation rates were proportional to the interval between onset of acute limb ischemia and exploration (6% within 12 h, 12% within 13–24 h, and 20% beyond 24 h), and earlier studies cited even higher amputation rates.

Anticoagulation with heparin reduces morbidity and mortality and is part of the overall treatment strategy that should begin prior to vascular intervention *(77,78)*, not only to prevent clot propagation but, in the case of arterial embolism, to mitigate against recurrent embolism. Administration of heparin may be briefly delayed in cases in which spinal or epidural anesthesia is important for overall patient management. Pain should be controlled by appropriate analgesia. Oxygen inhalation may be helpful, and there is some experimental evidence of its benefit *(79)*. Appropriate treatment for congestive cardiac failure or atrial or ventricular arrhythmias should be initiated immediately and continued through the intervention, rather than waiting until after it. There is no evidence that vasodilator drugs or sympathectomy are helpful in acute limb ischemia. Wherever possible, simple measures to improve existing perfusion should be undertaken, before or after revascularization, or occasionally as an attempt to avoid surgery in a high-risk patient with marginal viability. These include keeping the foot dependent, avoiding extrinsic pressure over the heel or bony prominence, avoiding temperature extremes (cold induces vasoconstriction, whereas heat raises the metabolic rate and circulatory demand), maximizing tissue oxygenation, and correcting hypotension.

Endovascular Procedures

THROMBOLYSIS

Angiography is performed when the severity of ischemia permits and in such cases catheter-directed thrombolytic therapy may be the initial treatment. The choice depends on location and anatomy of lesions, duration of the occlusion, the type of clot (embolus vs thrombosis), patient comorbidities, and the risk of the procedure. Contraindications to thrombolysis mainly involve conditions that increase the risk of bleeding complications, but this method of clot removal avoids or reduces the scope of surgery. Catheter-directed thrombolysis is performed following angiography for acute occlusion by passing a guidewire through the embolus or thrombus within the occluded artery. If the guidewire passes, then lytic therapy is initiated. If the catheter fails to pass, regional infusion with the catheter placed proximally may facilitate another attempt to cross the occluded segment. Regional infusion should not exceed 6 h before one attempts to achieve the optimum catheter position. Clinical deterioration during regional infusion signals the need to interrupt thrombolysis and proceed with surgical revascularization.

The advantages of catheter-directed thrombolysis over thromboembolectomy include decreasing endothelial trauma, uncovering underlying lesions, and visualizing the runoff vessels *(80)*. Its superiority over intravenously administered thrombolytic agents is well established, and the latter should not be used in acute limb ischemia. It has been suggested that gradual, low-pressure reperfusion may be superior to the abrupt high-pressure reperfusion that characterizes surgical revascularization *(81,82)*. After successful recanalization is achieved by intraarterial administration of streptokinase, tissue plasminogen activator, or urokinase, any underlying lesion should be identified and corrected by the most appropriate percutaneous or open surgical technique to increase the likelihood of long-term patency *(83,84)*.

OTHER ENDOVASCULAR TECHNIQUES

When thrombolysis reveals underlying localized disease (e.g., a discrete, short stenosis), catheter-based revascularization such as percutaneous transluminal angioplasty becomes an attractive option. Stenoses and occlusions are rarely the sole cause of acute limb ischemia or even severe chronic symptoms but commonly lead to superimposed thrombosis and therefore should be treated to avoid recurrent thrombosis *(85,86)*. Until recently, catheter-directed thrombolysis and open surgical thrombectomy were the only two basic options for dealing with arterial thromboembolism. Percutaneous aspiration thrombectomy and percutaneous mechanical thrombectomy provide an alternative non-surgical modality for the treatment of acute limb ischemia. In high-risk patients, in whom any form of surgery is highly dangerous, it has been suggested that these newer techniques of thrombus removal may be safer than emergency surgery *(131)*.

Percutaneous aspiration thrombectomy is a technique that uses thin-wall, large-lumen catheters and suction with a 50-mL syringe to remove embolus or thrombus from native femoropopliteal arteries, bypass grafts, and runoff vessels. It has been used together with fibrinolysis to reduce time and dose of the fibrinolytic agent or as a stand-alone procedure *(87–89)*.

Most mechanical thrombectomy devices are based on hydrodynamic recirculation, in which dissolution of thrombus occurs within a region of mixing known as the "hydro-dynamic vortex," which selectively traps and evacuates thrombotic material. Nonrecirculation devices function mainly by mechanical fragmentation of thrombus, and these are believed to carry a higher risk of peripheral embolization and vascular injury *(90)*. Studies of rotational *(91)* and hydraulic recirculation devices *(92,93)* have involved disparate patient populations; patients with acute graft occlusion predominated in some series *(92)*, while those with acute ischemia due to embolism predominated in others *(91)* and the duration of ischemia differed. In some studies, up to 90% of patients required adjunctive catheter treatments such as angioplasty, local intraarterial thrombolysis, or atherectomy *(93)*.

The effectiveness of percutaneous mechanical thrombectomy depends on the age of the thrombus; fresh thrombus is most amenable to intervention. In embolic occlusions, fragmentation devices show better results than hydraulic methods. Percutaneous aspiration and mechanical approaches may offer advantages over pharmacological thrombolysis in terms of time efficiency, safety, and cost, but formal trials are needed to compare these two percutaneous methods of thrombectomy with catheter-directed thrombolysis or surgical embolectomy.

Surgical Revascularization

For patients with a profoundly ischemic limb of level IIb and early level III severity, immediate surgical revascularization is indicated. In cases of embolism to a nonatherosclerotic limb, catheter embolectomy is usually preferred. Embolism in nonatherosclerotic limbs commonly produces severe ischemia (level IIb or III) that calls for surgical management. Time to intervention is a key determinant in the selection of operative vs percutaneous revascularization. Embolic occlusions are preferentially addressed surgically if they are located proximally in the limb or when they occur in a nonatherosclerotic limb. Once all accessible clot has been retrieved, distal vessels should be imaged carefully, as residual thrombus, identified in up to a third of cases, may compromise distal perfusion *(94–96)*. The most common method used to ensure the adequacy of clot removal is "completion" angiography before closure of the arteriotomy. Fiberoptic angioscopy may not provide comparable visualization of the distal vasculature.

Distal thrombus may be treated intraoperatively by brief administration of high doses of thrombolytic agents followed by additional attempts at balloon thromboembolectomy guided by repeated angiography and ultrasound examination. This will determine whether the procedure has been adequate or whether additional attempts at revascularization are warranted to ensure limb viability. Isolated limb perfusion has been advocated in extreme cases to reduce the systemic toxicity of thrombolysis *(97,98)*.

In cases of arterial thrombosis, residual thrombus and an underlying local lesion must be sought after clot extraction. Often this may be suspected from the tactile sensations and need for deflation at points during the withdrawal of the inflated balloon catheter. Completion angiography will help determine whether bypass or percutaneous catheter-based intervention is necessary. Arterial thrombosis superimposed on a narrowed artery ordinarily causes less severe ischemia because of collateral perfusion of the limb.

Comparison of Surgical Revascularization vs Thrombolysis

The first randomized study of surgery vs thrombolysis in patients with acute limb ischemia within 1–14 d of onset observed 1-mo limb salvage rates of 87% and 90%, respectively, for surgery and thrombolysis *(99)*, but additional procedures were required in a substantial proportion of cases. From 1994 to 1996, three large randomized trials compared catheter-directed thrombolysis with surgical revascularization for treatment of acute limb ischemia *(100,130,131)*; a number of other studies lacked randomization or suffered from other methodological deficiencies *(101–107)*. Comparisons are limited by differences in design, inclusion criteria, or endpoints, and it is worth keeping in mind that the most important outcomes of these procedures are limb salvage and survival rates.

In one study, patients with class II limb-threatening ischemia of < 7 d in duration were randomly assigned to either catheter-directed thrombolysis with urokinase or surgical revascularization *(100)*. Patients with both thrombotic and embolic occlusions of native arteries and bypass grafts were included. Following thrombolysis, anatomical lesions were treated with balloon angioplasty or bypass surgery. Although the cumulative limb salvage rates were identical in both groups (82%), 12-mo mortality was higher in the group treated surgically (42% vs 16%, $P = 0.01$), owing mainly to cardiopulmonary complications. This was the only randomized study to show a clear survival advantage of thrombolytic therapy for limb-threatening acute ischemia, based on primary endpoint analysis *(100)*.

In the STILE trial, patients with thrombotic native artery or bypass graft occlusions of less than 6 mo in duration were randomized to thrombolytic versus surgical management *(131)*. In most of the cohort, ischemia had been present for > 2 wk, but very few had class II limb-threatening ischemia. The trial was terminated when interim analysis showed a significantly higher rate of persistent or recurrent ischemia in the group treated with thrombolytic therapy than in the surgical group at 1 mo (54% vs 26%, $P < 0.001$), but overall clinical outcomes were similar, probably because of crossover to surgical treatment. The most frequent cause of failure of thrombolytic therapy (occurring in 28% of patients) was inability to pass a guidewire across the occlusion.

The TOPAS trial assessed angiographic evidence of recanalization and clot lysis in patients with limb ischemia of < 2 wk in duration after 4 h of infusion of recombinant urokinase, 2000, 4000 or 6000 IU/min *(108)*. The study found no significant difference among the three dose regimens in amputation-free survival, and no advantage of thrombolysis over surgery. The 4000 IU/min urokinase regimen was associated with the lowest rate of hemorrhage. Multivariate analysis found the length of occlusion a predictor of outcome; obstructions shorter than 30 cm favored surgery while those longer than 30 cm responded better to thrombolysis *(108)*.

Meta-analysis of three trials *(100,130,131)* suggests lower rates of the constellation of death or amputation at 6 mo in patients with limb ischemia for less than 2 wk when the initial management strategy involved catheter-directed thrombolysis rather than revascularization surgery (15% vs 38%, $P = 0.01$). The outcome was reversed in patients with ischemic symptoms of longer duration, but the difference was no longer statistically significant (18% vs 10%, $P = 0.08$). Among those with occlusions of native arteries, catheter-directed thrombolysis was associated with a greater incidence of persistent or recurrent ischemia at 1 mo (55% vs 24%, $P < 0.001$) compared with surgery. The survival benefit of catheter-directed thrombolysis was statistically significant in only one trial and was related mainly to cardiac disease *(100)*. Catheter-directed thrombolysis may be safer for such patients and can achieve limb salvage comparable to surgery, particularly because the extent of the surgical procedure was reduced in approximately half the patients in whom lytic therapy was initially used, even though surgery was ultimately required to address the underlying arterial lesion. The results were largely independent of the type of lytic agent (urokinase, recombinant urokinase, or recombinant tissue plasminogen activator). In patients treated with catheter-directed thrombolysis, bleeding complications developed in 5–20%, but were usually minor. The only significant predictor of major bleeding was a fibrinogen level < 150 mg/dL.

It thus appears that catheter-directed thrombolysis offers advantages compared with surgical revascularization in terms of mortality, the complexity of secondary revascularization, and reperfusion injury, despite a higher rate of persistent or recurrent ischemia, bleeding complications, and ultimate risk of amputation *(81,107)*. When a limb is not immediately or irreversibly jeopardized, catheter-directed thrombolysis may therefore be the preferred initial approach. Underlying lesions can then be defined angiographically to guide appropriate revascularization, if necessary.

OTHER ISSUES

Reperfusion Injury

Reperfusion injury is one of the most common complications leading to prolonged morbidity. The sudden return of oxygenated blood to acutely ischemic muscle causes the generation and release of oxygen free radicals and subsequent cellular injury. Failure to anticipate or recognize this complication can lead to the rapid development of compartment syndrome and myonecrosis. Treatment consists of fasciotomy. Prevention of reperfusion injury is the focus of much experimental research, but effective drug regimens have not been established for clinical practice. Other long-term complications include the persistence of sensory or motor impairment. Loss of sensation in the toes and foot increases the likelihood of development of neurotrophic ulceration. Such ulcers are more common in the setting of impaired motor function. A peripheral neuropathy is the most common form of residual nerve impairment, although selective damage to individual nerves has been reported. The manifestations of nerve damage include wasting of the small muscles of the foot associated with painful dysesthesias, leading to an alteration in gait. Treatment consists of attempts at pharmacological control of pain, bracing of the foot, and physical therapy until neuromuscular function improves, a process that may require many months.

Fasciotomy

Although fasciotomy in every case would produce unacceptable and unnecessary morbidity, in practice it is often undertaken too late. Compartment pressure measurements have been employed to some advantage, but there is disagreement on pressure criteria for proceeding with fasciotomy. After revascularization, fasciotomy also should be performed if there are signs of increased ischemia without evidence of reocclusion. A long skin incision and opening of all compartments, including the deep posterior compartment, are needed unless initial inspection shows no muscle death or swelling.

Treatment of the Underlying Lesion

Simply removing the occluding lesion, whether it is a thrombus or an embolus, is unlikely to be successful as the sole treatment. If the occlusion was caused by an embolus, the source has to be identified and treated. If the acute occlusion was caused by thrombosis superimposed on preexisting atherosclerosis, then this underlying lesion also has to be treated to avoid a recurrence of the acute occlusion. This may be accomplished by either an endovascular or an open surgical technique, depending on the balance between durable success and procedural risk. In the literature, the results of percutaneous catheter-based intervention are dependent on morphology of the lesion and patient selection and the criteria used to define technical and clinical success and patency. In general, the choice of treatment of an underlying lesion that caused the clot should be separated from the choice of method of clot removal. That is, thrombolysis should not necessitate catheter-based treatment of extensive atherosclerotic disease, which is better treated by surgery. Neither should thrombectomy be followed by bypass of a discrete underlying stenosis, which is amenable to percutaneous angioplasty.

Follow-Up Care and Anticoagulation

Patients with acute limb ischemia should be anticoagulated with heparin followed by oral anticoagulation to prevent recurrent ischemia. Heparin (20,000–40,000 IU/d) administered in the immediate postoperative period is usually safe *(109)*, and is generally continued for about a week, followed by warfarin for at least 3 mo *(110)*. In one series, the rate of recurrent in-hospital ischemia was as high as 31% in those not receiving anticoagulants compared with 9% in those treated with coumarin derivatives *(111)*, but other studies have been conflicting *(39,112)*. Whether to continue anticoagulant drugs beyond the first 3 mo is controversial in the absence of an embolic source. Series involving embolism tend to show benefit from protracted anticoagulation, while series in which arterial thrombosis predominates do not *(113)*. Long-term anticoagulation is therefore recommended for cases of arterial embolism, unless the source has been eliminated. Long-term anticoagulation should be considered in cases of arterial thrombosis when the risk of recurrent thrombosis persists.

GENERAL APPROACH TO MANAGEMENT

The selection of treatment for acute limb ischemia is based primarily on its severity at the time of presentation, determined by clinical evaluation and Doppler study. The timing of angiography and the method of clot removal are determined by the urgency of revascularization, which is directly related to the severity of ischemia. As soon as the diagnosis of acute arterial thromboembolism is established, virtually all patients benefit from early administration of heparin to avoid propagation of thrombus. Treatment any underlying lesion depends on its morphology and is independent of the method of clot removal.

In patients with a clearly viable leg (level I ischemia) revascularization may be delayed until a full evaluation is completed, and angiography is indicated if revascularization becomes necessary. Management is similar to that for patients who develop critical limb ischemia in the course of chronic peripheral arterial disease. In the case of a marginally threatened limb (level IIa severity), angiography should be performed promptly with the patient under close monitoring and catheter-directed thrombolytic therapy should be initiated based on the findings. Additional management depends on the response to the lytic agent, and the nature of any underlying lesion that might be disclosed.

Patients whose limbs are immediately jeopardized (level IIb severity) should undergo surgical thromboembolectomy and the outcome should be evaluated by intraoperative angiography. Depending on the adequacy of thrombus extraction, adjunctive lytic therapy, revascularization, or fasciotomy may be indicated. In patients with level III acute limb ischemia, in which irreversible changes preclude salvage of a functional foot, anticoagulation should be maintained while demarcation of the level of amputation becomes apparent. Systemic toxicity resulting from the metabolic complications of skeletal muscle ischemia may force an early amputation, especially when the clinical presentation has been protracted. Attempting revascularization under these circumstances is not only futile but also often hazardous owing to the hemodynamic and metabolic consequences of the reperfusion syndrome that include hyperkalemic acidosis, myoglobinuric renal failure, or central circulatory disturbances. Level IIa and level III ischemia may be difficult to distinguish early after the onset of acute arterial occlusion, however, and at this stage even those with profound ischemia may benefit from attempted thromboembolectomy.

OUTCOMES
Limb-Related Outcome

The risks and outcomes of acute limb ischemia are proportional to the severity of the reduction of distal perfusion. Patients in level IIa, IIb, or III face threats to both life and limb and benefit from restoration of blood flow. A late presentation typically requires major amputation because of extensive tissue necrosis. Limb hypoperfusion predisposes to systemic metabolic derangement that compromises cardiopulmonary function and elevated myoglobin levels may cause irreversible renal failure. Even successful revascularization may induce severe reperfusion injury, aggravating neuromuscular damage. Thirty-day operative mortality ranges from 10% to 17% (75,115–118) but may exceed 40% in the elderly (76) and the goals of therapy in such cases are more modest than in patients with lesser degrees of circulatory dysfunction.

The analysis of procedural outcomes in patients with acute lower extremity ischemia is often complicated by the absence of baseline assessment. The clinical urgency of advanced leg ischemia mandates expeditious intervention and may inhibit the acquisition of this baseline clinical information. Documentation of the presence or absence of peripheral pulses and sensory or motor function before treatment helps establish benchmarks to which postoperative status can be compared. The restoration of pulses, improvement in ABI, and patent arteries as visualized by duplex imaging or arteriography provide measures of technical success after treatment.

The duration of ischemia and symptoms before treatment are important determinants of the technical success of revascularization in patients with acute limb ischemia. Although thrombus extraction is relatively easy to document, this does not guarantee distal reperfusion because thrombus might have extended into smaller distal vessels rendered dysfunctional by spasm, edema, or thrombosis. And even complete clot removal may reveal underlying occlusive lesion or provoke reperfusion injury.

All patients with acute limb ischemia should undergo careful physical examination including assessment of capillary filling, sensory and motor functions, the presence or absence of pulses, and Doppler arterial studies. Preoperative duplex imaging or angiography is desirable when the patient's condition permits. For all patients, therefore, recording of postoperative ABI and appropriate imaging of the treated arterial segment are necessary to document anatomical and hemodynamic outcomes. The ABI can rarely be measured at the time of presentation, but tends to improve after intervention. Thus the change in ABI is a less useful measure of treatment success in acute than in chronic critical limb ischemia, but successful revascularization should lead to a segmental systolic arterial pressure above the critical range of 40–60 mmHg. Toe pressure measurements or pulse volume recordings may provide additional information about the hemodynamic status of the limb following intervention.

Procedural Mortality and Morbidity

Acute limb ischemia carries substantial mortality both because of associated underlying diseases and because metabolic derangement often arises as a result of deep tissue ischemia. Patients with acute limb ischemia are typically elderly and preexisting cardiac or cerebral problems are frequent. Despite advances in revascularization and cardiac support, the mortality of acute limb ischemia remains high (10–20%) and even higher in elderly subjects, and myocardial infarction or fatal arrhythmia account for most of the deaths (115–118). The following criteria on admission predict a high risk of cardiac death: mean arterial pressure <90 mmHg, clinical heart failure, ischemia extending to the thigh, hemoglobin >14 g/dL, and a history of myocardial infarction in the preceding 4 wk (119). Other complications of treatment include short-term procedural morbidity that prolongs hospitalization or requires specific therapy without affecting survival. Such procedural complications are common, occurring in more than 50% of patients (120–122).

Long-term procedural complications include not only those inflicting permanent disability but others that negatively impact or delay recovery. Limb loss represents treatment failure for patients with severity levels IIa and IIb ischemia and may be attributed to inability to extract sufficient thrombus or to treatment delay that results in myonecrosis. Limb loss is associated with a substantial and permanent alteration in patient lifestyle and often requires prolonged rehabilitation. When renal failure develops from myoglobinuria, long-term hemodialysis may be required.

Recurrence of Symptoms

In the absence of anticoagulation, recurrent ischemia caused by embolism occurs in as many as 43% of patients (123). Each episode reduces the likelihood of complete restoration of limb blood flow and increases the risk of death (124,125). Arterial thrombosis is also associated with a high incidence of reocclusion unless additional intervention is undertaken to address underlying occlusive lesions (126,127). Following thrombolytic therapy, the incidence of recurrent ischemia has been reported as high as 53% *(128,129)*, whereas following embolectomy the incidence of reocclusion is between 21% and 26% *(130,131)*.

The long-term success of surgical and endovascular reconstruction in patients with critical limb ischemia is limited by progression of atherosclerotic occlusive disease and by the development of restenosis at the site of reconstruction. One of the main causes of restenosis is neointimal hyperplasia, for which no reliably effective preventive treatment has been established. Various drugs and brachytherapy (localized radiation) are under investigation to limit or prevent restenosis. Therapeutic angiogenesis using vascular endothelial growth factor to promote relief of ischemia has been associated with encouraging experimental results that hold promise for eventual use in patients with acute limb ischemia. These modalities may allow treatment in the future of patients for whom surgical or endovascular reconstruction is not currently feasible.

SUMMARY

Acute ischemia arises when a rapid decrease in perfusion threatens limb viability. Its severity depends on the location and extent of arterial obstruction, collateral channels, and cardiac output. The principal mechanisms involve embolism and thrombosis. Embolism is suggested by sudden onset, a known embolic source, absence of prior arterial disease, and normal pulses elsewhere. Typical sources include cardiac disorders such as atrial fibrillation, valvular disease and ventricular mural thrombi, paradoxical embolism through right-to-left shunts, and thrombi in the proximal vasculature. Thrombosis is usually superimposed on atherosclerotic plaque, especially when flow is reduced by heart failure, myocardial infarction or extrinsic arterial compression.

The main symptoms are pain and dysfunction; classical clinical findings are pulselessness, pallor, coolness, and paralysis, but pulses may be normal in cases of atheromatous microembolism. Rigor, tenderness, or pain on passive movement are late signs of advanced ischemia that predict tissue loss. Emphasis is placed on distinguishing acute limb ischemia from vasospasm, low cardiac output, deep venous thrombosis, and compressive neuropathy and identifying atheroembolism, popliteal artery aneurysm thrombosis, arterial cysts and entrapment, vasculitis, trauma, dissection, and hypercoagulable syndromes. Doppler testing and imaging are used to evaluate the local and systemic circulation and to detect atherosclerotic involvement of other vascular regions. Severity is classified based on ischemic threat and limb viability, but definitive tests are lacking. Treatment challenges include reperfusion injury following revascularization and treatment of comorbidities, such that there is a 10–20% risk of limb loss or mortality. Because the risk increases with the duration of ischemia, prompt correction of arterial insufficiency is most important. Treatment is based primarily on its severity at the time of presentation, determined by clinical evaluation and Doppler study, and comparative trials suggest that catheter-directed thrombolysis offers advantages over surgical revascularization. Primary amputation is reserved for patients with prolonged irreversible ischemia or when the patient's life would otherwise be threatened. Patients with acute limb ischemia should be anticoagulated with heparin followed by oral anticoagulation to prevent recurrent ischemia. Long-term success is still limited by progression of vascular disease and restenosis at the site of reconstruction.

REFERENCES

1. Cerebral Embolism Task Force. Cardiogenic brain embolism: the second report of the Cerebral Embolism Task Force. Arch Neurol 1989; 46:727–743.
2. Kannel WB, Abbott RD, Savage DD, McNamara PM. Epidemiologic features of chronic atrial fibrillation: the Framingham Study. N Engl J Med 1982;306:1018–1022.
3. Wolf PA, Abbott RD, Kannel WB. Atrial fibrillation: a major contributor to stroke in the elderly: the Framingham Study. Arch Intern Med 1987;147:1561.
4. Halperin JL, Hart RG. Atrial fibrillation and stroke: new ideas, persisting dilemmas (Editorial). Stroke 1988;19:937–941.
5. Sherman DG, Dyken ML, Fisher M, Harrison MJG, Hart RG. Cerebral embolism. Chest 1986;89 (Suppl):82S–98S.
6. Fuster V, Halperin JL. Left ventricular thrombi and cerebral embolism. N Engl J Med 1989;320:392–394.
7. Natarajan D, Hotchandani RK, Nigam PD. Reduced incidence of left ventricular thrombi with intravenous streptokinase in acute anterior myocardial infarction: prospective evaluation by cross-sectional echocardiography. Int J Cardiol 1988;20:201–207.
8. Held AC, Gore JM, Paraskos J, et al. Impact of thrombolytic therapy on left ventricular mural thrombi in acute myocardial infarction. Am J Cardiol 1988;62:310–311.
9. Eigler N, Maurer G, Shah PK. Effect of early systemic thrombolytic therapy on left ventricular mural thrombus formation in acute anterior myocardial infarction. Am J Cardiol 1984;54:261–263.
10. Vaitkus PT, Barnathan ES. Do anticoagulants, thrombolytics or antiplatelet agents reduce the incidence of left ventricular thrombus after anterior myocardial infarction? J Am Coll Cardiol 1991;17 (Suppl 2):146A.
11. Virchow R. Gesammelte Abhandlungen zur Wissenschaftlichen Medicine. Frankfurt, Meidinger Sohn & Co, 1856, pp. 219–732.
12. Johnson RC, Crissman RS, Didio LJA . Endocardial alterations in myocardial infarction. Lab Invest 1979;40:183–193.
13. Hochman JS, Platia EB, Bulkley BH. Endocardial abnormalities in left ventricular aneurysms: a clinicopathologic study. Ann Intern Med 1984;100:29–35.
14. Roberts WC, Siegel RJ, McManus BM. Idiopathic dilated cardiomyopathy: analysis of 152 necropsy patients. Am J Cardiol 1987;60:1340–1355.
15. Mikell FL, Asinger RW, Elsperger KJ, Anderson WR, Hodges M. Regional stasis of blood in the dysfunctional left ventricle: echocardiographic detection and differentiation from early thrombosis. Circulation 1982;66:755–763.
16. Asinger RW, Mikell FL, Elsperger J, Hodges M. Incidence of left ventricular thrombosis after acute transmural myocardial infarction: serial evaluation by two-dimensional echocardiography. N Engl J Med 1981; 305:297-302.
17. Weinrich DJ, Burke JF, Pauletto FJ. Left ventricular mural thrombi complicating acute myocardial infarction: long term follow-up with serial echocardiography. Ann Intern Med 1984;100:789–794.
18. Shresta NK, Moreno FL, Narciso FV, Torres L, Calleja HB. Two-dimensional echocardiographic diagnosis of left atrial thrombus in rheumatic heart disease: a clinicopathologic study. Circulation 1983;67:341–347.
19. Fulton RM, Duckett K: Plasma-fibrinogen and thromboemboli after myocardial infarction. Lancet 1976;2:1161–1164.
20. Hagen PT, Scholz DG. Edwards WD. Incidence and size of patent foramen ovale during the first 10 decades of life: an autopsy study of 965 normal hearts. Mayo Clin Proc 1984;59:17–20.
21. Lechat P, Mas JL, Lascault, et al. Prevalence of patent foramen ovale as a risk factor for stroke. N Engl J Med 1988;318:1148–1152.
22. Cabanes L, Mas JL, Cohen A, et al. Atrial septal aneurysm and patent foramen ovale as risk factors for cryptogenic stroke in patients less than 55 years of age: a study using transesophageal echocardiography. Stroke 1993;24:1865–1873.
23. Wolf PA, Dawber TR, Thomas HE, Kannel WB. Epidemiologic assessment of chronic atrial fibrillation and risk of stroke: the Framingham Study. Neurology 1978;28:973–977.
24. Levine HJ, Pauker SG, Eckman MH. Antithrombotic therapy in valvular heart disease. Chest 1995; 108 (Suppl):360S–370S.

25. Sherman DG, Dyken ML, Gent, M, Harrison MJG, Hart RG, Mohr JP. Antithrombotic therapy for cerebrovascular disorders: an update. Chest 1995;108(Suppl):444S–456S.

26. Hart RG, Halperin JL. Atrial fibrillation and thromboembolism: a decade of progress in stroke prevention. Ann Intern Med 1999;131:688–695.

27. Hart RG, Benavente O, McBride R, Pearce LA. Antithrombotic therapy to prevent stroke in patients with atrial fibrillation: a meta-analysis. Ann Intern Med 1999;131:492–501.

28. Feinberg WM, Blackshear JL, Laupacis A, Kronmal R, Hart RG. Prevalence, age distribution, and gender of patients with atrial fibrillation. Arch Intern Med 1995;155:469–473.

29. Sudlow M, Thomson R, Thwaites B, Rodgers H, Kenny RA. Prevalence of atrial fibrillation and eligibility for anticoagulants in the community. Lancet 1998;352:1167–1171.

30. Fuster V, Rydén LE, Asinger RW, et al. ACC/AHA/ESC guidelines for the management of patients with atrial fibrillation: a report of the American College of Cardiology/American Heart Association Task Force on Practice Guidelines and the European Society of Cardiology Committee for Practice Guidelines and Policy Conferences (Committee to Develop Guidelines for the Management of Patients With Atrial Fibrillation). J Am Coll Cardiol 2001;38:1231–1266.

31. Atrial Fibrillation Investigators. The efficacy of aspirin in patients with atrial fibrillation: analysis of pooled data from three randomized trials. Arch Intern Med 1997;157:1237–1240.

32. Fairbairn JF, Joyce JW, Pairolero PC. Acute arterial occlusion of the extremities. In: Juergens JL, Spittell JA, Fairbairn JF, eds. Peripheral Arterial Diseases. Philadelphia: WB Saunders, 1980; p. 384.

33. Mercer KG, Berridge DC. Saddle embolus: the need for intensive investigation and critical evaluation: a case report. Vasc Surg 2001; 35:63–65

34. Ha JW, Chung N, Chang BC, Lee DY, Cho SY. Aortic saddle embolism. Clin Cardiol 1999; 22: 229–230.

35. Travis WD, Balogh K. Saddle embolism of the aorta. a complication of streptokinase therapy. Cardiology 1986;73:156–159.

36. Wells KE, Steed DL, Zajko AB, Webster MW. Recognition and treatment of arterial insufficiency from Cafergot. J Vasc Surg 1986;4:8–15.

37. Rosenkranz S, Deutsch HJ, Erdmann E. "Saint Anthony's fire:" ergotamine-induced vascular spasms as the cause of acute ischemic syndrome. Dtsch Med Wochenschr 1997;122:450–454.

38. Rutherford RB, Baker JD, Ernst C, et al. Recommended standards for reports dealing with lower extremity ischemia: revised version. J Vasc Surg 1997;26:517–538.

39. Jivegard L, Holm J, Bergqvist D, et al. Acute lower limb ischemia: failure of anticoagulant treatment to improve one month results of arterial thromboembolectomy: a prospective randomized multicentre study. Surgery 1991;109:610–616.

40. Flanigan DP, Burnham SJ, Goodreau JJ, Bergan JJ. Summary of cases of adventitial cystic disease of the popliteal artery. Ann Surg 1979;189:165–175.

41. Hierton T, Hemmingsson A. The autogenous vein graft as popliteal artery substitute: long term follow-up of cystic adventitial degeneration. Acta Chir Scand 1984;150:377–383.

42. Persky JM, Kempczinski RF, Fowl RJ. Entrapment of the popliteal artery. Surg Gynecol Obstet 1991; 173:84–90.

43. Hoelting T, Schuermann G, Allenberg JR. Entrapment of the popliteal artery and its surgical management in a 20-year period. Br J Surg 1997;84:338–341.

44. Klein RG, Hunder GG, Stanson AW, Sheps SG. Large artery involvement in giant cell (temporal) arteritis. Ann Intern Med 1975;83:806–812.

45. Shionoya S. Bueger's disease: patholology, diagnosis and treatment. Nagoya: The University of Nagoya Press, 1990:101–116.

46. Eldrup-Jorgensen J, Flanigan DP, Brace L, et al. Hypercoagulable states and lower limb ischemia in young adults. J Vasc Surg 1989;9:334–341.

47. Earnshaw JJ. Neurologic deficits more reliable than Doppler. Eur J Vasc Surg 1991;5:106–107.

48. Koelemay MJW, den Hartog D, Prins MH, Kromhout JG, Legemate DA, Jacobs MJHM. Diagnosis of arterial disease of the lower extremities with duplex ultrasonography. Br J Surg 1996;83:404–409.

49. De Vries SO, Hunink MGM, Polak JF. Summary receiver-operating characteristic curves as technique for meta-analysis of the diagnostic performance of duplex ultrasonography in peripheral arterial disease. Acad Radiol 1996;3:361–369.

50. Elsman BH, Legemate DA, van der Heyden FWHM, deVos HJ, Mali WP, Eikelboom BC. The use of color-coded duplex scanning in the selection of patients with lower extremity arterial disease for percutaneous transluminal angioplasty: a prospective study. Cardiovasc Interv Radiol 1996;19:313–316.

51. Elsman BHP, Legemate DA, van der Heyden FWHM, de Vos HJ, Mali WP, Eikelboom BC. Impact of ultrasonographic duplex scanning on therapeutic decision making in lower-limb arterial disease. Br J Surg 1995;82:6630–6633.

52. Hany TF, Debatin JF, Leung DA, Pfammatter T. Evaluation of the aortoiliac and renal arteries: comparison of breath-hold, contrast-enhanced, three-dimensional MR angiography with conventional catheter angiography. Radiology 1997;204:357–362.

53. Poon E, Yucel EK, Pagan-Marin H, Kayne H. Iliac artery stenosis measurements: comparison of two-dimensional time-of-flight and three-dimensional dynamic gadolinium-enhanced MR angiography. Am J Roentgenol 1997;169:1139-1144.

54. Ho KY, Leiner T, de Haan MW, Kessels AG, Kitslaar PJ, van Engelshoven JM. Peripheral vascular tree stenoses: evaluation with moving-bed infusion-tracking MR angiography. Radiology 1998;206: 683–692.

55. Cambria RP, Kaufman JA, L'Italien GJ, Gertler JP. Magnetic resonance angiography in the management of lower extremity arterial occlusive disease: a prospective study. J Vasc Surg 1997;25:380–389.

56. Quinn SF, Sheley RC, Semonsen KG, Leonardo VJ, Kojima K, Szumowski J. Aortic and lower-extremity arterial disease: evaluation with MR angiography versus conventional angiography. Radiology 1998;206:693–701.

57. Hoch JR, Tullis MJ, Kennell TW, McDermott J, Acher CW, Turnipseed WD. Use of magnetic resonance angiography for the preoperative evaluation of patients with infrainguinal arterial occlusive disease. J Vasc Surg 1996;23:792–800.

58. Rofsky NM, Johnson G, Adelman MA, Rosen RJ, Krinsky GA, Weinreb JC. Peripheral vascular disease evaluated with reduced-dose gadolinium-enhanced MR angiography. Radiology 1997;205: 163–169.

59. Huber TS, Back MR, Ballinger RJ, et al. Utility of magnetic resonance arteriography for distal lower extremity revascularization. J Vasc Surg 1997;26:415–423.

60. Blackshear JL, Pearce LA, Asinger RW, et al. Mitral regurgitation protects against thromboembolic events in patients with atrial fibrillation. Am J Cardiol 1993;72:840–843.

61. Wiener I. Clinical and echocardiographic correlates of systemic embolism in nonrheumatic atrial fibrillation. Am J Cardiol 1987;59:177.

62. Caplan LR, D'Cruz I, Hier DB, Reddy H, Shah S. Atrial size, atrial fibrillation and stroke. Ann Neurol 1986;19:158–161.

63. Tegeler CH, Hart RG: Atrial size, atrial fibrillation, and stroke. Ann Neurol 1987;21:315–316.

64. Rosenthal MS, Halperin JL. Thromboembolism in nonvalvular atrial fibrillation: The answer may be in the ventricle. Int J Cardiol 1992;37:277–282.

65. Kerr CR, Boone J, Connolly Sj. et al. The Canadian Registry of Atrial Fibrillation: a noninterventional follow-up of patients after the first diagnosis of atrial fibrillation. Am J Cardiol 1998;82:82N-5N.

66. Kannel WB, Abbott RD, Savage DD, McNamara PM. Epidemiologic features of chronic atrial fibrillation: the Framingham study. N Engl J Med 1982;306:1018–1022.

67. Daniel WG, Angermann C, Engberding, et al. Transesophageal echocardiography in patients with cerebral ischemic events and arterial embolism: a European multicenter study. Circulation 1989; 80(Suppl 4):II-473.

68. Manning WJ, Silverman DI, Gordon SP, Krumholz HM, Douglas PS. Cardioversion from atrial fibrillation without prolonged anticoagulation with use of transesophageal echocardiography to exclude the presence of atrial thrombi. N Engl J Med 1993;328:750–755.

69. Daniel WG, Nellessen U, Schroder E, et al. Left atrial spontaneous echo contrast in mitral valve disease: an indicator for an increased thromboembolic risk. J Am Coll Cardiol 1988;11:1204–1211.

70. Stroke Prevention in Atrial Fibrillation Investigators Committee on Echocardiography: Transesophageal echocardiography in atrial fibrillation: standards for acquisition and interpretation and assessment of inter-observer variability. J Am Soc Echocardiogr 1996;9:556–566.

71. Stroke Prevention in Atrial Fibrillation Investigators, Committee on Echocardiography. Transesophageal echocardiographic correlates of thromboembolism in high-risk patients with atrial fibrillation. Ann Intern Med 1998;128:639–647.

72. Dormandy JA, Rutherford RB, Bakal C, et al. Management of peripheral arterial disease (PAD). Transatlantic Inter-Society Consensus (TASC). Section C: acute limb ischaemia. Eur J Vasc Endovasc Surg 2000;19(Suppl A):S115–143.

73. Golledge J, Galland RB. Lower limb intra-arterial thrombolysis. Postgrad Med J 1995;71:146–150.

74. Golledge J. Lower-limb arterial disease. Lancet 1997;350:1459–1465.

75. Aune S, Trippestad A. Operative mortality and long-term survival of patients operated on for acute lower limb ischaemia. Eur J Vasc Endovasc Surg 1998;15:143–146.

76. Braithwaite BD, Davies B, Birch PA, Heather BP, Earnshaw JJ. Management of acute leg ischemia in the elderly. Br J Surg 1998;85:217–220.

77. Blaisdell FW, Steele M, Allen RE. Management of acute lower extremity ischemia due to embolism and thrombosis. Surgery 1978;84:822–834.

78. Jivegard L, Holm J, Schersten T. The outcome of arterial embolism misdiagnosed as arterial embolism. Acta Chir Scand 1986;152:251-256.

79. Berridge DC, Hopkinson BR, Makin GS. Acute lower limb arterial ischemia: a role for continuous oxygen inhalation. Br J Surg 1989;76:1021–1023.

80. Working Party on Thrombolysis in the management of limb ischemia. Thrombolysis in the management of lower limb peripheral arterial occlusion: a consensus document. Am J Cardiol 1998;81: 207–218.

81. Beyersdorf F, Matheis G, Kruger S, et al. Avoiding reperfusion injury after limb revascularization: experimental observations and recommendations for clinical application. J Vasc Surg 1989;9: 757–766.

82. Nilsson L, Albrechtsson U, Jonung T, et al. Surgical treatment versus thrombolysis in acute arterial occlusion: a randomised controlled study. Eur J Vasc Surg 1992;6:189–193.

83. McNamara TO, Bomberger RA. Factors affecting initial and six month patency rates after intra-arterial thrombolysis with high dose urokinase. Am J Surg 1986;152:709–712.

84. Gardiner GA, Harrington DP, Koltun W, Whittemore A, Mannick JA, Levin DC. Salvage of occluded bypass grafts by means of thrombolysis. J Vasc Surg 1989;9:426–431.

85. Isner JM, Rosenfield K. Redefining the treatment of peripheral artery disease: role of percutaneous revascularization. Circulation 1993;88:1534–1557.

86. Rosenfield K, Isner JM. Disease of peripheral vessels. In: Topol EJ, ed. Cardiovascular Medicine. Philadelphia: Lippincott-Raven, 1997.

87. Huettl EA, Soulen MC. Thrombolysis of lower extremity occlusions: a study of the results of the STAR registry. Radiology 1995;197:141–145.

88. Starck EE, McDermott JC, Crummy AB, Turnipseed WD, Acher CW, Burgess JH. Percutaneous aspiration thromboembolectomy. Radiology 1985;156:61–66.

89. Wagner HJ, Starck EE. Acute embolic occlusion of the infrainguinal arteries: percutaneous aspiration embolectomy in 102 patients. Radiology 1992;182:403–407.

90. Sharafuddin MJ, Hicks ME. Current status of percutaneous mechanical thrombectomy. Part 1 General principles. J Vasc Interv Radiol 1997;8:911–921.

91. Rilinger N, Gorich J, Scharrer-Pamler R, et al. Short term results with use of the Amplatz Thrombectomy Device in the treatment of lower limb occlusions. J Vasc Interv Radiol 1997;8:343–348.

92. Reekers JA, Kromhout JG, Spithoven HG, Jacobs MJHM, Mali WM, Schultz-Kool LJ. Arterial thrombosis below the inguinal ligament: percutaneous treatment with a thrombosuction catheter. Radiology 1996;198(1):49–56.

93. Wagner HJ, Mueller-Huelsbeck S, Pitton MB, Weiss W, Wess M. Rapid thrombectomy with a hydrodynamic catheter: results from a prospective, multicenter trial. Radiology 1997;205:675–681.

94. Gardiner GA, Harrington DP, Koltun W, Whittemore A, Mannick JA, Levin DC. Salvage of occluded bypass grafts by means of thromblysis. J Vasc Surg 1989;9:426–431.

95. Chester JF, Buckenham TM, Dormandy JA, Taylor RS. Perioperative t-PA thrombolysis. Lancet 1991; 337:861–862.

96. Bosma HW, Jorning PJ. Intra-operative arteriography in arterial embolectomy. Eur J Vasc Surg 1990;4: 469–472.

97. Goodman GR, Tersigni S, Li K, Lawrence PF. Thrombolytic therapy in an isolated limb. Ann Vasc Surg 1993;7:512–520.

98. Comerota AJ, White JV, Grosh JD. Intraoperative intra-arterial thrombolytic therapy for salvage of limbs in patients with distal arterial thrombosis. Surg Gynecol Obstet 1989;169:283–289.

99. Nehler MR, Moneta GL, Yeager RA, Edwards JM, Taylor LM, Porter JM. Surgical treatment of threatened reversed infrainguinal vein grafts. J Vasc Surg 1994;20:558–565.

100. Ouriel K, Shortell CK, De Weese JA, et al. A comparison of thrombolytic therapy with operative revascularization in the initial treatment of acute peripheral arterial ischemia. J Vasc Surg 1994;19: 1021–1030.

101. Clouse ME, Stokes KR, Perry LJ, Wheeler HC. Percutaneous intraarterial thrombolysis: analysis of factors affecting outcome. J Vasc Interv Radiol 1994;5:93–100.

102. De Maioribus CA, Mills TL, Fujitani RM, et al. A reevaluation of intraarterial thrombolytic therapy for acute lower limb ischemia. J Vasc Surg 1993;17:888–895.

103. Faggioli GL, Peer RM, Pedrini L, et al. Failure of thrombolytic therapy to improve long term vascular patency. J Vasc Surg 1994;19:289–296.

104. Leblang SD, Becker GJ, Benenati JF. Low dose urokinase regimen for the treatment of lower extremity arterial and graft occlusion: experience in 132 cases. J Vasc Interv Radiol 1992;3:475–483.

105. McNamara TO, Bombeger RA, Merchant RF. Intra-arterial urokinase as the initial therapy for acutely ischemic lower limbs. Circulation 1991;83(Suppl):106–119.

106. Schilling JD, Pond GD, Mulcahy MM. Catheter-directed urokinase thrombolysis: an adjunct to PTA/surgery for management of lower extremity thromboembolic disease. Angiology 1994;45: 851–860.

107. Diffin DC, Kandarpa K. Assessment of peripheral intraarterial thrombolysis versus surgical revascularization in acute lower limb ischemia: a review of limb-salvage and mortality statistics. J Vasc Interv Radiol 1996;7:57–63.

108. Ouriel K, Veith FJ, Sasahara AA, for the TOPAS Investigators. Thrombolysis or peripheral arterial surgery: phase I results. J Vasc Surg 1996;23:64–73.

109. Collins, GJ, Rich, NM, Clagett, GP, et al. Heparin: efficacy and safety after arterial operations. Arch Surg 1981;116:1077–1081.

110. Jackson MR, Clagett JP. Antithrombotic therapy in peripheral arterial occlusive disease. Sixth ACCP Consensus Conference on Antithrombotic Therapy. Chest 2001;119:283S–299S.

111. Green RM, DeWeese JA, Rob CG. Arterial embolectomy before and after the Fogarty catheter. Surgery 1975;77:24–33.

112. Silvers LW, Royster TS, Mulcare RJ. Peripheral arterial emboli and factors in their recurrence rate. Ann Surg 1980;192:232–236.

113. Elliott JP, Hageman JH, Szilagyi E, Ramakrishnan V, Bravo JJ, Smith RF. Arterial embolization: Problems of source, multiplicity, recurrence and delayed treatment. Surgery 1980;88:833–845.

114. Dawson I, Sie RB, van Bockel JH. Atherosclerotic popliteal aneurysm. Br J Surg 1997;84:293–299.

115. Nypaver TJ, Whyte BR, Endean ED, et al. Nontraumatic lower extremity acute arterial ischemia. Am J Surg 1998; 176:147–152.

116. Davies B, Braithwaite BD, Birch PA, Heather BP, Earnshaw JJ. Acute leg ischemia in Gloucestershire. Br J Surg 1997; 84:504–508.

117. Neuzil DF, Edwards WH, Mulherin JL, et al. Limb ischemia: surgical therapy in acute arterial occlusion. Am Surg 1997;63:270–274.

118. Kuukasjarvi P, Salenius JP. Perioperative outcome of acute lower limb ischemia on the basis of the national vascular registry: the Finnvasc Study Group. Eur J Vasc Endovasc Surg 1994;8:578–583.

119 Jivegard L, Bergqvist D, Holm J, et al. Preoperative assessment of the risk of cardiac death following thrombo-embolectomy for acute lower limb ischemia. Eur J Vasc Surg 1992;6:83–88.

120. Schina MJ, Atnip RG, Healy DA, Thiele BL. Relative risks of limb revascularization and amputation in the modern era. Cardiovasc Surg 1994;2:754–759.

121. Braithwaite BD, Birch PA, Poskitt KR, Heather BP, Earnshaw JJ. Accelerated thrombolysis with high dose bolus t-PA extends the role of peripheral thrombolysis but may increase the risks. Clin Radiol 1995;50:747–750.

122. Dawson KJ, Reddy K, Platts, AD, Hamilton G. Results of a recently instituted programme of thrombolytic therapy in acute lower limb ischaemia. Br J Surg 1991;78:409–411.

123. Elliott JP, Hageman JH, Szilagyi E, Ramakrishnan V, Bravo JJ, Smith RF. Arterial embolization: problems of source, multiplicity, recurrence, and delayed treatment. Surgery 1980;88:833–845.

124. Roy D, Marchand E, Gagne P, Chabot M, Cartier R. Usefulness of anticoagulant therapy in the prevention of embolic complications of atrial fibrillation. Am Heart J 1986;112:1039–1043.

125. Andersson B, Abdon NJ, Hammarsten J. Arterial embolism and atrial arrhythmias. Eur J Vasc Surg 1989;3:261–266.

126. Dregelid EB, Stangeland LB, Eide GE, Trippestad A. Patient survival and limb prognosis after arterial embolectomy. Eur J Vasc Surg 1987;1:263–271.

127. Jivegard L, Holm J, Scherstein T. The outcome of arterial thrombosis misdiagnosed as arterial embolism. Acta Chir Scand 1986;152:251–259.

128. Sicard GA, Schier JJ, Totty WG, et al. Thrombolytic therapy for acute arterial occlusion. J Vasc Surg 1985;2:65–78.
129. Belkin M, Donaldson MC, Whittemore AD, et al. Observations on the use of thrombolytic agents for thrombotic occlusion of infrainguinal vein grafts. J Vasc Surg 1990;11:289–296.
130. Ouriel K, Veith FJ, Sasahara AA. A comparison of recombinant urokinase with vascular surgry as initial treatment of acute arterial occlusion of the legs: thrombolysis or Peripheral Arterial Surgery (TOPAS) Investigators. N Engl J Med 1998;338:1105–1111.
131. Stile Investigators. Results of a prospective randomized trial evaluating surgery versus thrombolysis for ischemia of the lower extremity. Ann Surg 1994;220:251–268.

8

Exercise Rehabilitation for Intermittent Claudication

Timothy A. Bauer, MS and
William R. Hiatt, MD

INTRODUCTION

Intermittent claudication (IC), secondary to peripheral arterial disease (PAD), is an important cause of a reduced functional exercise capacity. In this population, peak exercise capacity is typically 50% of that measured in age-matched control subjects *(1–4)*. This severe reduction in functional capacity is significant and equivalent to those patients with the categorization of New York Heart Association class III heart failure. Owing to their limited ability to ambulate, this exercise disability affects all aspects of patients' lives including work and leisure time activities. Consequently, the reduction in walking capacity is associated with an impairment in measures of quality of life *(5,6)*. Therefore, the primary goal of exercise therapy is focused toward improving quality of life through relieving the symptoms of claudication and improving functional capacity. In addition, the modification of cardiovascular risk factors is an important secondary and long-term goal of PAD exercise rehabilitation.

EXERCISE REHABILITATION FOR PAD

Walking exercise has been recommended for nearly 50 yr as a therapy for improving claudication *(7)*. As a result, supervised exercise rehabilitation has become a well established and highly effective intervention for improving the walking ability of these patients. Recent reviews of the exercise training literature in PAD have revealed 28 studies examining the effect of training on exercise performance *(8–12)*. The data from all studies of exercise training in PAD report an increase in exercise performance and a

From: *Contemporary Cardiology: Peripheral Arterial Disease: Diagnosis and Treatment*
Edited by: J. D. Coffman and R. T. Eberhardt © Humana Press Inc., Totowa, NJ

reduction in leg pain severity with training. Of these, 12 studies employed a controlled design, although few were randomized. Meta-analyses of these studies indicate an average improvement in pain-free walking distance of approx 172% with an average increase in maximal walking distance of approx 125% (8–10). Thus, exercise training results in an increased ability to sustain walking exercise for longer duration and with less claudication pain. Additionally, studies using graded exercise testing to assess peak exercise capacity have reported improvements in peak exercise performance and peak oxygen consumption (2,3). These improvements in peak exercise capacity indicate that following training, patients can perform activities of higher intensity that may not have been possible prior to study entry. While some aspects of a physiological training effect occur similar to that observed in healthy subjects, the peripheral metabolic adaptations that occur with training in PAD differ from normal individuals (2,3,13,14). Clearly, the changes that occur with training may contribute to the improved ability to walk longer distances before claudication pain limits the activity.

Exercise training in PAD has effects on other important endpoints in addition to improving walking performance. In studies by Regensteiner and colleagues, functional assessment by questionnaires (Walking Impairment Questionnaire, WIQ; Medical Outcomes Study Short Form 36, MOS SF-36; Physical Activity Recall, PAR) over 12 wk of training demonstrated that trained subjects could walk further, at a faster speed, and perform greater levels of activities than nontrained patients (15–18). Thus, a supervised exercise-training program not only improved clinical laboratory measures but also facilitated a greater level of self-reported physical functioning in the community. Another important endpoint to consider is the potential effects of exercise training on cardiovascular risk factors. A recent study examined the effects of exercise training on cardiovascular risk factors in older PAD patients before and after a 6-mo walking exercise program (19). In addition to improvements in peak exercise capacity and time to maximal claudication pain, the exercise program reduced total cholesterol and low-density lipoprotein levels by 5.2% and 8%, respectively. These changes are consistent with favorable changes reported for patients with coronary artery disease (CAD) following cardiac rehabilitation programs (20–23). Thus, exercise training provides a significant potential for risk factor modification through exercise rehabilitation in the PAD population.

In comparison with other modes of exercise, treadmill walking is associated with the greatest improvement in functional capacity. A meta-analysis by Gardner and Poehlman sought to determine the components of exercise rehabilitation programs that were most effective in improving claudication symptoms (8). Their analysis of 21 studies indicated that programs consisting of walking exercise, supervised sessions of 6 mo or more, and exercise eliciting moderate to severe claudication symptoms were associated with the greatest improvement in walking distances. The results of this analysis have since been utilized to direct the components of exercise rehabilitation programs for successful treatment of intermittent claudication.

COMPONENTS OF EXERCISE REHABILITATION

Screening

Prior to beginning any exercise intervention, an evaluation of each patients' medical history, cardiovascular risk factors, and present medical and functional status should be completed. These measures allow for the identification of those patients who may require additional cardiac monitoring and integration of exercise therapy for functional walking improvement and cardiovascular disease management. Thus, the results of the initial evaluation identify key parameters useful in the determination of patient eligibility, initial functional disability, and concomitant disease processes that may affect the exercise rehabilitation plan. Importantly, identification and aggressive treatment of cardiovascular risk factors should occur prior to beginning an exercise program. An overview of the exercise rehabilitation process for PAD is shown in Fig. 1.

Baseline Assessment

Before a patient is enrolled into exercise rehabilitation, baseline assessments of peak exercise capacity and hemodynamics should be performed. These measures are particularly useful and important as they serve to verify the diagnosis of PAD, indicate the initial level of functional impairment, and establish a baseline for evaluation of the exercise treatment effectiveness.

The graded exercise treadmill test (GXT) is an effective method of measuring functional exercise capacity. There are several PAD-specific treadmill protocols available for use in the exercise assessment of PAD patients (24). GXT offers a useful method to determine pain-free (initial claudication time [ICT]) and maximal walking times (absolute claudication time [ACT]) as well as peak aerobic capacity and overall functional limitation. The results of this assessment also provide data for determining the initial exercise training session work rate. Unlike treadmill testing for CAD, GXT for PAD functional assessment typically requires a constant treadmill speed with modest increases in grade every few minutes. For example, in the Gardner treadmill test, speed is kept constant at 2.0 mph with increases in grade of 2 % every 2 min (24). One minute after exercise the ankle–brachial index (ABI) should be assessed. Patients with claudication symptoms due to PAD will demonstrate a decrease in the ABI after exercise, whereas patients with nonvascular causes of leg pain will not have a decrease in the ABI.

Because many patients with PAD have coexistent atherosclerotic disease in other vascular beds, it is particularly important to monitor the 12-lead electrocardiogram (EKG) and blood pressure responses during the GXT (25). Patients without clinical evidence of CAD may enter a PAD-focused exercise rehabilitation program. However, patients who demonstrate clinical manifestations of CAD with exercise testing should have their medical and/or revascularization therapy optimized *prior* to enrollment in an exercise program. The typical clinical signs and symptoms include angina or undue dyspnea on exertion, a drop in systolic blood pressure with increasing work loads, an excessive increase in systolic blood pressure (> 250 mmHg), ventricular arrhythmias, and ST segment changes (26). In our experience of performing several hundred exercise tests in the PAD population, approx 10–15% of patients will demonstrate evidence of silent cardiac ischemia that manifests as horizontal to downsloping ST segment depressions.

Once medical and/or revascularization therapy is optimized and stable baseline assessments are documented, patients with clinical evidence of CAD can be enrolled into supervised exercise rehabilitation. A combination of exercise therapies can then be utilized to address both the functional walking capacity and the cardiac exercise limitations. Typically, a circuit training approach is used consisting of non-weight-bearing exercises of large muscle mass (i.e., cycling) or unaffected muscle groups (i.e., arm ergometry) and treadmill walking for claudication symptoms.

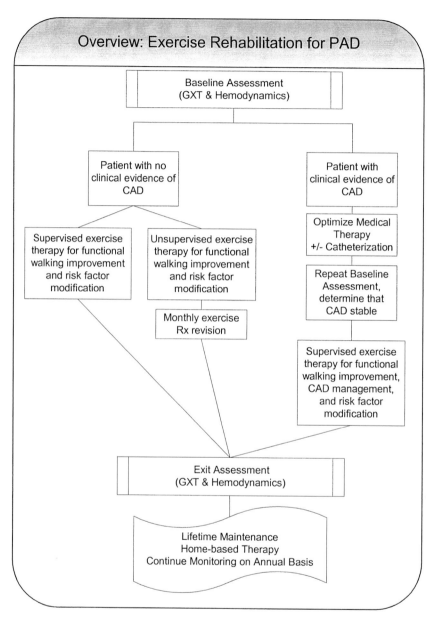

Fig. 1. Initial baseline assessments of exercise responses and limb hemodynamics are made prior to beginning an exercise program. PAD patients with no clinical evidence of CAD continue into either supervised (where available) or unsupervised exercise rehabilitation programs for the treatment of claudication. Patients in unsupervised programs should return to a rehabilitation facility monthly for exercise prescription modification. Patients with clinical evidence of CAD should have medical and/or revascularization therapy optimized prior to exercise program enrollment. Baseline assessments are repeated once patient CAD is stable. These patients may then continue into a supervised exercise rehabilitation program for exercise treatment of CAD and IC. Supervised exercise therapy for claudication and CAD combines non-weight-bearing exercises with treadmill walking. After a minimum of 12 wk of exercise training, exit assessment of exercise responses and hemodynamics occurs for evaluation of the training effect. Patients should continue exercise in a home-based or community setting for long-term training benefit. Monitoring of patient functional status should occur annually.

In summary, graded treadmill testing, hemodynamic measures of exercise heart rate, and blood pressure responses, as well as ABI, present a valuable profile of patient hemodynamic severity. In addition, a battery of questionnaires, such as the WIQ, PAR, and MOS SF-36, are useful for evaluating functional status, physical activity level, and quality of life. For practical considerations, use of the WIQ and MOS SF-36 may be adequate. Combined, these baseline measures of exercise testing, hemodynamic evaluation, and questionnaire assessment provide a powerful basis for exit assessment and follow-up comparisons.

Exclusion Criteria: For Whom Is Rehab Not Appropriate?

There are contraindications for enrollment into an exercise program for the treatment of IC. Essentially, patients should not exercise when there are comorbidities that limit exercise tolerance. These include, but are not limited to unstable angina, uncontrolled hypertension, moderate to severe aortic stenosis, uncontrolled arrhythmias, severe cardiac conduction abnormalities, uncontrolled congestive heart failure, uncontrolled diabetes, and orthopedic problems that prohibit exercise *(26,27)*. In addition, patients with severe peripheral hemodynamic compromise such as patients with ischemic rest pain or those with nonhealing lower limb ulcerations may also be excluded from participation in exercise rehabilitation programs.

Exercise Therapy

Essentially, the goals of supervised exercise rehabilitation for PAD are similar to those for all cardiovascular diseases: (1) improve functional capacity, (2) improve quality of life, and (3) improve survival (Fig. 2.). Specific to PAD, successful achievement of these goals is dependent on training-induced improvements in claudication symptoms, walking speed, and walking distance. These changes in basic functional walking capacity allow activities of greater intensity to be performed and assist in attaining the secondary goals of modifying cardiovascular risk factors and improving survival *(28)*. Walking exercise appears to have the most beneficial effect on functional capacity and comprises the predominant mode of exercise utilized in PAD rehabilitation programs. Every few weeks as training intensity is increased, patients will be able to perform exercise at higher workloads than at program entry. As increases in exercise tolerance are made, the ability to exercise at higher intensity (workloads) can potentially "unmask" underlying cardiac disease (i.e., angina) that was not apparent initially. In these patients, exercise training should be suspended until evaluation and optimization of medical therapy is achieved. As noted above, once stable, these patients may resume exercise rehabilitation following reassessment of exercise capacity. Thus, supervision and cardiac monitoring of patients during rehabilitation allows modification of the exercise plan for safety and in addressing additional targets of the exercise therapy.

The Exercise Prescription

CONCEPTS

The basic concepts of exercise prescription for patients with PAD were largely developed from methods utilized in the treatment of patients with or recovering from sequellae of CAD *(28)*. While the specific training methods used may differ from those traditionally used for CAD, these basic concepts still apply. Because patients vary greatly in health status, physical conditioning, age, and motivation, exercise rehabilitation needs

```
╭─────────────────────────────────────────────────────────────╮
│              Goals of Exercise Therapy                        │
├─────────────────────────────────────────────────────────────┤
│   1. Improve functional capacity                             │
│           - Relieve claudication symptoms                    │
│           - Improve walking speed to 3-4 mph                 │
│           - Improve walking distance by 50-100%              │
│                                                               │
│   2. Improve quality of life                                 │
│           - Increase activities of daily living              │
│           - Improve work potential                           │
│                                                               │
│   3. Improve survival                                         │
│           - Modify cardiovascular risk factors               │
│           - Prevent stroke, MI and death                     │
╰─────────────────────────────────────────────────────────────╯
```

Fig. 2. Goals of exercise therapy for IC.

to be *individualized* to meet each patient's unique needs. The individualization of exercise prescription allows the mode, frequency, intensity, duration, and progression of exercise training to be adjusted according to the appropriate level of patient conditioning. This is particularly important in the claudicant for whom the desired training effect is to improve functional walking ability. Here, the *specificity* of training (i.e., walking = treadmill exercise) can be used to great advantage in achieving the desired therapeutic goals. The active participation of patients in exercise rehabilitation programs highlights the concept that these programs are *participatory*, requiring the involvement of patients in regular, structured exercise sessions. The exercise program must also be *longitudinal,* as the effects of training occur over a period of weeks to months and require a long-term commitment for maintenance of the acquired training effects. Finally, the rehabilitation program is *preventive* and designed to favorably alter the risk of adverse events and cardiovascular risk factors.

SPECIFIC METHODS

The basic components of an exercise training session for patients with PAD are described in Figure 3. Following a brief warmup period consisting of light stretching and non-weight-bearing low-level exercise (i.e., cycling or arm cranking), the PAD patient walks on a treadmill at an intensity that elicits mild to moderate claudication pain (grade 3 or 4 on the five-point claudication scale, Fig. 4). On reaching the appropriate level of claudication pain, the exercise is stopped and the patient rests (seated) until the pain dissipates. The patient then resumes walking until a mild to moderate level of pain is again reached and then followed by another rest period. This process of walking exercise interspersed with rest (intermittent walking) continues until the total exercise period has elapsed. Initially, the treadmill workload (speed and grade) is determined from the GXT workload equivalent to the level of the ICT. For example, if the patient first experiences claudication pain at 2 mph 2% grade on the GXT (with a peak workload of 2 mph 6% grade), then the initial training workload is 2 mph 2% grade. This workload should elicit mild to moderate claudication pain within 3–5 min. At first, exercise sessions may constitute only 20–30 min of intermittent walking. As exercise tolerance improves, the length of exercise sessions may be increased to 40–50 min. At the end of

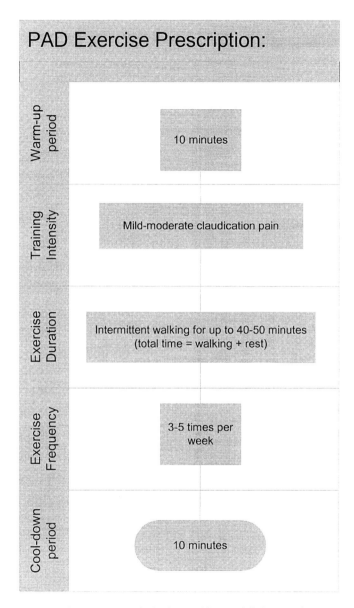

Fig. 3. Following a 10-min warmup period of stretching and light exercise, PAD patients walk on a treadmill set to a speed and grade that elicits mild to moderate claudication pain within 5–7 min of exercise. On achieving the appropriate level of claudication pain, the exercise is stopped and the patient sits until the pain dissipates. This process is repeated (intermittent walking) until the total exercise period has elapsed. A cool-down period of stretching and light exercise follows the walking portion of the session. Exercise sessions should occur three to five times per week for at least 12 wk.

```
┌─────────────────────────────────────────────────┐
│              PAD Claudication Scale               │
│                                                   │
│   ❑   Grade 1          No discomfort or leg pain  │
│                                                   │
│   ❑   Grade 2          Onset of claudication      │
│                                                   │
│   ❑   Grade 3          Mild claudication          │
│                                                   │
│   ❑   Grade 4          Moderate claudication      │
│                                                   │
│   ❑   Grade 5          Severe claudication        │
│                                                   │
└─────────────────────────────────────────────────┘
```

Fig. 4. A five-point scale is used during clinical treadmill testing and exercise training sessions to evaluate patient's perception of claudication pain.

the exercise session, a cool-down period of non-weight-bearing exercise and light stretching follows the walking exercise portion of the session. Each supervised exercise session should be held for up to 1 h, three to five times per week, and continue for a minimum of 12 wk (36 sessions).

RATE OF PROGRESSION

The progression of exercise training sessions for the PAD patient should increase gradually, with increases in exercise duration preceding increases in exercise intensity (speed and/or percent grade). The individualization of the program is accomplished by increasing the grade or speed when the patient can walk 8–10 min or longer without development of moderate claudication pain at the current work rate. Typically, each walking bout is kept between 5 and 7 min by adjusting speed and grade accordingly. As training workload increases, any clinical sign or symptoms of exercise intolerance should lead to individualized evaluation. In general, the intensity progression of patients who walk < 2.0 mph are made by increasing speed first. In those patients who can walk 2.0 mph or faster, either speed or percent grade are adjusted. Ultimately, a normal walking speed of 3.0–4.0 mph and an increase in percent grade are set as performance goals of the training program.

Home-Based Management

Home-based exercise programs for the treatment of claudication have been evaluated for PAD patients with variable results (29–35). However, the majority of available data appear to suggest that supervised exercise training programs are more effective than home-based therapy alone in improving claudication and maximal walking distances. The causes of the greater improvements in supervised settings are likely related to the group setting in promoting program compliance and more consistent regulation of exercise intensity and progression. In motivated patients, true compliance with home-based exercise training may produce results similar to those observed in a supervised setting. However, these observations are isolated and are largely subject to levels of patient motivation. The optimal method may be a combined approach of home-based exercise therapy with periodic monitored exercise sessions at an exercise rehabilitation center. For those patients without access to organized programs, exercise training in a health club setting may prove more effective than home-based training alone. Clearly, where a home-based program is required, regular feedback and evaluation of the patient remain important for successful participation.

Exit Assessment and Follow-up

On completion of the supervised exercise rehabilitation program, exit assessment should include GXT to define the functional improvement, describe the overall treatment effect, and provide a basis for effective patient follow-up. The primary endpoint of exit evaluation is maximal walking time (ACT). However, evaluation of ICT, questionnaires, and ECG may also provide useful information pertinent to functional evaluation and follow-up. The appropriate follow-up consists of recommendations for a maintenance exercise program through home or community-based settings and periodic treadmill tests to determine long-term compliance.

Special Considerations and Precautions

Supervised treadmill walking is well tolerated and associated with virtually no reported risk of morbidity or mortality from exercise rehabilitation *(9)*. However, the potential for adverse events exists. Because many patients with PAD have other concomitant forms of cardiovascular disease, supervised exercise rehabilitation programs should include routine cardiac telemetry monitoring for patients with clinical evidence or medical history of CAD. Blood pressure at rest and during exercise should also be recorded and monitored in all participants during these sessions. As noted earlier, functional capacity improvement may lead to an "unmasking" of central cardiac manifestations of atherosclerosis (i.e., angina). Other risks may include acute or exacerbation of musculoskeletal problems with exercise. These may be reduced by the incorporation of stretching and low-intensity, large muscle group warmup and cool-down exercises.

Reimbursement of Exercise Rehabilitation: The New CPT Code

Successful exercise treatment of claudication can be limited by a variety of factors. Patient motivation is an important limitation in terms of its effects on subject participation, compliance, and lifetime commitment to regular exercise for maintenance of the training benefit. Another important limitation is that although supervised exercise programs are proven to be effective, historically third party payers have not covered exercise rehabilitation for PAD. This has had an impact on the availability and access to supervised exercise programs to patients with PAD. Recently, the American Medical Association published a new Current Procedural Terminology code (CPT) for exercise rehabilitation of patients with PAD *(36)*. Code 93668 permits program reimbursement for supervised exercise rehabilitation of patients with PAD and is intended to cover the expenses related to providing the exercise program excluding physician costs. This development may provide new incentive for supervised exercise program development and availability for this patient population.

MECHANISMS OF BENEFIT

The mechanisms by which exercise training improves exercise performance in PAD are incompletely understood. In general, review of the improvements in exercise capacity are not well explained by any changes in peripheral blood flow *(37,38)*. Although some controversy exists, changes in limb blood flow that may occur with training are modest and do not correlate with increases in functional walking ability *(35,39–42)*. It is possible that exercise training may result in a better redistribution of blood flow to exercising muscle; however, this has not been specifically evaluated. Thus, although there may be modest increases in flow, current evidence does not support an increase in peripheral blood flow as the primary factor in the exercise improvement after training.

One important adaptation to training in PAD patients is an increase in walking efficiency. At a given submaximal workload, a certain level of oxygen consumption ($\dot{V}O_2$) is required to perform the exercise. After training, patients with PAD require a lower $\dot{V}O_2$ during walking for a given submaximal workload *(2,3,14)*. The reduction in oxygen consumption during submaximal exercise is consistent with an increase in walking efficiency. This is likely due to a change in gait that allows less motor unit recruitment (and thus oxygen consumption) to support a given level of ambulation. However, exercise training also improves peak exercise capacity (peak $\dot{V}O_2$) in patients by roughly 30%. In this context, not only is patient submaximal ambulation more efficient, but also the relative exercise intensity for a given submaximal workload is reduced. In consideration that claudication results from a metabolic supply and demand mismatch, the enhanced efficiency and reduced relative intensity following training may largely contribute to the ability of patients to sustain walking exercise for longer distances before claudication limits the activity.

There are other adaptations specific to the skeletal muscle that may also play a role in the training response. Several studies have reported an increased oxygen extraction across the affected limb after training *(43,44)*. The increased capability to extract and utilize oxygen following training suggests that an increase in oxidative metabolism may occur. Some studies have reported increases in some oxidative enzymes with training. However, these findings are inconsistent and no correlation to changes in exercise performance has been demonstrated *(45–47)*. A metabolic parameter that is associated with reduced exercise performance in PAD is the accumulation of acylcarnitines in skeletal muscle. Acylcarnitines are intermediates of oxidative metabolism that accumulate as a result of abnormal oxidative metabolism in the skeletal muscle of patients with claudication. With training, the accumulation of these metabolic intermediates is reduced, and their reduction is correlated with an improvement in peak exercise performance *(48,49)*. In addition, it has been observed that exercise training leads to a reduction in systemic markers of inflammation and an improvement in blood rheology in these patients *(50,51)*. To summarize, although exercise training is not associated with a large improvement in muscle blood flow, changes in walking economy, skeletal muscle metabolism, and blood rheology appear to contribute to the benefits of training.

SUMMARY

Exercise rehabilitation is an effective and well-tolerated treatment for intermittent claudication. The mechanisms of exercise training on the symptoms of claudication are only partially understood. Potential mechanisms for improvement include mild increases in peripheral blood flow or distribution, alterations in skeletal muscle metabolism, and changes in blood rheology. In addition, an improvement in walking efficiency may provide the greatest mechanism of benefit. Supervised exercise rehabilitation programs for PAD should consist of three 60-min exercise sessions per week. Improvements in walking capacity can be observed with 12 wk of training and further improvements in programs of 6 mo or longer. Where mandated by geographic location or patient access, home-based exercise therapy can be effective in improving walking ability although to a lesser degree. Home-based therapy should incorporate periodic monitoring sessions at an exercise rehabilitation facility to assist with patient compliance and modification of the exercise prescription. A new CPT code for exercise rehabilitation in patients with claudication should assist in increasing patient access and program availability in the future.

REFERENCES

1. Bauer TA, Regensteiner JG, Brass EP, Hiatt WR. Oxygen uptake kinetics during exercise are slowed in patients with peripheral arterial disease. J Appl Physiol 1999;87:809–816.
2. Hiatt WR, Regensteiner JG, Hargarten ME, Wolfel EE, Brass EP. Benefit of exercise conditioning for patients with peripheral arterial disease. Circulation 1990;81:602–609.
3. Hiatt WR, Wolfel EE, Meier RH, Regensteiner JG. Superiority of treadmill walking exercise vs. strength training for patients with peripheral arterial disease : implications for the mechanism of the training response. Circulation 1994;90:1866–1874.
4. Eldridge JE, Hossack KF. Patterns of oxygen consumption during exercise testing in peripheral vascular disease. Cardiology 1987;74:236–240.
5. McDermott MM, Liu K, Guralnik JM, Martin GJ, Criqui MH, Greenland P. Measurement of walking endurance and walking velocity with questionnaire: validation of the walking impairment questionnaire in men and women with peripheral arterial disease. J Vasc Surg 1998;28:1072–1081.
6. McDermott MM, Fried L, Simonsick E. Ling S,Guralnik JM. Aymptomatic peripheral arterial disease is independently associated with impaired lower extremity functioning : The Women's Health and Aging Study. Circulation 2001;101:1007–1012.
7. Foley WT. Treatment of gangrene of the feet and legs by walking. Circulation 1957;15:689–700.
8. Gardner AW, Poehlman ET. Exercise rehabilitation programs for the treatment of claudication pain: a meta-analysis. JAMA 1995;274:975–980.
9. Leng GC, Fowler B, Ernst E. Exercise for intermittent claudication (Cochrane Review). In: The Cochrane Library. Oxford: Update Software, 1999.
10. Brandsma JW, Robeer BG, van den HS, Smit B, Wittens CH, Oostendorp RA. The effect of exercises on walking distance of patients with intermittent claudication: a study of randomized clinical trials [published erratum appears in Phys Ther 1998 May;78:547]. Phys Ther 1998;78:278–286.
11. Girolami B, Bernardi E, Prins MH, et al. Treatment of intermittent claudication with physical training, smoking cessation, pentoxifylline, or nafronyl: a meta-analysis. Arch Intern Med 1999;159: 337–345.
12. Nehler MR, Hiatt WR. Exercise therapy for claudication. Ann Vasc Surg 1999; 13:109–114.
13. Dahllof A, Holm J, Schersten T, Sivertsson R. Peripheral arterial insufficiency: effect of physical training on walking tolerance, calf blood flow, and blood flow resistance. Scand J Rehab Med 1976;8: 19–26.
14. Tan KH, Cotterrell D, Sykes K, Sissons GR, de Cossart L, Edwards PR. Exercise training for claudicants: changes in blood flow, cardiorespiratory status, metabolic functions, blood rheology and lipid profile. Eur J Vasc Endovasc Surg 2000;20:72–78.
15. Regensteiner JG, Steiner JF, Panzer RJ, Hiatt WR. Evaluation of walking impairment by questionnaire in patients with peripheral arterial disease. J Vasc Med Biol 1990;2:142–152.
16. Tarlov AR, Ware JE, Jr., Greenfield S, Nelson EC, Perrin E, Zubkoff M. The Medical Outcomes Study: an application of methods for monitoring the results of medical care. JAMA 1989;262:925–930.
17. Sallis JF, Haskell WL, Wood PD, et al. Physical activity assessment methodology in the five-city project. Am J Epidemiol 1985;121:91–106.
18. Regensteiner JG, Steiner JF, Hiatt WR. Exercise training improves functional status in patients with peripheral arterial disease. J Vasc Surg 1996;23:104–115.
19. Izquierdo-Porrera AM, Gardner AW, Powell CC, Katzel LI. Effects of exercise rehabilitation on cardiovascular risk factors in older patients with peripheral arterial occlusive disease. J Vasc Surg 2000; 31:670–677.
20. Lavie CJ, Milani RV. Effects of cardiac rehabilitation and exercise training in obese patients with coronary artery disease. Chest 1996;109:52–56.

21. Lavie CJ, Milani RV. Effects of cardiac rehabilitation and exercise training programs in patients > or = 75 years of age. Am J Cardiol 1996;78:675–677.

22. Brubaker PH, Warner JG, Jr, Rejeski WJ, et al. Comparison of standard- and extended-length participation in cardiac rehabilitation on body composition, functional capacity, and blood lipids. Am J Cardiol 1996;78:769–773.

23. Warner JG, Jr, Brubaker PH, Zhu Y, et al. Long-term (5-year) changes in HDL cholesterol in cardiac rehabilitation patients: do sex differences exist? Circulation 1995;92:773–777.

24. Gardner AW, Skinner JS, Vaughan NR, Bryant CX, Smith LK. Comparison of three progressive exercise protocols in peripheral vascular occlusive disease. Angiology 1992;43:661–671.

25. Valentine R, Grayburn PA, Eichhorn EJ, Myers S, Clagett GP. Coronary artery disease is highly prevalent among patients with premature peripheral vascular disease. J Vasc Surg 1994;19:688–674.

26. American College of Sports Medicine. Guidelines for Exercise Testing and Prescription, 6 edit. Philadelphia: Lippincott Williams & Wilkins, 2000.

27. Katzel LI, Sorkin J, Bradham D, Gardner AW. Comorbidities and the entry of patients with peripheral arterial disease into an exercise rehabilitation program. J Cardiopulm Rehabil 2001;20:165–171.

28. Ades PA. Cardiac rehabilitation and secondary prevention of coronary heart disease. N Engl J Med 2001;345:892–902.

29. Regensteiner JG, Meyer TJ, Krupski WC, Cranford LS, Hiatt WR. Hospital vs home-based exercise rehabilitation for patients with peripheral arterial occlusive disease. Angiology 1997;48:291–300.

30. Jonason T, Ringqvist I, Oman-Rydberg A. Home-training of patients with intermittent claudication. Scand J Rehab Med 1981;13:137–141.

31. Larsen OA, Lassen NA. Effect of daily muscular exercise in patients with intermittent claudication. Lancet 1966;2:1093–1096.

32. Kasiske BL. Risk factors for accelerated atherosclerosis in renal transplant recipients. Am J Med 1988; 84:985–992.

33. Clifford PC, Davies PW, Hayne JA, Baird RN. Intermittent claudication: is a supervised exercise class worth while? Br Med J 1980;280:1503–1505.

34. Patterson RB, Pinto B, Marcus B, Colucci A, Braun T, Roberts M. Value of a supervised exercise program for the therapy of arterial claudication. J Vasc Surg 1997;25:312–318.

35. Alpert JS, Larsen OA, Lassen NA. Exercise and intermittent claudication.: blood flow in the calf muscle during walking studied by the xenon-133 clearance method. Circulation 1969;39:353–359.

36. American Medical Association. Current Procedural Terminology (CPT). Chicago. 2001. Ref Type: Catalog

37. Remijnse-Tamerius HCM, de Buyzere M, Oeseburg B, Clement DL. Why is training effective in the treatment of patients with intermittent claudication? Internat Angio 2001;18:103–112.

38. Tan KH, de Cossart L, Edwards PR. Exercise training and peripheral vascular disease. Br J Surg 2000; 87:553–562.

39. Hiatt WR, Regensteiner JG. Exercise rehabilitation in the treatment of patients with peripheral arterial disease. J Vasc Med Biol 1990;2:163–170.

40. Ericsson B, Haeger K, Lindell SE. Effect of physical training on intermittent claudication. Angiology 1970;21:188–192.

41. FitzGerald DE, Keates JS, MacMillan D. Angiographic and plethysmographic assessment of graduated physical exercise in the treatment of chronic occlusive arterial disease of the leg. Angiology 1971;22:99–106.

42. Lundgren F, Dahllof A, Lundholm K, Schersten T, Volkmann R. Intermittent claudication - surgical reconstruction or physical training? A prospective randomized trial of treatment efficiency. Ann Surg 1989;209:346–355.

43. Sorlie D, Myhre K. Effects of physical training in intermittent claudication. Scand J Clin Lab Invest 1978;38:217–222.

44. Zetterquist S. The effect of active training on the nutritive blood flow in exercising ischemic legs. Scand J Clin Lab Invest 1970;25:101–111.

45. Hiatt WR, Regensteiner JG, Wolfel EE, Carry MR, Brass EP. Effect of exercise training on skeletal muscle histology and metabolism in peripheral arterial disease. J Appl Physiol 1996;81:780–788.

46. Lundgren F, Dahllof AG, Schersten T, Bylund-Fellenius AC. Muscle enzyme adaptation in patients with peripheral arterial insufficiency: spontaneous adaptation. Clin Sci 1989;77:485–493.

47. Holm J, Dahllof A, Bjorntorp P, Schersten T. Enzyme studies in muscles of patients with intermittent claudication: effect of training. Scand J Clin Lab Invest 1973;(Suppl 128)31:201–205.

48. Hiatt WR, Regensteiner JG, Wolfel EE, Ruff L, Brass EP. Carnitine and acylcarnitine metabolism during exercise in humans: dependence on skeletal muscle metabolic state. J Clin Invest 1989;84: 1167–1173.
49. Hiatt WR, Wolfel EE, Regensteiner JG, Brass EP. Skeletal muscle carnitine metabolism in patients with unilateral peripheral arterial disease. J Appl Physiol 1992;73:346–353.
50. Tisi PV, Shearman CP. The evidence for exercise-induced inflammation in intermittent claudication: should we encourage patients to stop walking? Eur J Vasc Endovasc Surg 1998;15:7-17.
51. Ernst EE, Matrai A. Intermittent claudication, exercise, and blood rheology. Circulation 1987;76: 1110–1114.

9

Treatment of Risk Factors and Antiplatelet Therapy

Emile R. Mohler III, MD

INTRODUCTION

The factors that predispose to atherosclerotic disease of the lower extremity arteries have been evaluated in numerous case-control and prospective studies. Data continue to accumulate that modification of these risk factors is essential to prevent progression of disease, not only in the lower extremities, but also in the coronary and cerebrovascular systems. The following sections detail these risk factors and medical strategies for modification of atherosclerotic disease risk.

TRADITIONAL RISK FACTORS (FIG. 1)

Smoking

The association between peripheral arterial disease (PAD) and cigarette smoking was reported as early as 1911 by Erb, who found that his patients who smoked were three to six times more likely to have intermittent claudication (IC) compared to nonsmokers *(1)*. Since then, there have been numerous studies evaluating the prevalence of smoking in patients with PAD *(2–10)*. Data collected from the Framingham Study indicate that heavy smokers have a fourfold increased risk of having IC compared with nonsmokers *(11,12)*. A study in Iceland, the Reykhaviak Study, found in a prospective investigation of men that smoking predicted the incidence of IC with an increased risk of 8- to 10-fold compared with nonsmokers *(13)*. The PAD Awareness, Risk, and Treatment: New Resources for Survival (PARTNERS) program was a multicenter study conducted in the United States that evaluated the ankle–brachial index in patients aged 70 yr or older, or aged 50–69 yr with history of smoking or diabetes *(14)*. In this study, the prevalence of

From: *Contemporary Cardiology: Peripheral Arterial Disease: Diagnosis and Treatment*
Edited by: J. D. Coffman and R. T. Eberhardt © Humana Press Inc., Totowa, NJ

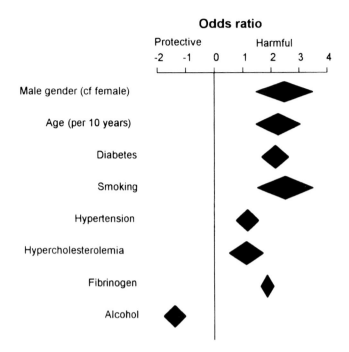

Fig. 1. Range of odds ratios for risk factors for developing intermittent claudication. (Reproduced with permission of Mosby, Inc. from J Vasc Surg 2000:31:136 [49]).

smoking was 60% in patients known to have PAD and 62% in those with both PAD and cardiovascular disease (CVD).

Numerous other studies conducted throughout the world have supported this strong association between PAD and smoking *(15–19)*. It is estimated that the relative risk for developing claudication is 2.11 if a person smokes more than 20 cigarettes per day and 1.75 if a person smokes 11–20 cigarettes per day *(20)*. Data from the Framingham Study indicate that there is a doubling of the risk, at all ages, for PAD compared to coronary artery disease (CAD) in those who smoke *(5)*. Environmental smoke is also thought to increase the relative risk of cardiovascular events and likely increases the risk of developing PAD and claudication.

Smoking has an impact not only on the development of PAD but also on the expression of its manifestations. Gardner and colleagues evaluated the exercise capacity of 138 patients with PAD and stable claudication *(21)*. Cigarette smokers experienced claudication more quickly in this study and the discomfort took longer to subside after discontinuation of exercise compared to nonsmokers ($p < 0.05$). Cigarette smoking also seems to hasten the progression of saphenous or prosthetic lower extremity bypass graft disease *(22)*. The results from a retrospective study indicate that patients with PAD requiring surgical revascularization who continue to smoke more than 15 cigarettes per day increased the probability of losing the affected limb approximately five times at 2 yr and three times at 5 yr, compared with nonsmokers and smokers of up to 15 cigarettes per day *(22)*.

Only nonrandomized (level 3) studies are available regarding the impact of smoking cessation on PAD and its manifestations *(23)*. Quick and colleagues found that smoking cessation can result in an improvement in maximal treadmill walking distance up to 46.7

m *(24)*. Jonason and colleagues found that patients who continued to smoke were more likely to develop ischemic rest pain compared to those who quit smoking *(17)*. Specifically, rest pain occurred in 18% of those with claudication who continued to smoke for more than 7 yr, compared with 9% in those who quit smoking tobacco. Smoking cessation may also reduce the risk of cardiovascular events in the PAD population *(17)*.

The therapeutic approach to smoking cessation can include several strategies to alter behavior including educational materials, behavioral counseling, and pharmacological treatment. Fortunately, a majority of patients with PAD, according to published data, are able to successfully quit smoking. It is estimated that only 30–40% of individuals with stable claudication are current smokers *(17,25)*. Unfortunately, approx 80–90% of patients presenting for surgical or percutaneous revascularization, due to severe PAD continue to smoke *(25)*.

The most efficacious approach to smoking cessation is usually a combination of education, counseling, and pharmacologic therapies. Patients with PAD who smoke should be informed that they have a 40–50% risk of death over the next 10 yr primarily due to myocardial infraction (MI) and stroke *(4,26)*. With adequate counseling, patients will understand that it is never too late to quit smoking and that the risk of cardiovascular events falls relatively rapidly compared to the risk of oncological disease. The pharmacological therapies are either nicotine or nonnicotine based. Nicotine is available as a patch, gum, spray, or oral inhalant. The use of nicotine does not seem to increase cardiovascular or cerebrovascular events. However, an investigation by Heeschen and colleagues found that nicotine might actually cause increased angiogenesis *(27)*. Some investigators have speculated that acceleration of atherosclerosis may be a result of angiogenesis that occurs within the atherosclerotic plaque. It is unclear whether long-term nicotine treatment may cause progression of atherosclerotic disease. Nonnicotine pharmacotherapies include bupropion hydrochloride (Zyban®, Welbutrin®). In one study, a 12-mo abstinence rate of 23% was noted with sustained-release bupropion at a dose of 150–300 mg daily compared with 12% in the placebo group *(28)*.

Diabetes

It is estimated that 16 million people or close to 6% of the population in the United States has diabetes mellitus *(29)*. Each day approximately 2200 people are diagnosed with diabetes mellitus. There are at least 5.4 million people who are not aware that they have the disease. This relatively high number of diabetic patients increases the prevalence of PAD and its complications, as diabetes has been found to be an important risk factor for the development and progression of PAD *(5,7,11,30,31)*. The presence of diabetes is associated with a two- to threefold increased risk for the development of IC *(7,31)*. The prevalence of diabetes in the PARTNERS study was 38% among those with PAD only and 44% for those with both PAD and CVD *(14)*. Diabetes is a contributing factor in half of all lower extremity amputations in the United States; the relative risk for leg amputation is 40 times higher in patients with diabetes *(32)*.

The components of atherosclerotic intimal lesions of the diabetic patient are the same as those of patients without diabetes. However, diabetic individuals have an increased risk for medial artery calcification and a more distal distribution of the atherosclerotic lesions *(33–35)*. There is a common misconception that diabetics have occlusive disease in the arteriolar microcirculation, the so-called "small-vessel disease." This notion of nonatheromatous vascular disease of the lower extremities was proposed in the past and probably originated from a retrospective study demonstrating the presence of periodic acid-Schiff (PAS)-positive material occluding the arterioles in amputated limb specimens from diabetic patients *(36)*. However, subsequent studies with prospective study design *(37,38)*, as well as some physiologic studies *(39)*, have demonstrated no arteriolar occlusive lesions in patients with diabetes.

A difference between the diabetic and nondiabetic patient is that diabetics experience accelerated atherosclerosis. Beach and colleagues found that patients with type 2 diabetes mellitus had PAD more commonly than age- and gender-matched controls *(40)*. It is estimated that the risk for amputation is increased 16% in diabetic patients compared to the risk in nondiabetic individuals with arterial disease *(41)*.

Patients predisposed to diabetes with the insulin resistance syndrome, first described by Reaven and colleagues, are also likely to be at increased risk for macrovascular disease *(42)*. This syndrome involves impaired glucose tolerance, dyslipidemia (low level of high-density lipoprotein, elevated triglycerides), and hypertension. There also appear to be prothrombotic risk factors that accompany the insulin-resistance syndrome, including a suppression of fibrinolysis due to high plasma concentrations of plasminogen activator inhibitor type 1 (PAI-1), as well as alteration of other clotting factors *(43,44)*.

Therapies to alter peripheral arterial and cardiovascular outcomes in patients with diabetes mellitus have focused on glycemic control and more recently the use of angiotensin-converting enzyme (ACE) inhibitors. The United Kingdom Prospective Diabetes Study (UKPDS) was conducted primarily to determine if intensive blood glucose control reduces microvascular and macrovascular complications *(45)*. A total of 3867 newly diagnosed patients with type 2 diabetes mellitus were randomized to intensive control with a sulfonylurea or insulin, or to conventional therapy with diet. The patients were then followed for 10 yr for the development of microvascular complications (retinopathy, vitreous hemorrhage, or renal failure) or macrovascular complications (cardiovascular events). The results from the study confirmed that tight control of blood glucose reduced microvascular complications (i.e., retinopathy and nephropathy); however, there was only a borderline reduction in the risk for MI ($p = 0.052$). Clinical evidence indicates that large-vessel atherosclerosis can precede the development of microvascular complications in patients with diabetes mellitus.

The Heart Outcomes Prevention Evaluation (HOPE) trial was a double-blind, randomized multinational clinical trial of ACE inhibitor use in a population at high risk for cardiovascular events *(46)*. The study enrolled patients 55 yr or older with a history of either CAD, stroke, or PAD, or diabetes and at least one additional cardiovascular disease risk factor. Exclusion criteria included heart failure, known depressed ejection fraction (<0.40), uncontrolled hypertension, overt nephropathy, MI or stroke within 4 wk of study entry, and current use of an ACE inhibitor or vitamin E. The primary endpoint in the HOPE study was a composite outcome that included MI, stroke, or death from cardiovascular causes. Of the 4645 patients randomized to ramipril, 651 (14%) reached the primary endpoint compared with 826 (17.8%) of the 4652 randomized to placebo. There was a 22% reduction in the risk of reaching the composite endpoint in the ramipril group as compared to the placebo group (relative risk of 0.78 with a 95% confidence interval of 0.70–0.86, $p = 0.0001$) *(46)*. A substudy of the HOPE study, the Microalubminuria, Cardiovascular and Renal Outcomes (MICRO-HOPE) study, found a significant reduction in vascular death, MI, heart failure, revascularization, and nephropathy, as well as a 30% reduction in the development of new-onset diabetes with ACE inhibitor treatment *(47)*. Thus, all diabetic patients should be carefully screened for macrovascular and microvascular disease and treated with tight glycemic control and ACE inhibition.

Hypertension

Hypertension is a frequent finding in patients with PAD. The Framingham Study results indicate that hypertension is a significant risk factor in the development of IC *(5)*. Specifically, stage II or greater hypertension (with a systolic blood pressure > 160 mmHg or a diastolic blood pressure > 100 mmHg) was more prevalent in patients with IC than in patients without this symptom *(8,48)*. The Edinburgh Artery Study also showed an association between PAD and hypertension *(30)*. However, all the available evidence is not concordant. Other studies have found that hypertension is not an independent risk factor for PAD *(4,19)*. This lack of association in these reports may be attributable to the multifactorial nature of atherosclerotic plaque development and a complex interaction between hypertension and claudication *(49)*. The majority of studies support hypertension as an independent risk factor for development of PAD.

Several prospective studies found that a reduction of blood pressure in hypertensive patients yields a reduction of cardiovascular events. The UKPDS Blood Pressure Study was done to determine whether tight control of blood pressure prevents macrovascular and microvascular complication in patients with type 2 diabetes *(50)*. The group assigned to tight blood pressure control had a 24% risk reduction in any diabetes-related endpoint and a 37% reduction in microvascular endpoints. When all macrovascular diseases were combined (MI, sudden death, stroke, and PAD), the tight blood pressure control group had 34% risk reduction compared to the less tight control group ($p = 0.019$) *(50)*. Patients with PAD should be treated similarly to other patients with hypertension according to current guidelines *(51,52)*. In addition, the results from the HOPE study indicated that patients with PAD, both with and without hypertension, gain benefit from ACE inhibitor treatment—independent of its blood pressure lowering effects *(46)*. Of note, there is no convincing data that β-blocker treatment adversely affects symptoms in patients with mild to moderate claudication *(49)*.

Dyslipidemia

Patients with dyslipidemia are at increased risk for the development of PAD and its manifestations including IC, as well as graft occlusion. Several lipid fractions confer an increased risk of PAD including elevations of total cholesterol *(3,6,20)*, low-density lipoprotein cholesterol (LDL-C), triglycerides *(3)*, and lipoprotein(a) [Lp(a)] *(53,54)*. It is estimated that for every 10 mg/dL increase in total cholesterol concentration, the risk for developing PAD increases approx 10% *(55)*. Similarly, results from epidemiological studies indicate that elevated LDL-C increases the likelihood of developing PAD. Patients with relative elevation in high-density lipoprotein cholesterol (HDL-C) and apolipoprotein A-1 have a reduced incidence of PAD *(54)*. Mowat and colleagues found that in their population, PAD patients had higher levels of triglycerides and very low density lipoprotein (VLDL) concentrations, as well as low HDL-C *(56)*. Patients with familial dysbetalipoproteinemia (familial type III hyperlipidemia) have a structural defect in apo E and accumulate remnants of VLDL and chylomicrons in plasma owing to defective binding to receptors within the liver *(57)*. Tendinous and tuberous xanthomas can develop and the lipid profile is typically such that the cholesterol and triglycerides are elevated to the same degree. These individuals have a propensity for early onset PAD. Thus, in addition to elevated total cholesterol, study results suggest that elevated triglycerides and low HDL-C contribute to the development of peripheral atherosclerosis.

Unfortunately, there is no published prospective, randomized controlled study of cholesterol reduction and evaluation of cardiovascular events in patients with PAD. However, there is a large amount of published data indicating a reduction of LDL-C in this patient population is likely beneficial. Blankenhorn and colleagues conducted a prospective study that evaluated femoral atherosclerosis by angiography (performed at baseline and 1 yr later) in patients receiving cholesterol-reducing therapy with a combination of colestipol and niacin *(58)*. The annual rate of change in computer-estimated atherosclerosis, a measure of lumen abnormality, was evaluated between treatment groups. There was a significant treatment effect in segments with moderately severe atherosclerosis ($p < 0.04$) and in proximal segments ($p < 0.02$) *(58)*. Another human angiographic study, the Probucol Quantitative Regression Swedish Trial (PQRST), was designed to evaluate if the addition of probucol to a diet low in cholesterol and treatment with cholestyramine retarded progression of femoral atherosclerosis *(59)*. In this study, the addition of probucol did not result in significant regression of atherosclerosis compared to the cholestyramine-treated group.

The Program On Surgical Control of Hyperlipidemia (POSCH) Study revealed that ileal bypass surgery reduced LDL-C levels in patients who had suffered an MI. Patients who received ileal bypass surgery had a reduced incidence of hemodynamically significant PAD compared to the control group, 44% vs 30%, respectively *(60)*.

The Scandinavian Simvastatin Survival Study (4S) was a secondary prevention trial in patients who had a MI and was aimed at demonstrating whether statin therapy can reduce both total mortality and cardiovascular mortality *(61)*. In this trial, simvastatin reduced LDL-C by 35%, increased HDL-C by 8%, and reduced major coronary events and total mortality by 42% and 30%, respectively. A *posthoc* analysis of the data revealed that patients treated with statin therapy had less new or worsening IC (38%) than patients who received placebo ($p = 0.008$) *(62)*.

A study by Kroon and colleagues evaluated patients with CAD and elevations in total cholesterol and Lp(a) after receiving treatment with simvastatin therapy alone or simvastatin with biweekly apheresis *(63)*. The group that received simvastatin alone had no effect on Lp(a) levels, whereas the combination of simvastatin with apheresis reduced Lp(a) levels by 20%. Simvastatin therapy alone did not prevent an increase in the number of occlusive lesions in leg vessels over time. In contrast, simvastatin plus apheresis decreased the accumulation of atherosclerotic lesions. This study suggests that lowering Lp(a) concentrations reduces the progression of PAD.

Thus, patients with PAD are at high risk for cardiovascular events and lipid-modifying therapy likely will reduce the progression of PAD and cardiovascular events. The National Cholesterol Education Program III (NCEP-III) guidelines recommend the target goal of LDL-C reduction to < 100 mg/dL for patients with PAD *(64)*. Therapy may include a combination of diet, exercise, and lipid-modifying agents, although statin drugs are usually required to achieve the target LDL-C level.

EMERGING RISK FACTORS

Hyperhomocysteinemia

Homocysteine is an intermediate metabolite in the processing of methionine to cysteine. The results from case-control studies indicate that elevated homocysteine levels are associated with vascular disease, and several prospective studies indicate that hyperhomocystinemia is an independent risk factor for PAD *(65–67)*. The metabolism of this protein requires folic acid, vitamin B_6, and vitamin B_{12}. Patients with hyperhomocystinemia may benefit from increased folate and B vitamin intake. Clinical trials are underway to determine if vitamin supplementation will improve prognosis in patients with PAD.

Inflammatory Markers of Disease

Recent data indicate that low-grade inflammation is present among patients at risk for future atherothrombotic disease in the coronary and cerebral circulations. Ridker and colleagues investigated whether C-reactive protein (CRP) was predictive of the development of PAD *(68)*. Using a prospective, nested, case-controlled design, CRP was measured in 144 apparently healthy men participating in a physician's health study, who subsequently developed PAD (IC or the need for revascularization) and in an equal number of control subjects. The median CRP levels at baseline were significantly higher among those who developed PAD (1.34 mg/L compared with controls, 0.99 mg/L [$p = 0.04$]). Also, the risk of developing PAD increased significantly with each increasing quartile of baseline CRP concentration such that the relative risks of PAD from the lowest to highest CRP were 1.0, 1.3, 2.0, and 2.1. These data indicate that baseline levels of CRP may predict future risk of developing symptomatic PAD and provide further support that chronic inflammation is an important component of the pathogenesis of peripheral atherosclerosis.

A study by Blann and colleagues evaluated whether treatment of hypercholesterolemia with a statin drug in patients with PAD would be associated with concurrent reduction of plasma markers of platelet activity (such as soluble P-selectin), endothelial cell function (such as von Willebrand factor), and inflammation (such as CRP and soluble intercellular adhesion molecule-1 [sICAM-1]) *(69)*. The study was a randomized, double-blind, placebo-controlled trial of 40 mg of pravastatin daily in patients with PAD and hypercholesterolemia. They found that patients taking pravastatin had a significant reduction in CRP (45%), sICAM-1 (24%), and von Willebrand factor (18%) (all $p < 0.05$). Another study by Ridker and colleagues found that patients treated with pravastatin have a reduction in CRP levels in the 18% range. These data suggest that the anti-inflammatory effects of statins may contribute to the delay in progression of atherosclerosis in patients with PAD.

Infection

Chronic inflammation, recognized more than 125 yr ago by Virchow, is an integral component of atherosclerosis *(70)*. However, the pathophysiological processes that fuel this inflammation, perhaps including chronic infection, are only now being discovered. Infectious agents such as *Chlamydia pneumoniae* and cytomegalovirus are associated with atherosclerosis in the coronary, cerebrovascular, and peripheral arteries *(71–73)*.

The mechanism by which infection predisposes to atherosclerosis is unclear. Some investigators speculate that chronic inflammation can be fueled by direct toxic influence of a blood-borne infectious agent on the vessel wall from the bloodstream or indirectly due to production of autoantibodies directed toward specific epitopes to molecules within the artery wall *(74,75)*.

Infection with *Chlamydia pneumoniae* accelerates development of atherosclerosis and treatment with azithromycin prevents it in a rabbit model *(76)*. Observations such as this in animal models have led to human clinical trials of antibiotics aimed at prevention of cardiovascular events with mixed results *(77)*. The results from two small studies were promising *(78,79)* but results from the larger Azithromycin in Coronary Artery Disease: Elimination of Myocardial Infection with Chlamydia (ACADEMIC) study found no difference in antibody titers or clinical events *(80)*. Further clinical trials are needed before antibiotics can be recommended as treatment for PAD *(77,81)*.

Hemostatic Factors

There is strong evidence to support the hypothesis that there are individuals with atherosclerotic disease who are prone to thrombosis as evidenced from epidemiologic studies of impaired fibrinolysis and cardiovascular risks. Fibrinogen has been identified in several studies as a marker of increased risk of cardiovascular events *(3,82,83)*. A polymorphism of the fibrinogen gene (455AA) was more common in patients with peripheral atherosclerosis in the Edinburgh Artery Study *(84)*. Testing for fibrinogen, although intriguing, is not generally recommended to the community-practicing physician primarily because of variation in assays and lack of standardization.

A homeostatic balance exists between the intrinsic fibrinolytic system with endothelial-derived proteins capable of dissolving thrombi (such as tissue-type plasminogen activator [TPA]) and those capable of inhibiting the clot-dissolving process (such as plasminogen activator inhibitor type I). The results from several studies indicate that elevated levels of both these substances are associated with increased thrombotic risk *(85)*. However, both of these factors are acute phase reactants and are influenced by environmental factors such as cigarette smoking. Recent studies indicate a potentially important interaction between TPA, PAI-I, and the renin–angiotensin system *(86)*. The beneficial effect of ACE inhibitors may be partly explained by a favorable effect on the hemostatic balance. The increased levels of other molecules such as TPA antigen and fibrin D-dimer are associated with an increased risk of cardiovascular events *(87)*. Further investigation is needed before measurement of these factors can be recommended in routine clinical practice.

ANTIPLATELET THERAPY

Patients with atherosclerotic disease are at risk for *in situ* thrombosis or embolism downstream to the microvasculature because of numerous factors. Fundamentally, there is an alteration in the normal balance and regulation of intravascular thrombosis creating an inherently prothrombotic environment wherein previously inhibited stimuli for thrombosis can provoke clot formation. An atherothrombosis (white clot) can be divided into a platelet-dominant phase and a coagulation-dominant or growth phase. The former is generally divided into four categories including platelet adhesion, platelet activation, platelet secretion, and platelet aggregation. The goal of currently approved antiplatelet therapy is to inhibit platelet aggregation.

The presence of an atherosclerotic plaque may cause thrombus formation due to either plaque ulceration or rupture. Adhesive proteins such as collagen and von Willebrand Factor (vWF) may be exposed, leading to platelet adhesion. Interestingly, higher levels of vWF are associated with an increased risk of developing PAD *(83,88)*. Platelets may then become activated through a cascade of steps that involve different agonists, including collagen, thrombin, serotonin, and epinephrine, which bind to specific platelet receptors. These agonists act in concert to trigger the release of aggregating agents, such as adenosine diphosphate (ADP) and thromboxane A_2 (TXA_2). ADP and TXA_2 bind to specific receptor sites on the platelets and activate the glycoprotein IIb/IIIa (GpIIb/IIIa) receptor complex. Once activated, GpIIb/IIIa undergoes a conformational change that enables fibrinogen to bind. Fibrinogen links platelets together to form the platelet aggregate. The coagulation cascade (or secondary hemostasis) is then activated to stabilize the thrombus, which can then expand and cause occlusion of the vessel, leading to ischemic events such as heart attack, stroke, or lower extremity arterial occlusion.

Numerous studies have been conducted to evaluate the effectiveness of different antiplatelet agents in the prevention of thrombus formation and subsequent acute ischemic events. The Antiplatelet Trials Collaboration (ATC) is a retrospective meta-analysis of 145 randomized trials of antiplatelet agents in approximately 100,000 patients at risk of vascular events *(89)*. Antiplatelet therapy was associated with a 25% odds reduction in the cluster of MI, stroke, or vascular death in all trials, including both high- and low-risk patients. The odds reduction ranged from 22% to 32% depending on the patient population. The most widely used agent in these studies was aspirin at dosages of 75–325 mg daily, and thus the results essentially reflect its efficacy. There was no clear evidence that doses of aspirin higher than 325 mg daily had any benefit. The exact dose of aspirin is not known owing to lack of prospective studies, but the ATC meta-analysis supports the use of 325 mg daily. The benefit conferred by taking antiplatelet therapy was present at 2 yr and probably extends beyond this time frame.

Dipyridamole is another agent that reduces platelet aggregation, presumably by stimulation of prostacyclin synthesis and increasing intraplatelet levels of cyclic adenosine monophosphate, which potentiates the antiplatelet activity of prostacyclin. Dipyridamole is usually used in conjunction with aspirin and is approved in one formulation for the prevention of cerebrovascular events in those with cerebral ischemic events based on results of the European Stoke Prevention Study 2 *(90)*. Of note, several studies have been conducted using the combination of aspirin and dipyridamole that did not show a benefit of the combination of aspirin and dipyridamole over aspirin alone *(89)*. Dipyridamole alone or in combination is not approved for reduction of cardiovascular events in patients with PAD. The side effects of aspirin are well known and include gastrointestinal intolerance and ulcer formation. Of course, with any antiplatelet agent there is a risk of bleeding including gastrointestinal bleeding and hemorrhagic stroke.

The thienopyridines are ADP antagonists, such as ticlopidine and clopidogrel, which ultimately inhibit platelet aggregation. The ATC meta-analysis demonstrated a 33% reduction in vascular events when ticlopidine was compared to controls, in patients with atherosclerotic disease. However, concern regarding the development of severe neutropenia with ticlopidine (in about 0.8% of patients) has limited its clinical utility. The neutropenia seen with this agent tended to occur in the first 12 wk of therapy. Common side effects of ticlopidine that prompt a discontinuation of the drug include diarrhea and rash. Ticlopidine is given twice daily with food. Because of these safety concerns, white blood cell count monitoring is required with ticlopidine.

Clopidogrel, also a thienopyridine, is given in daily doses of 75 mg. This daily administration of clopidogrel results in a steady-state level between d 3 and 7. However, anti-aggregating effects are measurable within 2 h. Clopidogrel is extensively and reversibly bound to human plasma proteins in vitro and undergoes metabolism in the liver to active and inactive metabolites. The Clopidogrel vs Aspirin in Patients at Risk of Ischemic Events (CAPRIE) Study was a large randomized trial that involved more than 19,000 patients from 16 countries that compared clopidogrel to aspirin in the prevention of ischemic events (91). The patients were randomized into one of two treatment groups: clopidogrel, 75 mg once daily or aspirin, 325 mg once daily. Patients received treatment for as long as 3 yr, with a mean treatment duration of 1.6 yr. The CAPRIE Study population included patients with ischemic stroke within 1 wk to 6 mo, MI within 35 d, or current IC and ankle–brachial index of ≤ 0.85 on two readings on separate days or previous interventions, including amputation, reconstructive surgery, or angioplasty. The primary analysis of this study was the composite endpoint of a first occurrence of ischemic stroke, MI, or vascular death. Deaths not attributable to stroke or MI (e.g., congestive heart failure, sudden death) were classified as other vascular death. Clopidogrel was associated with a lower incidence of outcome events including fatal and nonfatal strokes and MI. The overall risk reduction was 8.7%, $p = 0.045$ by intention to treat analysis. A *posthoc* analysis of the CAPRIE data indicated that patients with PAD significantly benefited with treatment of clopidogrel.

The safety profile of clopidogrel was also evaluated in the CAPRIE study. Clopidogrel was associated with a lower incidence of gastrointestinal hemorrhage ($p < 0.05$) and related hospitalizations ($p = 0.012$) than aspirin. The observed frequency of severe neutropenia (< 450 neutrophils/μL) was 0.04% (four patients) with clopidogrel and 0.02% (two patients) with aspirin. Of note, one of the four clopidogrel patients was receiving cytotoxic chemotherapy, and another recovered and returned to the trial after temporary interruption of treatment with clopidogrel. Because of this low incidence of neutropenia, no hematological monitoring is required. However, because myelotoxicity is possible, patients with fever or other sign of infection should be carefully evaluated for neutropenia.

Thrombotic thrombocytopenic purpura (TTP) has been reported rarely following use of clopidogrel, sometimes after a short exposure (< 2 wk). It is estimated that TTP occurs at a rate of about four cases per million patients exposed (92). This rare hematological disorder is characterized by sudden onset of microangiopathic hemolytic anemia (schistocytes on blood smear), thrombocytopenia, and the presence of platelet-rich thrombi. Most patients present with initial nonspecific complaints of fatigue, weakness, anorexia, nausea, diarrhea, and abdominal pain that is usually accompanied by fever, neurological findings, and renal dysfunction. Prompt treatment with plasma exchange can result in survival rates of up to 90%. TTP is also associated with the use of ticlopidine, quinolone antibiotics, and cyclosporine as well as a variety of conditions such as connective tissue disorders, advanced cancer, and severe infections.

The data are overwhelming in support of using an antiplatelet therapy to prevent cardiovascular events in patients with PAD. There are no "primarily" antiplatelet drugs approved for the treatment of claudication symptoms. Thus, all patients with PAD should be treated with antiplatelet therapy to reduce the risk of cardiovascular events unless otherwise contraindicated.

SUMMARY

The well established risk factors for developing PAD are male gender, age, diabetes mellitus, smoking, hypertension, and hypercholesterolemia (Fig. 1). The lipoprotein fractions including LDL-C, low HDL-C, as well as triglycerides and Lp(a) also confer increased risk. Emerging risk factors for PAD include hemostatic factors (i.e., fibrinogen) and homocysteine. The modification of atherosclerotic risk factors and treatment with antiplatelet agents will improve prognosis in patients with PAD. Patients with PAD but without claudication symptoms are at a similar risk of cardiovascular events as those with symptoms and therefore risk factors should be addressed in this population as well.

REFERENCES

1. Erb W. Beiträge zur Pathologie des intermittierenden Hinkens. Münch Med Wschr 1911; 2:2487.
2. Schroll M, Munck O. Estimation of peripheral arteriosclerotic disease by ankle blood pressure measurements in a population study of 60-year-old men and women. J Chronic Dis 1981;34:261–269.
3. Hughson WG, Mann JI, Garrod A. Intermittent claudication: prevalence and risk factors. Br Med J 1978;1:1379–1381.
4. Reunanen A, Takkunen H, Aromaa A. Prevalence of intermittent claudication and its effect on mortality. Acta Med Scand 1982;211:249–256.
5. Kannel WB, McGee DL. Update on some epidemiologic features of intermittent claudication: the Framingham Study. J Am Geriatr Soc 1985;33:13–18.
6. Gofin R, Kark JD, Friedlander Y, et al. Peripheral vascular disease in a middle-aged population sample: the Jerusalem Lipid Research Clinic Prevalence Study. Isr J Med Sci 1987;23:157–167.
7. Kannel WB, McGee DL. Diabetes and cardiovascular disease: the Framingham study. JAMA 1979; 241:2035–2038.
8. Murabito JM, D'Agostino RB, Silbershatz H, Wilson WF. Intermittent claudication: a risk profile from the Framingham Heart Study. Circulation 1997;96:44–49.
9. Kannel WB. Risk factors for atherosclerotic cardiovascular outcomes in different arterial territories. J Cardiovasc Risk 1994;1:333–339.
10. Criqui MH, Browner D, Fronek A, et al. Peripheral arterial disease in large vessels is epidemiologically distinct from small vessel disease: an analysis of risk factors. Am J Epidemiol 1989;129: 1110–1119.
11. Gordon T, Kannel WB. Predisposition to atherosclerosis in the head, heart, and legs: the Framingham study. JAMA 1972;221:661–666.
12. Freund KM, Belanger AJ, D'Agostino RB, Kannel WB. The health risks of smoking: the Framingham Study: 34 years of follow- up. Ann Epidemiol 1993;3:417–424.
13. Ingolfsson IO, Sigurdsson G, Sigvaldason H, Thorgeirsson G, Sigfusson N. A marked decline in the prevalence and incidence of intermittent claudication in Icelandic men 1968–1986: a strong relationship to smoking and serum cholesterol—the Reykjavik Study. J Clin Epidemiol 1994;47:1237–1243.
14. Hirsch AT, Criqui MH, Treat-Jacobson D, et al. Peripheral arterial disease detection, awareness, and treatment in primary care. JAMA 2001;286:1317–1324.
15. Weiss NS. Cigarette smoking and arteriosclerosis obliterans: an epidemiologic approach. Am J Epidemiol 1972;95:17–25.
16. Lepantalo M, Lassila R. Smoking and occlusive peripheral arterial disease. Clinical review. Eur J Surg 1991;15783–15787.
17. Jonason T, Bergstrom R. Cessation of smoking in patients with intermittent claudication: effects on the risk of peripheral vascular complications, myocardial infarction and mortality. Acta Med Scand 1987;221:253–260.
18. Powell JT, Edwards RJ, Worrell PC, Franks PJ, Greenhalgh RM, Poulter NR. Risk factors associated with the development of peripheral arterial disease in smokers: a case-control study. Atherosclerosis 1997;129:41–48.

19. Smith GD, Shipley MJ, Rose G. Intermittent claudication, heart disease risk factors, and mortality: the Whitehall Study. Circulation 1990;82:1925–1931.

20. Bowlin SJ, Medalie JH, Flocke SA, Zyzanski SJ, Goldbourt U. Epidemiology of intermittent claudication in middle-aged men. Am J Epidemiol 1994;140:418–430.

21. Gardner AW. The effect of cigarette smoking on exercise capacity in patients with intermittent claudication. Vasc Med 1996;1:181–186.

22. Ameli FM, Stein M, Provan JL, Prosser R. The effect of postoperative smoking on femoropopliteal bypass grafts. Ann Vasc Surg 1989;3:20–25.

23. Girolami B, Bernardi E, Prins MH, et al. Treatment of intermittent claudication with physical training, smoking cessation, pentoxifylline, or nafronyl: a meta-analysis. Arch Intern Med 1999;159: 337–345.

24. Quick CR, Cotton LT. The measured effect of stopping smoking on intermittent claudication. Br J Surg 1982;69(Suppl):S24–S26.

25. Hirsch AT, Treat-Jacobson D, Lando HA, Hatsukami DK. The role of tobacco cessation, antiplatelet and lipid-lowering therapies in the treatment of peripheral arterial disease. Vasc Med 1997;2: 243–251.

26. Faulkner KW, House AK, Castleden WM. The effect of cessation of smoking on the accumulative survival rates of patients with symptomatic peripheral vascular disease. Med J Aust 1983;1:217–219.

27. Heeschen C, Jang JJ, Weis M, et al. Nicotine stimulates angiogenesis and promotes tumor growth and atherosclerosis. Nat Med 2001;7:833–839.

28. Hurt RD, Sachs DP, Glover ED, et al. A comparison of sustained-release bupropion and placebo for smoking cessation. N Engl J Med 1997;337:1195–1202.

29. Anonymous. American Diabetes Association Website. www.diabetes.org/ada/facts.asp, editor. 2001.

30. Fowkes FG, Housley E, Riemersma RA, et al. Smoking, lipids, glucose intolerance, and blood pressure as risk factors for peripheral atherosclerosis compared with ischemic heart disease in the Edinburgh Artery Study. Am J Epidemiol 1992;135:331–340.

31. Brand FN, Abbott RD, Kannel WB. Diabetes, intermittent claudication, and risk of cardiovascular events: the Framingham Study. Diabetes 1989;38:504–509.

32. Nathan DM. Long-term complications of diabetes mellitus. N Engl J Med 1993;328:1676–1685.

33. Everhart JE, Pettitt DJ, Knowler WC, Rose FA, Bennett PH. Medial arterial calcification and its association with mortality and complications of diabetes. Diabetologia 1988;31:16–23.

34. Mozes G, Keresztury G, Kadar A, et al. Atherosclerosis in amputated legs of patients with and without diabetes mellitus. Int Angiol 1998; 17:282–286.

35. Edmonds ME. Medial arterial calcification and diabetes mellitus. Z Kardiol 2000;89(Suppl 2): 101–104.

36. Goldenberg S, Alex M, Joshi RA, Blumenthal HT. Nonatheromatous peripheral vascular disease of the lower extremity in diabetes mellitus. Diabetes 1959;8:261–273.

37. Strandness DE, Priest RE, Gibbons GE. A combined clinical and pathologic study of diabetic and nondiabetic peripheral arterial disease. Diabetes 1964;13:366–372.

38. Conrad MC. Large and small artery occlusion in diabetics and nondiabetics with severe vascular disease. Circulation 1967;36:83–91.

39. Barner HB, Kaiser GC, Willman VL. Blood flow in the diabetic leg. Circulation 1971;43:391–394.

40. Beach KW, Brunzell JD, Strandness DE Jr. Prevalence of severe arteriosclerosis obliterans in patients with diabetes mellitus: relation to smoking and form of therapy. Arteriosclerosis 1982;2:275–280.

41. McDaniel MD, Cronenwett JL. Basic data related to the natural history of intermittent claudication. Ann Vasac Surg 1989;3:273–277.

42. Reaven GM. Banting lecture 1988. Role of insulin resistance in human disease. Diabetes 1988;37: 1595–1607.

43. Juhan-Vague I, Alessi MC, Vague P. Increased plasma plasminogen activator inhibitor 1 levels: a possible link between insulin resistance and atherothrombosis. Diabetologia 1991;34:457–462.

44. Juhan-Vague I, Roul C, Alessi MC, Ardissone JP, Heim M, Vague P. Increased plasminogen activator inhibitor activity in non insulin dependent diabetic patients—relationship with plasma insulin. Thromb Haemost 1989;61:370–373.

45. UK Prospective Diabetes Study Group. The UK Prospective Diabetes Study. Lancet 1998;352: 837–853.

46. Fegan G, Ward D, Clarke L, MacLeod K, Hattersley A. The HOPE study and diabetes: Heart Outcomes Prevention Evaluation. Lancet 2000;355:1182–1183.

47. Heart Outcomes Prevention Evaluation Study Investigators. Effects of ramipril on cardiovascular and microvascular outcomes in people with diabetes mellitus: results of the HOPE study and MICRO-HOPE substudy. Lancet 2000;355:253–259.

48. Jelnes R, Gaardsting O, Hougaard JK, Baekgaard N, Tonnesen KH, Schroeder T. Fate in intermittent claudication: outcome and risk factors. Br Med J (Clin Res Ed) 1986;293:1137–1140.

49. Dormandy JA, Rutherford RB for the TransAtlantic Inter-Society Concensus (TASC) Working Group. Management of peripheral arterial disease (PAD). J Vasc Surg 2000;31:S1–S296.

50. UK Prospective Diabetes Study Group. UKPDS Blood Pressure Study. Br Med J 1998;317:703–713.

51. The sixth report of the Joint National Committee on prevention, detection, evaluation, and treatment of high blood pressure. Arch Intern Med 1997;157:2413–2446.

52. O'Brien E, Staessen JA. Critical appraisal of the JNC VI, WHO/ISH and BHS guidelines for essential hypertension. Expert Opin Pharmacother 2000;1:675–682.

53. Cantin B, Moorjani S, Dagenais GR, Lupien PJ. Lipoprotein(a) distribution in a French Canadian population and its relation to intermittent claudication (the Quebec Cardiovascular Study). Am J Cardiol 1995;75:1224–1228.

54. Johansson J, Egberg N, Johnsson H, Carlson LA. Serum lipoproteins and hemostatic function in intermittent claudication. Arterioscler Thromb 1993;13:1441–1448.

55. Hiatt WR, Hoag S, Hamman RF. Effect of diagnostic criteria on the prevalence of peripheral arterial disease: the San Luis Valley Diabetes Study. Circulation 1995;91:1472–1479.

56. Mowat BF, Skinner ER, Wilson HM, Leng GC, Fowkes FG, Horrobin D. Alterations in plasma lipids, lipoproteins and high density lipoprotein subfractions in peripheral arterial disease. Atherosclerosis 1997;131:161–166.

57. Brewer HB, Jr., Zech LA, Gregg RE, Schwartz D, Schaefer EJ. NIH conference. Type III hyperlipoproteinemia: diagnosis, molecular defects, pathology, and treatment. Ann Intern Med 1983;98: 623–640.

58. Blankenhorn DH, Azen SP, Crawford DW, et al. Effects of colestipol–niacin therapy on human femoral atherosclerosis. Circulation 1991;83:438–447.

59. Walldius G, Erikson U, Olsson AG, et al. The effect of probucol on femoral atherosclerosis: the Probucol Quantitative Regression Swedish Trial (PQRST). Am J Cardiol 1994;74:875–883.

60. Buchwald H, Bourdages HR, Campos CT, Nguyen P, Williams SE, Boen JR. Impact of cholesterol reduction on peripheral arterial disease in the Program on the Surgical Control of the Hyperlipidemias (POSCH). Surgery 1996;120:672–679.

61. Scandinavian Simvistatin Survival Study Group. Randomised trial of cholesterol lowering in 4444 patients with coronary heart disease: the Scandinavian Simvastatin Survival Study (4S). Lancet 1994; 344:1383–1389.

62. Pedersen TR, Kjekshus J, Pyorala K, et al. Effect of simvastatin on ischemic signs and symptoms in the Scandinavian simvastatin survival study (4S). Am J Cardiol 1998;81:333–335.

63. Kroon AA, van Asten WN, Stalenhoef AF. Effect of apheresis of low-density lipoprotein on peripheral vascular disease in hypercholesterolemic patients with coronary artery disease. Ann Intern Med 1996; 125:945–954.

64. Executive Summary of The Third Report of The National Cholesterol Education Program (NCEP) Expert Panel on Detection, Evaluation, and Treatment of High Blood Cholesterol in Adults (Adult Treatment Panel III). JAMA 2001;285:2486–2497.

65. Malinow MR, Kang SS, Taylor LM, et al. Prevalence of hyperhomocyst(e)inemia in patients with peripheral arterial occlusive disease. Circulation 1989;79:1180–1188.

66. Kang SS, Wong PW, Malinow MR. Hyperhomocyst(e)inemia as a risk factor for occlusive vascular disease. Annu Rev Nutr 1992;12:279–298.

67. Fermo I, Vigano' DS, Paroni R, Mazzola G, Calori G, D'Angelo A. Prevalence of moderate hyperhomocysteinemia in patients with early-onset venous and arterial occlusive disease. Ann Intern Med 1995;123:747–753.

68. Ridker PM, Cushman M, Stampfer MJ, Tracy RP, Hennekens CH. Plasma concentration of C-reactive protein and risk of developing peripheral vascular disease. Circulation 1998;97:425–428.

69. Blann AD, Gurney D, Hughes E, Buggins P, Silverman SH, Lip GY. Influence of pravastatin on lipoproteins, and on endothelial, platelet, and inflammatory markers in subjects with peripheral artery disease. Am J Cardiol 2001;88:89–92.

70. Virchow R. Cellular Pathology: As Based upon Physiological and Pathological Histology. New York: Dover, 1863.

71. Elkind MS, Lin IF, Grayston JT, Sacco RL. *Chlamydia pneumoniae* and the risk of first ischemic stroke: the Northern Manhattan Stroke Study. Stroke 2000;31:1521–1525.

72. Siscovick DS, Schwartz SM, Corey L, et al. *Chlamydia pneumoniae*, herpes simplex virus type 1, and cytomegalovirus and incident myocardial infarction and coronary heart disease death in older adults : the Cardiovascular Health Study. Circulation 2000;102:2335–2340.

73. Muhlestein JB. Chronic infection and coronary artery disease. Med Clin North Am 2000;84:123–148.

74. Bachmaier K, Neu N, de la Maza LM, Pal S, Hessel A, Penninger JM. Chlamydia infections and heart disease linked through antigenic mimicry. Science 1999;283:1335–1339.

75. Benitez RM. Atherosclerosis: an infectious disease? Hosp Pract (Off Ed) 1999;34:79-6, 89.

76. Muhlestein JB, Anderson JL, Hammond EH, Zhao L, Trehan S, Schwobe EP, Carlquist JF. Infection with *Chlamydia pneumoniae* accelerates the development of atherosclerosis and treatment with azithromycin prevents it in a rabbit model. Circulation 1998;97:633–636.

77. Grayston JT. Secondary prevention antibiotic treatment trials for coronary artery disease. Circulation 2000;102:1742–1743.

78. Gupta S, Leatham EW, Carrington D, Mendall MA, Kaski JC, Camm AJ. Elevated *Chlamydia pneumoniae* antibodies, cardiovascular events, and azithromycin in male survivors of myocardial infarction. Circulation 1997;96:404–407.

79. Gurfinkel E, Bozovich G, Daroca A, Beck E, Mautner B. Randomised trial of roxithromycin in non-Q-wave coronary syndromes: ROXIS Pilot Study. ROXIS Study Group. Lancet 1997;350:404–407.

80. Muhlestein JB, Anderson JL, Carlquist JF, et al. Randomized secondary prevention trial of azithromycin in patients with coronary artery disease: primary clinical results of the ACADEMIC study. Circulation 2000;102:1755–1760.

81. Dunne M. WIZARD and the design of trials for secondary prevention of atherosclerosis with antibiotics. Am Heart J 1999;138(5 Pt 2):S542–S544.

82. Kannel WB, Wolf PA, Castelli WP, D'Agostino RB. Fibrinogen and risk of cardiovascular disease: the Framingham Study. JAMA 1987;258:1183–1186.

83. Smith FB, Lee AJ, Hau CM, Rumley A, Lowe GD, Fowkes FG. Plasma fibrinogen, haemostatic factors and prediction of peripheral arterial disease in the Edinburgh Artery Study. Blood Coagul Fibrinolysis 2000;11:43–50.

84. Lee AJ, Fowkes FG, Lowe GD, Connor JM, Rumley A. Fibrinogen, factor VII and PAI-1 genotypes and the risk of coronary and peripheral atherosclerosis: Edinburgh Artery Study. Thromb Haemost 1999; 81:553–560.

85. Smith FB, Lee AJ, Rumley A, Fowkes FG, Lowe GD. Tissue-plasminogen activator, plasminogen activator inhibitor and risk of peripheral arterial disease. Atherosclerosis 1995;115:35–43.

86. Vaughan DE. Angiotensin, fibrinolysis, and vascular homeostasis. Am J Cardiol 2001;87(8A): 18C–24C.

87. Smith FB, Rumley A, Lee AJ, Leng GC, Fowkes FG, Lowe GD. Haemostatic factors and prediction of ischaemic heart disease and stroke in claudicants. Br J Haematol 1998;100:758–763.

88. Blann AD, Seigneur M, Steiner M, Boisseau MR, McCollum CN. Circulating endothelial cell markers in peripheral vascular disease: relationship to the location and extent of atherosclerotic disease. Eur J Clin Invest 1997;27:916–921.

89. Antiplatelet Trialists' Collaboration. Collaborative overview of randomised trials of antiplatelet therapy. I. Prevention of death, myocardial infarction, and stroke by prolonged antiplatelet therapy in various categories of patients. Br Med J 1994;308:81–106.

90. Diener HC, Cunha L, Forbes C, Sivenius J, Smets P, Lowenthal A. European Stroke Prevention Study. 2. Dipyridamole and acetylsalicylic acid in the secondary prevention of stroke. J Neurol Sci 1996;143: 1–13.

91. CAPRIE Steering Committee. A randomised, blinded, trial of clopidogrel versus aspirin in patients at risk of ischaemic events (CAPRIE). Lancet 1996;348:1329–1339.

92. Bennett CL, Connors JM, Carwile JM, et al. Thrombotic thrombocytopenic purpura associated with clopidogrel. N Engl J Med 2000;342:1773–1777.

10 Pharmacotherapy for Intermittent Claudication

Robert T. Eberhardt, MD

CONTENTS

INTRODUCTION

Despite extensive clinical investigations over the past several decades, the development of effective pharmacotherapy for the treatment of intermittent claudication (IC) has been elusive. No pharmacologic agent has become established as the paramount therapy to alleviate the symptoms of IC. Numerous agents are available for the treatment of atherosclerosis risk factors and antiplatelet therapy to prevent cardiovascular events (*see* Chapter 9). For improvement in symptoms, exercise has been advocated in the treatment of IC for > 40 yr (*see* Chapter 8). Supervised exercise programs have been shown to improve walking distances up to 200% compared with control therapy *(1)*. The available pharmacologic armamentarium to provide relief of symptoms is limited to a few agents, most with uncertain benefit. The growth in knowledge about the pathophysiology of limb ischemia has not translated into finding a site to direct therapy that has had clinical utility. Agents have been targeted to dilate blood vessels, improve blood rheology, enhance oxidative muscle metabolism, and inhibit platelet function.

This chapter reviews the agents that have been approved for the symptomatic treatment of IC, those agents still undergoing investigation, and finally those agents with minimal or no established benefit. Considering the potential effectiveness of a pharmacologic agent for the treatment of IC requires a careful review of the clinical trials performed. The primary endpoint of claudication trials has been a change in the absolute claudicant distance (ACD), also known as the maximal walking distance, or the maximal walking time on a standardized treadmill test. The initial claudicant distance (ICD), also known as the pain-free walking distance, or the claudicant onset time, is a secondary endpoint with changes tending to parallel those seen in the ACD. Subjective

From: *Contemporary Cardiology: Peripheral Arterial Disease: Diagnosis and Treatment*
Edited by: J. D. Coffman and R. T. Eberhardt © Humana Press Inc., Totowa, NJ

response and functional assessment using standardized questionnaires are essential features of clinical trials. The use of a placebo control is the most important aspect, as nearly all claudication trials have shown a 15–30% improvement in the treadmill walking distances with placebo compared with the baseline. Clinicians should be skeptical evaluating trials if the placebo fails to show any improvement over baseline.

APPROVED AGENTS (IN THE UNITED STATES AND ABROAD)

Pentoxifylline

Pentoxifylline was approved by the United States Food and Drug Administration (US FDA) in 1984 for the symptomatic treatment of IC. It is a dimethylxanthine derivative that increases cyclic adenosine monophosphate (cAMP) by inhibiting 3,5-monophosphate diesterase. The proposed mechanism of action involves decreased whole blood viscosity, in part due to improved erythrocyte deformability, diminished platelet aggregation, and decreased fibrinogen levels.

Numerous small studies evaluating pentoxifylline for the symptomatic treatment of IC have yielded equivocal results. An early trial conducted in the United States demonstrated an improvement in ICD of 23% (21 m) and ACD of 13% (27 m) in subjects with IC with pentoxifylline over placebo at 24 wk *(2)*. However, a comparison of the mean difference during wk 2–24 was required to reach statistical significance, rather than the result at 24 wk compared to baseline. Supporting this was an improvement in ACD with pentoxifylline over placebo during wk 16–24 compared with baseline *(3)*. It was suggested that the benefit of pentoxifylline was the greatest in those with moderate disease and longer duration. In the target population defined by an ankle–brachial index (ABI) of < 0.8 and duration of symptoms of > 1 yr, a 33% improvement in ACD was seen with pentoxifylline over placebo *(3)*.

Initial attempts to analyze the aggregate data from the pentoxifylline studies concluded that the data were inadequate to reach a reliable conclusion regarding its efficacy *(4)*. Two more recent meta-analyses concluded that pentoxifylline had a modest effect on treadmill walking distance with an improvement of approx 20–30 m in the ICD and 40–50 m in the ACD compared with placebo *(1,5)*. This finding has come into question as a recent trial comparing pentoxifylline to cilostazol or placebo found no significant improvement compared to placebo *(6)*.

The clinical relevance of this magnitude of an effect on walking distance has been questioned by many clinicians. However, others have concluded that its is highly relevant, allowing greater daily function *(7)*. This treadmill distance is equivalent to walking 90 m on level ground, which may minimize the disability in these patients, enabling engagement in social activities and employment *(5)*.

There is limited (or discouraging) information regarding the impact of pentoxifylline on functional status or quality of life. An early study found some improvement in paresthesias but no improvement in other subjective variables *(8)*. The use of quality of life questionnaires had not been employed in the clinical trials with pentoxifylline until recently, in comparison to cilostazol. There was no demonstrable improvement in daily functional status in subjects with IC treated with pentoxifylline as assessed using the Walking Impairment Questionnaire (WIQ) or Medical Outcome Scale Health Survey (SF-36) *(6)*.

In addition to its effects on walking performance, it has been suggested that pentoxifylline may alter the natural history of peripheral arterial disease. Continuous use of pentoxifylline reduced the number of invasive vascular procedures within the first year in a small group of patients with IC *(9)*. Although there was no difference in the risk of peripheral arterial disease (PAD)-related hospitalization, the use of pentoxifylline was associated with a reduction in hospital costs without a greater overall cost of PAD-related care *(7)*.

The dose of pentoxifylline is 400 mg three times a day, preferably with meals or food. Important pharmacokinetic issues with pentoxyfylline include nearly complete absorption with some first-pass metabolism, biotransformation by erthyrocytes and hepatic tissue, and elimination by the renal route. Precaution needs to be used in those with renal impairment as metabolites of pentoxifylline may accumulate. Side effects are infrequent and include stomach discomfort, nausea, vomiting, headache, and dizziness. Pentoxifylline is well tolerated, as only a small percentage of patients need to discontinue the medication because of intolerable side effects.

There is still considerable uncertainty and skepticism regarding the clinical utility of pentoxifylline. Many clinicians will give a 6- to 12-wk trial of pentoxifylline to assess its efficacy after other measures (including exercise) have failed to diminish symptoms.

Cilostazol

Cilostazol became the second agent approved by the US FDA for the symptomatic treatment of IC in 1999. Cilostazol is a type III phosphodiesterase inhibitor, inhibiting proteolysis of intracellular cAMP, leading to increased levels. The proposed mechanisms of therapeutic action are vasodilation, due to direct smooth muscle relaxation and perhaps enhanced effect of prostacyclin, inhibition of platelet activity, and inhibition of smooth muscle proliferation *(10–12)*.

The efficacy of cilostazol in the treatment of IC has been shown in an extensive clinical development program, including a number of controlled trials. A randomized, double-blind, placebo-controlled trial involving 239 subjects with mild to moderate IC found that cilostazol, at a dose of 100 mg twice daily for 16 wk, improved walking distance *(13)*. Cilostazol increased ACD by 65 m (34%) and ICD by 28 m (27%) compared with placebo ($p < 0.05$) on a variable-grade treadmill protocol. Another trial of cilostazol involving subjects with moderately severe IC found significant improvements, by estimated treatment effects, in ICD (35%) and ACD (41%) on a fixed-incline treadmill protocol *(14)*. Several other studies have reported similar beneficial effects of cilostazol on walking distance *(6,15–17)*.

A comparison of cilostazol with pentoxifylline for the treatment of IC demonstrated a greater improvement in walking distance with cilostazol *(6)*. After 24 wk of treatment, the increase in the ACD of 107 m (54%) with cilostazol was larger than that seen with pentoxifylline of 64 m (30%) or placebo of 65 m (34%). The beneficial effect of cilostazol on walking in claudication patients rapidly dissipates on withdrawal of the drug *(18)*. There was a decline in walking distance with crossover to placebo within 6 wk, providing support that the initial improvement with cilostazol was due to the drug's action.

Further evidence of clinical benefit is a subjective improvement in the functional status and walking performance. There was significant improvement in the physical component scale score of the Medical Outcome Scale Health Survey (SF-36) with cilostazol relative to placebo *(13,17)*. Using the Walking Impairment Questionnaire there was an improvement in the walking speed and walking distance and in specific measures of walking difficulty with cilostazol *(13,17)*. More investigators and patients judged claudication symptoms to have improved at the end of treatment with cilostazol than with placebo. A global therapeutic assessment found that significantly more patients rated their outcome as "better" or "much better" with cilostazol compared with placebo *(14,17)*.

Additional findings from the clinical trails that deserve to be mentioned are an improvement in the ankle pressure and alteration in the lipid profile with cilostazol. Two trials demonstrated an approx 9% increase in ABI with cilostazol *(13,15)*. Although the clinical significance of this finding remains uncertain, some have suggested that this provides evidence of the vasodilator properties *(13,15)*. It has also been reported that cilostazol may favorably modify plasma lipoproteins with an increase in high-density lipoprotein (HDL) cholesterol (by 10%) and reduction of triglycerides (by 15%) (15).

The recommended dose of cilostazol is 100 mg twice daily but it may be used at a dose from 50 to 150 mg twice daily. A trial involving 516 patients with moderately severe IC found that 50 mg of cilostazol given twice daily also improved walking distance with a possible dose response *(17)*. Important pharmacokinetic issues of cilostazol include rapid oral absorption, extensive binding to plasma proteins (95%), hepatic metabolism by cytochrome P450 isoenzymes (especially CYP3A4 and CYP2C19) with the formation of active metabolites, and elimination primarily by the renal route (74%) *(11)*. Pharmacokinetic studies have suggested that dose adjustment is not required in renal insufficiency or mild hepatic impairment but caution should be exercised in those with moderate or severe hepatic impairment *(19,20)*. Dose adjustment should be made during coadministration of inhibitors of CYP3A4 or CYP2C19 such as ketoconazole, erythromycin, diltiazem, and omeprazole.

Although there are clear benefits, the use of cilostazol requires some consideration, careful instructions, and close monitoring. Side effects of cilostazol are reported frequently ($> 25–30\%$ of patients), including gastrointestinal complaints with loose stools or diarrhea, headaches, dizziness, and palpitations *(11)*. The side effects reported are often transient and some appear to be dose dependent *(17)*. The most common of these side effects was headaches, which were mild and responded to nonprescription analgesics. Despite these side effects, in the clinical trials the rates of withdrawal among patients taking cilostazol were similar to those among patients receiving placebo or pentoxifylline *(18)*.

Cilostazol contains a "black-box" warning that it is contraindicated in patients with congestive heart failure of any severity. This is a result of adverse findings with other agents in this pharmacologic category, type III phosphodiesterase inhibitors, in a subpopulation of patients with heart failure. Oral milrinone with significant inotropic properties had a detrimental effect on mortality in patients with New York Heart Association class III–IV heart failure *(21)*. Cilostazol has not been shown to have such adverse effects but has been inadequately studied in those with heart failure. Cilostazol does increase heart rate significantly by five to eight beats per minute depending on dose, as reflected in the adverse events of tachycardia and palpitations. The long-term effects of type III phosphodiesterase inhibitors are unknown. Such concerns have led some to recommend routine screening for signs or symptoms of congestive heart failure prior to initiating therapy, regular reassessment of the risk–benefit ratio based on interval ischemic events, and close monitoring for tachycardia during initiation of therapy *(22)*.

In the clinical trials conducted in the United States, involving more than 2000 subjects, there was no appreciable detrimental effect as evidenced by myocardial infarction or mortality with the use of cilostazol for up to 6 mo *(10)*.

Naftidrofuryl

Naftidrofuryl is a serotonin receptor antagonist that reduces erythrocyte and platelet aggregation and enhances aerobic metabolism in oxygen-depleted tissue. This agent is not available in the United States, but has been used in Europe for the symptomatic treatment of IC for > 20 yr. A number of randomized, controlled trials have shown a moderate beneficial effect of naftidrofuryl in the treatment of IC. There was an improvement in walking distance with 12–24 wk of treatment with naftidrofuryl in subjects with mild to moderate symptoms (Fontaine's classification stage II) *(23–28)*. These studies have shown a fairly consistent improvement in the ICD but an inconsistent effect on the ACD. A recent meta-analysis of four selected randomized trials involving 409 patients found naftidrofuryl increased ICD by 59 m and ACD by 71 m compared with placebo *(1)*. A randomized trial involving 188 patients with severe IC failed to confirm an improvement with no change in ICD or ACD *(29)*. There has been limited information regarding the effect of naftidrofuryl on functional status or quality of life. Subjectively there was a delay in the deterioration of symptoms while the patient was on naftidrofuryl compared with placebo (7% vs 22% with placebo) *(28)*. The recommended dose of naftidrofuryl is 600–800 mg daily (in two or three divided doses). Naftidrofuryl is well tolerated, with the most common side effects being mild gastrointestinal symptoms.

Buflomedil

Buflomedil acts through adrenolytic and weak calcium antagonistic effects to promote vasodilation. It improves blood rheology, facilitating erythrocyte deformability and promoting platelet disaggregation. This agent has been used in selected countries for over 10 yr, although it has not been adequately studied and is not available in the United States. The results of clinical investigations evaluating its efficacy in the treatment of IC have been conflicting. In a randomized trial involving 93 patients with IC, treatment with buflomedil for 12 wk improved ICD by 100% and ACD by 97%, compared with placebo (38% and 42%, respectively) *(30)*. A small study comparing buflomedil to pentoxifylline failed to show an improvement in treadmill walking distance, although some subjective improvement was noted in hypothermia and paresthesia *(31)*. Another small study comparing buflomedil to pentoxifylline or nifedipine found the improvement in ICD with buflomedil and nifedipine was less than that noted with pentoxifylline *(32)*. The dose of buflomedil is 600 mg daily; side effects include gastrointestinal symptoms, headache, dizziness, erythema, and pruritus.

INVESTIGATIONAL AGENTS

Carnitine

Although the principal disturbance in PAD is hypoperfusion with relative tissue hypoxemia, metabolic dysfunction contributes to its pathophysiology. Carnitine is an important cofactor for skeletal muscle metabolism during exercise, facilitating the transfer of fatty acids into the mitochondria for β-oxidation *(33)*. Persons with PAD have impaired muscle energetics and abnormalities in carnitine metabolism *(33,34)*. There is a deficiency of carnitine and accumulation of acylcarnitine in PAD that correlates with the exercise impairment *(34)*. The potential feasibility of restoring carnitine homeostasis and normalizing energy metabolism with carnitine supplementation has been suggested as a therapeutic target for PAD *(33)*.

Initial studies with L-carnitine suggested some biochemical and clinical improvement. In a small group of subjects with IC, L-carnitine at a dose of 2 g twice daily for 3 wk appeared to improve muscle energetics and walking distance *(35)*. There was an improvement in pyruvate utilization and oxidative phosphorylation efficiency in ischemic skeletal muscle. On treadmill testing the ACD rose 306 m with L-carnitine compared to 174 m with placebo ($p < 0.01$). Subsequent studies have focused on the analog of carnitine, propionyl-L-carnitine (PLC), owing to the "superiority" of this compound when administered in an equimolar dose *(36)*. A single intravenous dose of PLC (600 mg) had a beneficial effect on walking distances with an improvement in both ICD and ACD compared with placebo.

A double-blind, placebo-controlled trial involved 245 subjects with IC treated with escalating doses of PLC for 24 wk *(37)*. The dose was titrated from 1 g/d to 3 g/d at 2-mo intervals. There was a modest increase in ACD of 73% (140 m) in subjects receiving PLC compared with 46% (90 m) in those receiving placebo *(37)*. There was a doubling in the ICD compared with placebo, which failed to reach significance. Another study involved 485 patients with IC treated with 1 g twice daily for at least 12 m. There was a slight improvement in ACD of 62% with PLC compared with 46% with placebo by intention-to-treat analysis. This study identified a potential target population, those with an ACD of < 250 m, who may benefit from PLC therapy *(38)*. In this group, representing 114 of the patients enrolled, there was an improvement in walking distances with PLC with an increase in ACD of 98% (155 m) compared with a 54% (95 m) increase with placebo ($p < 0.05$) *(38)*.

Corroborating the treadmill testing results has been a subjective improvement in functional status and quality of life. This was first reported among individuals with the most severely impaired walking capacity, assessed using the McMaster Health Index Questionnaire (MHIQ) *(39)*. There was an improvement in the physical function, emotional function, and global MHIQ score with PLC compared to placebo among those with the poorest walking ability (<250 m) *(39)*. In the more recent trial similar improvement was noted in functional status using the Walking Impairment Questionnaire and the Medical Outcome Scale Health Survey (SF-36) *(40)*. There was an improvement in walking distance and walking speed and enhanced physical function, reduced body pain, and better health transition score *(40)*.

The optimal dose of PLC is still under investigation, but the maximal benefit appears to occur at 2 g/d. Side effects reported with the use of PLC include occasional headache and gastrointestinal symptoms. PLC is well tolerated with minimal adverse events requiring drug discontinuation. PLC may improve exercise performance and functional status; however, further clarification is required. This agent is not approved in the United States for the treatment of IC.

Prostaglandins

Prostaglandins have potent vasodilator and antiplatelet properties that may be useful in the treatment of PAD. Investigations evaluating the role of prostaglandins, including prostaglandin I_2 (PGI_2), prostaglandin E_1 (PGE_1), and several analogs, have primarily been in the management of critical limb ischemia (*see* Chapter 6). Daily intravenous infusions of PGE_1 in patients with chronic critical leg ischemia improved tissue perfusion with diminished ongoing ischemia and reduced need for amputation at hospital discharge *(41)*. Additional investigations have sought to evaluate the benefit of prostaglandins in the treatment of intermittent claudication.

Several studies have suggested a benefit of PGE_1 in the treatment of IC, with an improvement in treadmill walking distance and perhaps an improvement in the quality of life. A surprising finding in one open-label study was a marked beneficial effect when PGE_1 infusion was added to an exercise program *(42)*. The exercise program alone resulted in a 99% increase in ACD; however, there was a 371% increase when PGE_1 was added for 4 wk. These results have not been confirmed in a rigorously conducted manner. A prodrug of PGE_1 (AS-013) was studied in 80 patients with IC, randomized to placebo or one of three dosage regimens given intravenously 5 d per week for 8 wk *(43)*. There was an improvement in ACD of 53% (35 m) in the combined active treatment groups compared to a decrease of 14% (11 m) with placebo *(43)*. The decrease in walking distance in the placebo group is most unusual. There was, however, a dose-related improvement in the pain-free walking distance and quality of life. Another study compared PGE_1 for 8 wk (given 5 d/wk for 4 wk then 2 d/wk for 4 wk) to placebo in a group of 213 patients with IC *(44)*. At the end of the 8 wk, there was a significant improvement in the pain-free walking distance of 101% in the treated group compared with 60% in the placebo group *(44)*.

Other trials have suggested a benefit of PGI_2 in the treatment of IC. A recent trial evaluated the effect of an oral PGI_2 analog, beraprost sodium (40 µg three times daily for 6 mo), on treadmill walking distance in 549 patients with severe IC *(45)*. There was an improvement in ICD of 82% in the beraprost sodium group compared with an increase of 53% in the placebo group, providing a 36-m increase in ICD over placebo compared with baseline ($p = 0.001$) *(45)*. Similarly there was an improvement in ACD of 60% in the beraprost sodium group compared with an increase of 35% in the placebo group, providing a 70-m increase in the ACD over placebo compared with baseline ($p = 0.04$) *(45)*.

Side effects reported with these agents include headache, flushing, and gastrointestinal intolerance. Although the use of prostaglandins by daily intravenous infusion may be useful in the management of critical limb ischemia, establishing their role in the treatment of IC is in the early stages. With the development and refinement of newer oral prostaglandin analogs, these agents may be useful in the management of IC. These agents are not available in the United States for the treatment of IC or critical limb ischemia.

L-Arginine

Nitric oxide is a critical vasoregulatory mediator released from the endothelium and participates in control of vascular tone and regulation of blood flow. Nitric oxide is generated during the conversion of L-arginine to L-citrulline by the action of nitric oxide synthase. Nitric oxide has multiple actions that may be beneficial in the treatment of limb ischemia including vasodilation, and antiplatelet and antiproliferative actions.

L-Arginine and nutritional supplements that enhance nitric oxide generation have been gaining interest as a potential therapy for PAD. Experimentally, L-arginine administered intravenously increased limb perfusion and nutritive capillary flow, as determined by positron emission tomography, in ischemic human limbs *(46)*. A trial involving 39 patients with IC found that both L-arginine and PGE_1 improved walking distance compared with placebo *(47)*. In this study, 8 g of L-arginine administered by daily infusion for 3 wk increased ICD by 147 m (230%) and ACD by 216 m (155%) *(47)*. These effects lasted for 6 wk after the discontinuation of therapy and were associated with improved endothelium-dependent vasodilation, supporting enhanced nitric oxide generation. Similar benefits on walking distance have been reported with a nutritional supplement designed to enhance nitric oxide metabolism *(48)*. After 2 wk there was an improvement in the ICD of 66% and ACD of 23% in the group receiving the supplement twice daily that was not observed in the group receiving placebo or supplement once daily *(48)*. These initial studies with L-arginine are promising and provide support for further investigations.

Growth Factors

The use of growth factors to stimulate the growth of new blood vessels, in an approach known as therapeutic angiogenesis, is an area of research that has gained widespread attention for the treatment of ischemic vascular disorders. In the area of PAD these agents have primarily been studied in critical limb ischemia (*see* Chapter 11) *(49)*. Vascular endothelial growth factor (VEGF) has been found to augment collateral development and improve tissue perfusion in experimental models of hind limb ischemia *(50)*. However, the use of growth factors has also been considered in the management of IC. In a phase I trial 19 patients with IC were randomized to receive by intraarterial infusion one of three doses of basic fibroblast growth factor (bFGF) or placebo *(51)*. There was an improvement in resting calf blood flow measured by plethysmography in the two higher doses of bFGF at 1 mo by 66% and 6 mo by 153% *(51)*. The use of recombinant FGF-2 has been evaluated in a phase II trial, the Therapeutic Angiogenesis with FGF-2 for Intermittent Claudication (TRAFFIC) study, in patients with PAD and IC. Preliminary findings reported an improvement in the ACD at 90 d with a single infusion of recombinant FGF-2 compared with placebo *(52)*. However, this benefit was no longer seen at 180 d and there was no additional benefit of repeat infusions *(52)*. Although intriguing as potential therapeutic targets, these agents are in the early stages of development.

Defibrotide

Defibrotide is a polydeoxyribonucleotide that modulates endothelial function, enhancing the release of tissue plasminogen activator, decreasing the release of tissue plasminogen inhibitor, stimulating the release of prostacyclin and other prostanoids, and perhaps inhibiting platelet aggregation. In a double-blind, placebo-controlled trial involving 227 patients with IC, defibrotide increased ACD by about 50% compared with 17% in the placebo group *(53)*. A trend toward improvement in ABI was reported, although this may be explained by a reduction in systolic blood pressure. In another small open study, defibrotide improved walking distance and rest pain *(54)*. A meta-analysis of 10 placebo-controlled trials involving 743 subject found a 73-meter improvement in the ACD with defibrotide compared to placebo *(55)*. Defibrotide is dosed 200–400 mg twice daily. This agent deserves further investigation but is at present unavailable for use.

INEFFECTIVE AGENTS
Vasodilators

In theory, vasodilators may be beneficial in treatment of IC by improving muscle blood flow and decreasing tissue ischemia. However, there have been no adequate controlled studies to demonstrate their efficacy in the treatment of IC. The lack of benefit may be explained by failure of these agents to dilate a fixed lesion in the peripheral vessels that limit blood flow in PAD and near maximal dilation of resistance vessels in ischemic limbs. As a result, most vascular specialists agree there is no role for vasodilators in the treatment of IC *(10,56)*. A single trial suggested a benefit of verapamil in the treatment of IC, with an improvement in ICD of 29% and ACD of 49% compared with placebo *(57)*.

Antiplatelet Drugs

The increase in cardiovascular events among individuals with PAD warrants some form of antiplatelet therapy, given the benefit of these agents in prevention of coronary events (*see* Chapter 9). There is no evidence to support the use of aspirin alone or in combination with other antiplatelet agents for the symptomatic treatment of claudication *(58,59)*. The only agent with some suggestion of a benefit has been the adenosine diphosphate (ADP) receptor antagonist ticlopidine. In 151 subjects with IC, ticlopidine was reported to significantly improve walking distance with an increase in both ICD and ACD compared with placebo *(60)*. In contrast, another randomized trial involving 169 patients failed to find an effect of ticlopidine on treadmill walking distance *(61)*. The aggregate data on the use of antiplatelet agents for the symptomatic treatment of IC indicate that there is no improvement. However, because of the cardioprotective benefit of these drugs, antiplatelet therapy should be part of the medical regimen of nearly every patient with PAD (provided there are no absolute contraindications) *(62)*.

α-Tocopherol

α-Tocopherol, the most active form of vitamin E, is a lipid-soluble antioxidant that participates in the defense against oxygen-derived free radicals. Vitamin E has been advocated for the treatment of claudication since the 1950s, when several small studies suggested some improvement *(63,64)*. Since that time, the data supporting the use of vitamin E have been limited. In a large cancer prevention study, α-tocopherol (50 mg daily) did not prevent the development of claudication in male smokers, as assessed by the Rose questionnaire *(65)*. The results of The Heart Outcome Prevention Evaluation trial were disappointing with regard to the effect of vitamin E use on cardiovascular events in a high-risk group of patients, many with established PAD *(66)*.

Ketanserin

Ketanserin is a selective S_2-serotonin receptor antagonist with actions including vasodilation, decreased blood viscosity, and perhaps dilation of collateral vessels. Clinical trials evaluating the effect of ketanserin in the treatment of IC have been controversial. Although a small placebo-controlled study found an improvement in walking distance, ketanserin failed to improve treadmill walking distance compared to placebo in a multicenter trial involving 179 patients with IC *(67,68)*.

In this study a serendipitous discovery of a higher incidence of cardiovascular complications in the placebo group was made, which was subsequently confirmed in a pooled analysis *(69)*. This led to the PACK trial (Prevention of Atherosclerotic Complications with Ketanserin), which was designed to determine the effect of ketanserin on cardiovascular events during 1 yr of treatment *(70)*. In the PACK trial, 3899 patients with IC were randomized to receive ketanserin or placebo; however, many patients were withdrawn prematurely owing to excessive mortality in the ketanserin group. This has since been attributed to QT interval prolongation in association with hypokalemia caused by potassium wasting diuretic agents *(70)*. Furthermore, in the Claudication Substudy of the PACK trial involving 436 subjects, there was no effect of ketanserin on treadmill walking distances after 1 yr of treatment *(71)*. Ketanserin is not available in the United States and its role in the treatment of IC remains undefined.

Hemodilution

Hemodilution involves the removal of blood and replacement with a colloid solution such as hydroxyethyl starch (HES) or a low-molecular-weight dextran. Hemodilution may decrease plasma viscosity and erythrocyte aggregation and increase resting limb blood flow. This approach may have a modest effect on walking distance in patients with IC. In one study of 75 patients, HES was superior to Ringer's lactate plus exercise or exercise alone in increasing the ICD (44% vs 20% and 14%, respectively) *(72)*. Another study found a 50% improvement in walking distance with both 10% HES and dextran 40 infusions *(73)*. Current data do not support the routine use of this therapy, which is likely to be unacceptable to most patients.

Chelation Therapy

Chelation therapy has been advocated for the treatment of IC as well as other atherosclerotic disorders. Chelation therapy involves the administration of agents, such as ethylenediamine tetraacetic acid (EDTA), that are theorized to mobilize calcium within atherosclerotic lesions and promote regression of existing lesions. There are limited controlled data to suggest a benefit from this type of therapy. A randomized, double-blind, placebo-controlled trial of 153 patients with IC found that chelation therapy did not improve walking distance, angiographic findings, tissue oxygen tension, ABIs, or subjective assessments of symptoms *(74,75)*. Despite its supporters, this type of treatment is of dubious benefit and has significant potential side effects, such as hypoglycemia and renal failure.

Other Agents

Many other agents have been evaluated for the symptomatic relief of IC without encouraging initial findings. These have included cinnarizine *(76)*, aminophylline *(77)*, inositol niacinate *(78)*, testosterone *(79)*, and low-molecular-weight heparin *(80)*. Although controversial, a recent meta-analysis of eight randomized, controlled trails found ginkgo biloba improved ICD by 33 m compared with placebo *(81)*.

SUMMARY

Despite years of intense investigation, effective drug therapy for the symptomatic treatment of manifestations of arteriosclerosis obliterans remains elusive. The current focus remains on the treatment of modifiable risk factors for atherosclerosis (including smok-

Table 1

Drug Therapy for Intermittent Claudication: A Comparison of the Effect on Walking Distance of Various Treatments

Drug/study	N	Daily dose	Duration (wk)	Change in ACD Placebo %	M	Drug %	M	p value
Cilostazol								
Dawson 1998 (14)	81	200 mg	12	−10	−17	63	90	<0.001
Money 1998 (13)	239	200 mg	16	13	31	47	96	<0.001
Beebe 1999 (17)	516	200 mg	24	15	27	51	129	<0.001
Dawson 2000 (6)	698	200 mg	24	34	65	54	107	<0.001
Pentoxifylline								
Porter 1982 (2)	128	1.2 g	24	25	69	38	96	0.19
Lindgarder 1989 (3)	150	1.2 g	24	29	66	50	132	0.09
Dawson 2000 (6)	698	1.2 g	24	34	65	30	64	0.82
Naftidrofuryl								
Moody 1994 (29)	188	600 mg	24	29	47	40	73	0.27
Trubestein 1984 (28)	104	600 mg	12	40	90	55	122	0.02
Adhoute 1990 (26)	94	600 mg	24	26	69	74	200	<0.001
Buflomedil								
Trubestein 1984 (30)	113	600 mg	12	42	60	97	141	<0.01
Propionyl-L-carnitine								
Brevetti 1995 (37)	245	1–3 g	24	46	90	73	140	<0.03
Brevetti 1999 (38)	485	2 g	52	46	111	62	146	<0.05
Prostaglandins								
Beraprost								
Lievre 2000 (45)	424	120 µg	24	53	108	82	197	0.004
PGE₁ Prodrug: AS-013								
Diehm 1997 (44)	213	60 µg	8	60	161	101	186	<0.005
Belch 1997 (43)	80	varied	8	−14	−11	53	35	<0.001
L-Arginine								
Maxwell 2000 (48)	41	8 g	2	4	7	20	69	NS
Defibrotide								
Strano 1991 (53)	227	400–800 mg	24	17	41	47–52	109–113	<0.01

ing cessation) and exercise regimens. Only two agents, pentoxifylline and cilostazol, are available in the United States for the symptomatic treatment of IC. Despite its approval in the 1980s the clinical utility of pentoxifylline is doubtful. The more recently approved cilostazol has beneficial effects on walking performance and quality of life by questionnaires. Side effects are frequent but cilostazol is usually well tolerated. It is contraindicated in patients with heart failure. Two other agents, naftidrofuryl and buflomedil, are approved in select countries but not in the United States. These agents have been inadequately studied. Investigational agents involving nitric oxide metabolism, carnitine metabolism, growth factors, and prostaglandins remain viable therapeutic targets in the management of IC. Propionyl-L-carnitine improves energetics in ischemic muscle and may improve symptoms and walking ability in those with severe IC. Prostaglandins hold promise in the treatment of critical limb ischemia and now oral prostaglandins are being evaluated in the treatment of claudication. L-Arginine supplementation has been shown in small studies to improve vascular function and walking distance but its clinical utility is uncertain. The exciting field of angiogenesis is expanding to evaluate functional outcomes in ischemic limbs and claudication, but remains in its infancy. A great number of agents have proven to be ineffective in the symptomatic treatment of IC including vasodilators, antiplatelet drugs (such as aspirin and ticlopidine), ketanserin, vitamin E, chelation therapy, and hemodilution.

REFERENCES

1. Girolami B, Bernardi E, Prins MH, et al. Treatment of intermittent claudication with physical training, smoking cessation, pentoxifylline, or nafronyl: a meta-analysis. Arch Intern Med 1999;159: 337–345.
2. Porter JM, Cutler BS, Lee BY, Reich T, Reichle FA, Scogin JT. Pentoxifylline efficacy in the treatment of intermittent claudication: multicenter controlled double-blind trial with objective assessment of chronic occlusive arterial disease patients. Am Heart J 1982;104:66–72.
3. Lindgarde F, Jelnes R, Bjorkman H, et al. Conservative drug treatment in patients with moderately severe chronic occlusive peripheral arterial disease. Scandinavian Study Group. Circulation 1989;80: 1549–1556.
4. Radack K, Wyderski RJ. Conservative management of intermittent claudication. Ann Intern Med 1990;113:135–146.
5. Hood SC, Moher D, Barber GG. Management of intermittent claudication with pentoxifylline: meta-analysis of randomized controlled trials. Can Med Assoc J 1996;155:1053–1059.
6. Dawson DL, Cutler BS, Hiatt WR, et al. A comparision of cilostazol and pentoxifylline for treating intermittent claudication. Am J Med 2000;109:523–530.
7. Gillings DB. Pentoxifylline and intermittent claudication: review of clinical trials and cost-effectiveness analyses. J Cardiovasc Pharmacol 1995;25(Suppl 2):S44–S50.
8. Reich J, Cutler BC, Lee BY, et al. Pentoxifylline in the treatment of intermittent claudication of the lower limbs. Angiology 1984;35:389–395.
9. Stergachis A, Sheingold S, Luce BR, Psaty BM, Revicki DA. Medical care and cost outcomes after pentoxifylline treatment for peripheral arterial disease. Arch Intern Med 1992;152:1220–1224.
10. Sorkin EM, Markham A. Cilostazol: new drug profile. Drugs Aging 1999;14:63–71.
11. Hiatt WR. Medical treatment of peripheral arterial disease and claudication. N Engl J Med 2001;344:1608–1621.
12. Ishizaka N, Taguchi J, Kimura Y, et al. Effects of a single local administration of cilostazol on neointimal formation in balloon-injured rat carotid artery. Atherosclerosis 1999;142:41–46.
13. Money SR, Herd JA, Isaacsohn JL, et al. Effect of cilostazol on walking distances in patients with intermittent claudication caused by peripheral vascular disease. J Vasc Surg 1998;27:267–274.
14. Dawson DL, Cutler BS, Meissner MH, Strandness DE. Cilostazol has beneficial effects in treatment of intermittent claudication: results from a multicenter, randomized, prospective, double-blind trial. Circulation 1998;98:678–686.
15. Elam MB, Heckman J, Crouse JR, et al. Effect of the novel antiplatelet agent cilostazol on plasma lipoproteins in patients with intermittent claudication. Arterioscler Thromb Vasc Biol 1998;18: 1942–1947.
16. Strandness DE, Dalman R, Panian S, et al. Two doses of cilostazol versus placebo in the treatment of claudication: results of a randomized, multicenter trial. Circulation 1998;98:I–12.
17. Beebe HG, Dawson DL, Cutler BS, et al. A new pharmacological treatment for intermittent claudication: Results of a randomized, multicenter trial. Arch Intern Med 1999;159:2041–2050.

18. Dawson DL, DeMaioribus CA, Hagino RT, et al. The effect of withdrawal of drugs treating intermittent claudication. Am J Surg 1999;178:141–146.

19. Bramer SL, Forbes WP. Effect of hepatic impairment on the pharmacokinetics of a single dose of cilostazol. Clin Pharmacokinet 1999:37(Suppl 2):25–32.

20. Mallikaarjun S, Forbes WP, Bramer SL. Effect of renal impairment on the pharmacokinetics of cilostazol and its metabolites. Clin Pharmacokinet 1999;37(Suppl 2):33–40.

21. Packer M, Carver JR, Rodeheffer RJ, et al. Effect of oral milrinone on mortality in severe congestive heart failure. N Engl J Med 1991;325:1468–1475.

22. Hiatt WR. Medical treatment of claudication: IV: Morbidity of PAD: medical approaches to claudication. In: Hirsh AT, Hiatt WR, eds. An Office-Based Approach to the Diagnosis and Treatment of Peripheral Arterial Disease. Continuing Education Monograph Series from the American Journal of Medicine, Bellemead, NJ: Excerpta Medica, 1999; pp.6–15.

23. Waters KJ, Craxford AD, Chamberlain J. The effect of naftidrofuryl (Praxilene) on intermittent claudication. Br J Surg 1980;67:349–351.

24. Clyne CA, Galland RB, Fox MJ, et al. A controlled trial of naftidrofuryl (Praxilene) in the treatment of intermittent claudication. Br J Surg 1980;67:347–348.

25. Adhoute G, Bacourt F, Barral M, et al. Naftidrofuryl in chronic arterial disease: results of a six month controlled multicenter study using naftidrofuryl tablets 200 mg. Angiology 1986;37:160–169.

26. Adhoute G, Andreassian B, Boccalon H, et al. Treatment of stage II chronic arterial disease of the lower limbs with the serotonergic antagonist naftidrofuryl: results after 6 months of a controlled, multicenter study. J Cardiovasc Pharmacol 1990;16(Suppl 3):S75–S80.

27. Kriessman A, Neiss A. Demonstration of the clinical effectiveness of naftidrofuryl in the intermittent claudication. VASA 1988;24:27–32.

28. Trübestein G, Bohme H, Heidrich H, et al. Naftidrofuryl in chronic arterial disease: results of a controlled multicenter study. Angiology 1984;35:701–708.

29. Moody AP, al-Khaffaf HS, Lehert P, Harris PL, Charlesworth D. An evaluation of patients with severe intermittent claudication and the effect of treatment with naftidrofuryl. J Cardiovasc Pharmacol 1994;23(Suppl 3):S44–S47.

30. Trubestein G, Balzer K, Bisler H, et al. Buflomedil in arterial occlusive disease: results of a controlled multicenter study. Angiology 1984;35:500–505.

31. Pignoli P, Ciccolo F, Villa V, Longo T. Comparative evaluation of bluflomedil and pentoxifylline in patients with peripheral arterial occlusive disease. Curr Ther Res 1985;37:596–606.

32. Chacon-Quevedo A, Eguaras MG, Calleja F, et al. Comparative evaluation of pentoxifylline, buflomedil, and nifedipine in the treatment of intermittent claudication of the lower limbs. Angiology 1994;45:647–653.

33. Brevetti G, Angelini C, Rosa M, et al. Muscle carnitine deficiency in patients with severe peripheral vascular disease. Circulation 1991;84:1490–1495.

34. Hiatt WR, Wolfel EE, Regensteiner JG, Brass EP. Skeletal muscle carnitine metabolism in patients with unilateral peripheral arterial disease. J Appl Physiol 1992;73:346–353.

35. Brevetti G, Chiariello M, Ferulano G, et al. Increases in walking distance in patients with peripheral vascular disease treated with L-carnitine: a double-blind cross-over study. Circulation 1988;77: 767–773.

36. Brevetti G, Perna S, Sabba C, Martone VD, Condorelli M. Superiority of L-propionyl carnitine vs L-carnitine in improving walking capacity in patients with peripheral vascular disease: an acute, intravenous, double-blind, cross-over study. Eur Heart J 1992;13:251–255.

37. Brevetti G, Perna S, Sabba C, Martone VD, Condorelli M. Propionyl-L-carnitine in intermittent claudication: double-blind, placebo-controlled, dose titration, multicenter study. J Am Coll Cardiol 1995; 26:1411–1416.

38. Brevetti G, Diehm C, Lambert D. European multicenter study on propionyl-L-carnitine in intermittent claudication. J Am Coll Cardiol 1999;34:1618.

39. Brevetti G, Perna S, Sabba C, Martone VD, Di Iorio A, Barletta G. Effect of propionyl-L-carnitine on quality of life in intermittent claudication. Am J Cardiol 1997;79:777–780.

40. Hiatt WR. Medical treatment of peripheral arterial disease and claudication. N Engl J Med 2001;344: 1608–1621.

41. The ICAI study group. Prostanoids for chronic critical leg ischemia: a randomized, controlled, open-label trial with prostaglandin E1. Ann Intern Med 1999;130:412–421.

42. Scheffler P, de la Hamette D, Gross J, Mueller H, Schieffer H. Intensive vascular training in stage IIb of peripheral arterial occlusive disease: the additive effects of intravenous prostaglandin E1 or intravenous pentoxifylline during training. Circulation 1994;90:818–822.

43. Belch JJ, Bell PR, Creissen D, et al. Randomized, double-blind, placebo-controlled study evaluating the efficacy and safety of AS-013, a prostaglandin E1 prodrug, in patients with intermittent claudication. Circulation 1997;95:2298–2302.

44. Diehm C, Balzer K, Bisler H, et al. Efficacy of a new prostaglandin E1 regimen in outpatients with severe intermittent claudication: results of a multicenter placebo-controlled double-blind trial. J Vasc Surg 1997;25:537–544.

45. Lièvre M, Morand S, Besse Bi, et al. Oral beraprost sodium, a prostaglandin I_2 analogue, for intermittent claudication: a double-blind, randomized multicenter controlled trial. Circulation 2000;102: 426–431.

46. Schellong SM, Boger RH, Burchert W, et al. Dose-related effect of intravenous l-arginine on muscular blood flow of the calf in patients with peripheral vascular disease: a $H_2^{15}O$ positron emission tomography study. Clin Sci 1997;93:159–165.

47. Boger RH, Bode-Boger SM, Thiele W, et al. Restoring vascular nitric oxide formation by L-arginine improves the symptoms of intermittent claudication in patients with peripheral arterial occlusive disease. J Am Coll Cardiol 1998;32:1336–1344.

48. Maxwell AJ, Anderson B, Cooke JP. Nutritional therapy for peripheral arterial disease: a double-blind, placebo-controlled, randomized trial of HeartBar®. Vasc Med 2000;5:11–19.

49. Baumgartner I, Pieczek A, Manor O, et al. Constitutive expression of phVEGF165 after intramuscular gene transfer promotes collateral vessel development in patients with critical limb ischemia. Circulation 1998;97:1114–1123.

50. Tsurumi Y, Takeshita S, Chen D, et al. Direct intramuscular gene transfer of naked DNA encoding vascular endothelial growth factor augments collateral development and tissue perfusion. Circulation 1996;94:3281–3290.

51. Lazarous DF, Unger EF, Epstein SE, et al. Basic fibroblast growth factor in patients with intermittent claudication: results of a phase I trial. J Am Coll Cardiol 2000;36:1239–1244.

52. Lederman RT. TRAFFIC (Therapeutic Angiogenesis with rFGF-2 for Intermittent Claudication). Presentation at the American College of Cardiology 50th Scientific Session. Progress in Clinical Trials. Clin Cardiol 2001;24:481.

53. Strano A, Fareed J, Sabba C, et al. A double-blind, multicenter, placebo-controlled, dose comparison study of orally administered defibrotide: preliminary results in patients with peripheral arterial disease. Semin Thromb Hemost 1991;17(Suppl 2):228–234.

54. Sabba C, Zupo V, Dina F, Nazzari M, Albano O. A pilot evaluation of the effect of defibrotide in patients affected by peripheral arterial occlusive disease. Int J Clin Pharmacol Ther Toxicol 1988;26: 249–252.

55. Ferrari PA. Defibrotide versus placebo in the treatment of intermittent claudication: a meta-analysis. Drug Invest 1994;7:157–160.

56. Coffman JD. Drug therapy: vasodilator drugs in peripheral vascular disease. N Engl J Med 1979;300: 713–717.

57. Bagger JP, Helligsoe P, Randsbaek F, Kimose HH, Jensen BS. Effect of verapamil in intermittent claudication: a randomized, double-blind, placebo–controlled, cross-over study after individual dose-response assessment. Circulation 1997;95:411–414.

58. Libretti A, Catalano M. Treatment of claudication with dipyridamole and aspirin. Int J Clin Pharm Res 1986;6:59–60.

59. Giansante C, Calabrese S, Fisicaro M, Fiotti N, Mitri E. Treatment of intermittent claudication with antiplatelet agents. J Int Med Res 1990;18:400–407.

60. Balsano F, Coccheri S, Libretti A, et al. Ticlopidine in the treatment of intermittent claudication: a 21-month double-blind trial. J Lab Clin Med 1989;114:84–91.

61. Arcan JC, Panak E. Ticlopidine in the treatment of peripheral occlusive arterial disease. Semin Thromb Hemost 1989;15:167–170.

62. Jackson MR, Clagett GP. Antithrombotic therapy in peripheral arterial occlusive disease. Chest 2001;119(Suppl):283S–299S.

63. Hamilton M, Wilson GM, Armitage P, Boyd JT. The treatment of intermittent claudication with vitamin E. Lancet 1953;1:367–370.

64. Livingstone PD, Jones C. Treatment of intermittent claudication with vitamin E. Lancet 1958;2: 602–604.
65. Tornwall M, Virtamo J, Haukka JK, et al. Effect of alpha-tocopherol (vitamin E) and beta-carotene supplementation on the incidence of intermittent claudication in male smokers. Arterioscler Thromb Vasc Biol 1997;17:3475–3480.
66. The Heart Outcome Prevention Evaluation Study Investigators. Vitamin E supplementation and cardiovascular events in high-risk patients. N Engl J Med 2000;342:154–160.
67. De Cree J, Leempoels J, Geukens H, Verhaegen H. Placebo-controlled double-blind trial of ketanserin in treatment of intermittent claudication. Lancet 1984;2:775–779.
68. Thulesius O, Lundvall J, Kroese A, et al. Ketanserin in intermittent claudication: effect on walking distance, blood pressure, and cardiovascular complications. J Cardiovasc Pharmacol 1987;9:728–733.
69. Clement DL, Duprez D. Effect of ketanserin in the treatment of patients with intermittent claudication: results from 13 placebo-controlled parallel group studies. J Cardiovasc Pharmacol 1987;10(Suppl 3):S89–S95.
70. Prevention of Atherosclerotic Complications with Ketanserin Trial Group. Prevention of atherosclerotic complications: controlled trial of ketanserin. Br Med J 1989;298:424–430.
71. PACK Claudication Substudy. Randomized placebo-controlled, double-blind trial of ketanserin in claudicants. Changes in claudication distance and ankle systolic pressure. Circulation 1989;80: 1544–1548.
72. Kiesewetter H, Blume J, Jung F, Spitzer S, Wenzel E. Haemodilution with medium molecular weight hydroxyethyl starch in patients with peripheral arterial occlusive disease stage IIb. J Intern Med 1990;227:107–114.
73. Ernst E, Kollar L, Matrai A. A double-blind trial of dextran-haemodilution vs. placebo in claudicants. J Intern Med 1990;227:19–24.
74. Sloth-Nielsen J, Guldager B, Mouritzen C, et al. Arteriographic findings in EDTA chelation therapy on peripheral arteriosclerosis. Am J Surg 1991;162:122–125.
75. Guldager B, Jelnes R, Jorgensen SJ, et al. EDTA treatment of intermittent claudication: a double-blind, placebo-controlled study. J Intern Med 1992;231:261–267.
76. Donald JF. A mulitcenter general practice study of cinnarizine in the treatment of peripheral vascular disease. J Int Med Res 1979;7:502–506.
77. Picano E, Testa R, Pogliani M, Lattanzi F, Gaudio V, L'Abbate A. Increase of walking capacity after acute aminophylline administration in intermittent claudication. Angiology 1989;40:1035–1039.
78. Kiff RS, Quick CRG. Does inositol nicotinate (hexapol) influence intermittent claudication? A controlled trial. Br J Clin Pract 1988;42:141–145.
79. Price JF, Leng GC. Steroid sex hormones for lower limb atherosclerosis. Cochrane Data Syst Rev 2000:CD000188.
80. Mannarino E, Pasqualini L, Innocente S, et al. Efficacy of low-molecular-weight heparin in the management of intermittent claudication. Angiology 1991;42:1–7.
81. Pittler MH, Ernst E. Ginkgo biloba extract for the treatment of intermittent claudication: a meta-analysis of randomized trials. Am J Med 2000;108:276–81.

11

Angiogenesis and Gene Therapy

Iris Baumgartner, MD and
Jeffrey M. Isner, MD

Contents

INTRODUCTION

Angiogenic growth factors constitute a potentially novel form of therapy for patients with ischemic vascular disease. The feasibility of using recombinant formulations of angiogenic growth factors to augment collateral artery development by stimulation of capillary growth in animal models of myocardial and hind limb ischemia has now been well established. This novel strategy for the treatment of vascular insufficiency, depicted schematically for peripheral vascular disease in Fig. 1, has been termed *therapeutic angiogenesis*. Studies have suggested that three angiogenic growth factors in particular—acidic fibroblast growth factor (aFGF), basic fibroblast growth factor (bFGF), and vascular endothelial growth factor (VEGF)—are sufficiently potent to merit further investigation. In the case of VEGF and aFGF, bioavailability and meaningful angiogenic bioactivity were also shown to be achievable by intramuscular gene transfer, with clinical phase I trials in patients with chronic critical limb ischemia (CLI) cautiously interpreted to support both the strategy of somatic gene therapy and the concept of therapeutic angiogenesis.

VASCULAR DEVELOPMENT

Vascular development can be categorized into vasculogenesis, angiogenesis, and arteriogenesis. Vasculogenesis is confined to the embryonic phase of development and consists of the initial process of *in situ* differentiation of endothelial cells from mesodermal

From: *Contemporary Cardiology: Peripheral Arterial Disease: Diagnosis and Treatment*
Edited by: J. D. Coffman and R. T. Eberhardt © Humana Press Inc., Totowa, NJ

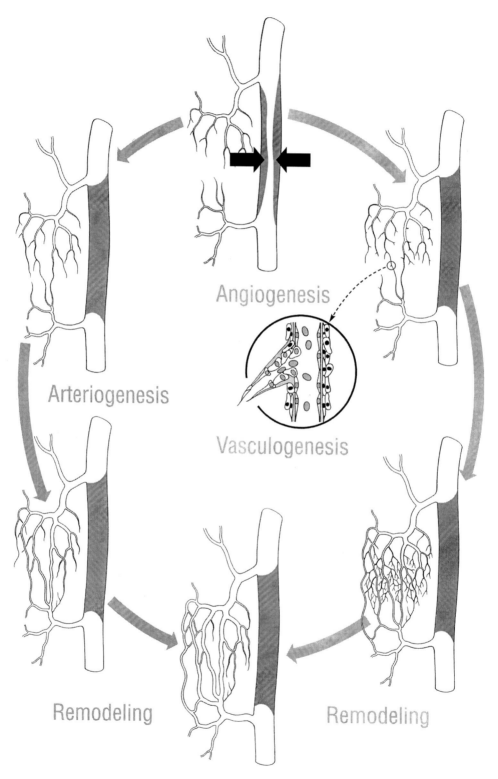

Fig. 1. Schematic depiction of postnatal vasculogenesis, angiogenesis, and arteriogenesis linked to each other.

precursors (angioblasts), and their subsequent organization into a primary capillary plexus *(1)*. VEGF and its receptor Flk-1/KDR seem to have a key function emphasized by the fact that removal of their genes is lethal early in embryogenesis in animals heterozygous for the mutation *(2)*. After the vascular plexus is formed, endothelial cells form new capillaries by sprouting from their vessel of origin in a process termed *angiogenesis*. This process, in which endothelial cells from a quiescent, nonproliferative microvasculature with a turnover of thousands of days are activated to undergo rapid proliferation and migration *(3)*, can be initiated by a variety of cytokines. Families of angiogenic growth factors investigated most extensively are VEGF and FGF *(4)*. Other cytokines in or near the blood vessel wall involved in the process of angiogenesis include transforming growth factor (TGF)-α, hepatocyte growth factor (HGF), and in microvascular endothelial cells, platelet-derived growth factor (PDGF), each interacting with specific receptors on the endothelial and/or smooth muscle cell surface. Recent discovery of angiopoietin-1, which mediates recruitment of vascular smooth muscle cells by developing vessels, and of angiopoietin-2, which counteracts angiopoietin-1, will also need to be included in future models of vessel formation and remodeling *(5,6)*.

Formation of new capillaries by sprouting from existing capillaries or venules occurs in a series of steps. Stationary, nonproliferative endothelial cells of the vascular intima are activated by cytokines, followed by release of extracellular proteinases (plasminogen activators, metalloproteinases) required to degrade basement membrane and matrix constituents underlying the endothelium. Thereafter, endothelial cells actually migrate, reattach, and proliferate beyond the vessel of origin. The newly originated column of endothelial cells lengthens, forms a three-dimensional tubular structure (branch), and individual branches fuse to loops through which blood can flow. Loops generate new sprouts and the process is repeated until a network of new capillaries is formed, which is capped and inactivated by reciprocal interaction with pericytes *(7)*. For vessels larger than capillaries, vascular smooth muscle cells must migrate as well. Pericytes and smooth muscle cells are attracted by chemotactic factors upregulated in association with an active capillary sprouting (i.e., PDGF-BB, angiopoietin-1, degraded extracellular matrix). Intra- and extraluminal factors are involved in further modification of blood vessels, which can mature or regress along with demands of the tissue or organs they supply.

THERAPEUTIC ANGIOGENESIS

Nature has created mechanisms to partially adapt to regional ischemia through compensatory development of a functional collateral circulation, which is driven by angiogenic factors (Fig. 2). Main components involved are *arteriogenesis*, the *in situ* enlargement of preexisting arterioles and arteries into larger sized muscular arteries *(8)*, and *angiogenesis*, the formation of new capillary networks by capillary sprouting, intussusception, and pruning from existing parent vessels. Hypoxia is generally considered to represent a fundamental stimulus for angiogenesis, although angiogenesis can occur in areas with normal oxygen tension. Arteriogenesis, in contrast, is dependent on a pressure gradient with resultant increase of flow and shear stress. Hence, angiogenesis can affect arteriogenesis by enlargement of the vascular bed and reduction of vascular resistance distal to an obstruction. In any case, it is true that collaterals develop by either pathway only when angiogenic growth factors are present and their receptors are expressed.

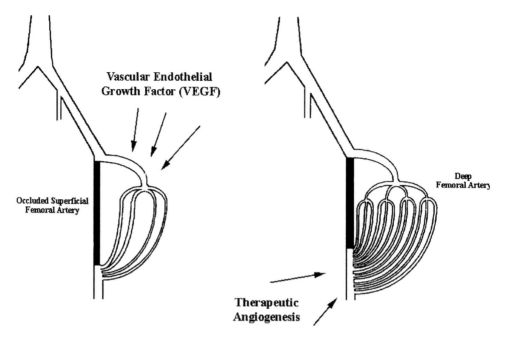

Fig. 2. Collateral vessel development in the peripheral circulation.

The adaptive development of collaterals, however, is rather slow and often unable to compensate fully for the effects of ischemia. Why the collateral flow does not usually increase to the point that it can restore normal flow is not clear; it may result from a combination of time lag of collateral development in case of rapid progression of the occlusive process, and either insufficient local generation of necessary cytokines or other factors needed for angiogenesis to occur, or perhaps a decreased responsiveness of endothelial cells to growth factors involved in neovascularization *(9)*. At least in a subset of patients it seems logical to supply angiogenic growth factors. This novel strategy for the treatment of vascular insufficiency has been termed therapeutic angiogenesis and has been demonstrated for recombinant formulations of aFGF, bFGF, and VEGF in animal models of myocardial and hindlimb ischemia, respectively *(10–13)*.

VASCULAR ENDOTHELIAL GROWTH FACTOR (A SECRETED, ENDOTHELIAL CELL SPECIFIC MITOGEN)

VEGF (or VEGF-A) was discovered in the early 1980s by Dvorak and co-workers as a factor that made blood vessels "leaky"; hence, it was given the name vascular permeability factor *(14)*. Then in the late 1980s, several groups showed that VEGF stimulated endothelial cell migration and replication, and was a potent angiogenic factor in vivo *(15)*. VEGF differs from other angiogenic growth factors by some features. First, high-affinity binding sites (Flk-1/KDR) are restricted to endothelial cells, making the direct proliferative action of VEGF endothelial cell specific *(16)*. Second, in contrast to other growth factors, the gene possesses a secretory signal sequence, so that the protein is naturally secreted by intact cells *(17)*. Third, expression of VEGF and its receptors KDR/Flk-1 and Flt-1 are highly regulated by hypoxia, providing a physiological feedback mechanism to accommodate the angiogenic effect to tissue oxygenation. Mechanisms of hypoxia-mediated regulation have been unraveled recently. Analogous to other hypoxia-inducible genes, the VEGF gene has a hypoxia recognition site (hypoxia inducible factor, HIF-1) in its promoter *(18)*. Furthermore, mRNA stability is increased under hypoxic conditions (posttranscriptional regulation) *(19)*, and the KDR/Flk-I receptor is upregulated in response to factors released from hypoxic tissues *(20,21)*.

Evidence that VEGF stimulates angiogenesis in vivo had been developed in experiments performed on rat and rabbit cornea, the chorioallantoic membrane, and the rabbit bone graft model. The concept that the angiogenic activity of VEGF is sufficiently potent to achieve augmented neovascularization in ischemic tissues was established using a rabbit ischemic hind limb model (the inferior epigastric, deep femoral, lateral circumflex, and superficial epigastric arteries ligated and the femoral artery completely excised). In these experiments physiological evidence of an increased downstream perfusion was documented by serial measurements of the lower limb blood pressure ratio (ischemic/nonischemic limb). The pressure ratio was significantly greater in animals receiving VEGF compared to controls (0.75 ± 0.14 vs 0.48 ± 0.19, $p < 0.05$), consistent with the stimulation of more mature collaterals. Direct anatomic evidence of an augmented collateral circulation was demonstrated by the increased number of angiographically visible collaterals 10 and 30 d after VEGF administration. Complementary flow studies (intraarterial flow wire measurements) provided proof of an increase in maximum blood flow *(22)* and restored vasoreactivity *(23)*. Necropsy examination showed a significant higher capillary density in ischemic muscles and increased endothelial cell proliferative activity *(24)*, consistent with the classic definition of angiogenesis. Despite the fact that the mitogenic effects of VEGF previously have been shown to be limited to endothelial cells, the proliferative activity of smooth muscle cells in small sized so-called midzone collaterals was also increased. The ability to induce vascular permeability is a well-known feature of VEGF, responsible in fact for its alternate designation as vascular permeability factor. It is possible that extravasation of certain antigenic growth factors from circulating blood might result in activation of smooth muscle cell proliferation. Endothelial cells stimulated by VEGF may secrete factor(s) that promote smooth muscle proliferation. VEGF-induced chemotaxis of monocytes (Flt-1 receptor) represents another source of growth factor secretion stimulating smooth muscle cell proliferation *(25)*, and recent studies have documented direct effects of VEGF on smooth muscle cells (Flt-1 receptor) *(26)*.

The fact that the VEGF gene encodes a secretory signal sequence was more recently exploited as part of a strategy designed to accomplish therapeutic angiogenesis by somatic gene transfer. Gene products that are secreted may have profound paracrine effects, even when the number of transduced cells remains low. In contrast, for genes such as FGFs, which do not encode a secretory signal sequence, transfection of a much larger cell population might be required for that intracellular gene product to express its biological effects *(27)*. The first technique tested was arterial gene transfer using naked plasmid DNA encoding VEGF driven by a cytomegalovirus promoter (phVEGF$_{165}$). For delivery a hydrogel-coated standard angioplasty balloon was utilized (28). The polymer surface of the balloon acts like a sponge onto which concentrated DNA can be applied ex vivo, and subsequently be delivered into the vessel wall at the time of inflation (Fig. 3). Site-specific transfection of phVEGF$_{165}$ was confirmed by analysis of transfected arteries using the reverse transcriptase-polymerase chain reaction *(29)*. Arterial gene transfer

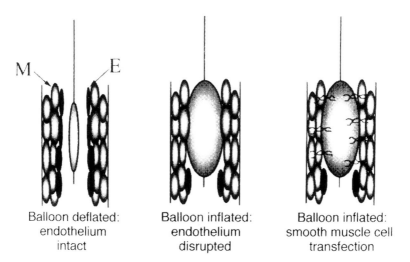

Balloon deflated: endothelium intact

Balloon inflated: endothelium disrupted

Balloon inflated: smooth muscle cell transfection

Fig. 3. Intraarterial gene transfer.

was followed by testing intramuscular gene transfer. Wolff and colleagues *(30)* demonstrated evidence of transgene expression with direct intramuscular injection of nonviral, covalently closed plasmid DNA. In the rabbit hind limb model, intramuscular injection of phVEGF$_{165}$ into ischemic muscles showed a significantly augmented development of collateral vessels compared to control animals documented by serial angiograms in vivo and increased capillary density at necropsy. Amelioration of the hemodynamic deficit in the ischemic limb was shown by improvement in the limb blood pressure ratio in VEGF-transfected animals (0.70 ± 0.08) vs controls (0.50 ± 0.18, $p < 0.05$). Regarding the therapeutic target, it has been demonstrated that VEGF-induced angiogenesis is not indiscriminative or widespread but rather restricted to sites of ischemia *(31)*.

At least four isoforms—VEGF$_{121}$, VEGF$_{165}$, VEGF$_{189}$, and VEGF$_{206}$—have been identified and shown to result from alternative splicing of the VEGF transcript. These isoforms all share the important biological property of mitogenicity for endothelial cells, but differ markedly in solubility: the longer the isoform, the more basic amino acid residues, the greater is the acidity for cell-surface heparan sulfates and proteoglycans of the extracellular matrix. More recently, other VEGF-related factors have been identified: VEGF-B, VEGF-C, and placenta growth factor. VEGF-C was initially characterized by its lymphangiogenic potency induced by autophosphorylation of the tyrosine kinase receptor Flt-4 located on lymphatic cells. A VEGF-C signaling pathway via the endothelial cell specific receptor Flk-1 was documented by Joukov and colleagues *(32)* and stimulation of endothelial cell migration in vitro as well as augmented angiogenesis in vivo was shown by Witzenbichler and colleagues *(33)*.

GENE TRANSFER VS RECOMBINANT PROTEIN

Despite encouraging results with recombinant protein, it can be argued that transferring the gene encoding the protein is a better choice. Perhaps most notably, gene transfer offers the potential advantage of a reservoir of continuous protein synthesis; the gene provides a concentrated amount of protein in a relatively low dose at the site where it is needed. It may be preferable to deliver a low dose of an angiogenic growth factor over a period of several days from an actively expressing gene rather than from a single, high-dose intraarterial bolus of recombinant protein. Clearly, further clinical investigation of both recombinant protein and alternative dosing regimens for gene therapy will be necessary to define the optimal therapeutic strategy. It remains to be seen whether the slow-release aspect of gene therapy, administered in site-specific manner and concentrated according to local pathology, will produce outcomes superior to those achieved with bolus or continuous intraarterial administration of recombinant protein.

MOLECULAR AND MECHANICAL ASPECTS OF GENE THERAPY

The use of gene transfer as a potential therapeutic approach represents a rapidly emerging field of basic and applied medical research, which has recently matured into clinical trials for a substantial variety of inherited as well as acquired diseases. The field of cardiovascular medicine is no exception to this. The goal of gene transfer is protein expression, a process brought about by the insertion of a gene coding for a protein into target cells resulting in synthesis of the protein. The use of viral vectors is based on the fact that viruses have evolved highly efficient mechanisms to transfer their genetic material to target cells (34) and both DNA and RNA recombinant viruses have been employed. Viral-based systems are more efficient to transfect target cells compared to plasmid-based systems. However, they have general limitations: restricted size of the inserted gene due to packaging constraints, potential tumorigenesis (e.g., retroviruses), potential for insertional mutagenesis (greater than in plasmid-based systems), potential immunogenicity (e.g., adenoviruses), and quality control considerations. Effective plasmid-based approaches must provide mechanisms to accomplish what viruses do by nature: target the desired host, penetrate the cell membrane, pass through the cytoplasm avoiding degradation, and enter the nucleus and be translated into a functional protein. Plasmid expression vectors contain the gene of interest, and a transcriptional promoter, as well as sequences that impart stability and functionality to the mRNA. Promoters such as cytomegalovirus or the Rous sarcoma virus promoter are mostly used to turn on transcription of DNA to mRNA. The desired gene can be transfected into mammalian cells grown in culture (ex vivo), with reintroduction of modified cells to the host after transfer of foreign DNA, or gene transfer can be achieved in vivo by transfection of cells in the intact host. No single delivery system is likely to be universally appropriate, as the optimal treatment for each disease is different. The delivery method selected will depend, in part, on the proportion of cells to be transfected, and the cell type and location. Current methodologies are divided among three distinct categories: physical (direct injection, electroporation), chemical (liposomes, receptor-mediated endocytosis), and biological (viral vectors). Most recent developments combine both cytotoxic and cytostatic gene transfer strategies to modify cell growth in arterial injury models using local catheter-based delivery systems; however, clinical feasibility and safety studies are necessary.

CLINICAL TRIALS IN PATIENTS WITH CLI

VEGF

Striking advantages of VEGF gene transfer in particular were its confinement to the target organ, with minimal expression of the transgene in other organs, and low systemic effect due to a half-life of a few minutes in the circulation (35). In 1994, the first clinical

Table 1
Clinical Therapeutic Angiogenesis Trials in Peripheral Arterial Occlusive Disease

Treatment specification	Application	Dose	No. of patients	Reference
Plasmid DNA VEGF$_{165}$	Intraarterial	100–1000 µg	12	37,38
Plasmid DNA VEGF$_{165}$	Intramuscular	200–8000 µg[b]	51	38–40
Plasmid DNA VEGF-C	Intramuscular	200–8000 µg	31 (43)	Unpublished
Plasmid DNA acidic FGF	Intramuscular	500–4000 µg	51	47
Recombinant basic FGF	Intraarterial	1 × 10 µg/kg and 2 × 30 µg/kg	13 (19)	49
Recombinant basic FGF	Intraarterial	1 × 30 µg/kg and 2 × 30 µg/kg	128 (190)	48

[a]including placebo controls.
[b]One patient with bilateral gene transfer, each limb was injected with 4000 µg of phVEGF$_{165}$.

trial of human gene therapy involving percutaneous arterial gene transfer of phVEGF$_{165}$ was initiated. This was a prospective, nonrandomized, open phase I trial for patients with CLI *(36)*. Although surgical or endovascular revascularization offers relief in the majority of these patients, there is still a considerable portion in whom the anatomic extent and distribution of arterial obstructions prohibit such procedures; lack of available medical therapy implies that many of them face amputation *(37)*.

As tested in preclinical studies, plasmid DNA encoding VEGF$_{165}$ was applied to the hydrogel coating of a standard angioplasty balloon covered with a sheath to prevent washoff of the genetic material. Under fluoroscopic guidance, the balloon was subsequently advanced and inflated within an artery supplying the ischemic limb. Dose-escalating treatment was initiated with 100 µg of phVEGF$_{165}$. Three patients presenting with rest pain and treated with 1000 µg were subsequently shown at 1-yr follow-up to have improved blood flow to the ischemic limb and remained free of rest pain *(unpublished data)*. With the increase in dose of phVEGF$_{165}$ to 2000 µg, the first evidence of new blood vessel formation became apparent *(38,39)*. One month after treatment angiography revealed newly visible vessels at the calf level. Angiogenesis was even apparent by clinical inspection, for one patient developed three spider angiomas over the ankle and forefoot. However, it was considered that low, unreliable transfection efficiency would occur in atherosclerotic, calcified arteries, and there is also the potential risk of arterial injury at the site of transfection. Therefore, the administration technique was changed in a second clinical trial. Treatment was performed at the patients bedside, injecting the plasmid DNA solution directly into ischemic muscles of the affected limbs (Fig. 4). There were 51 patients with 55 critically ischemic limbs treated. For therapeutic use, four aliquots, each consisting of 500–4000 µg of naked plasmid DNA, were injected using a 27-gauge needle. The identical treatment was repeated 4 wk later *(40)*. Gene expression at the protein level was documented by a transient peak of VEGF serum levels 1–3 wk after each treatment (enzyme-linked immunosorbent assay [ELISA]). Ankle or toe brachial artery systolic pressure index increased from 0.33 at baseline to 0.48 at 12 wk follow-up and serial angiograms at 4, 8, and 16 wk showed newly visible small sized (200–800 µm) collateral vessels (Fig. 5). These promising hemodynamic and angiographic findings correlated with clinical improvement. In the 55 limbs followed for a mean of 19 mo after treatment,

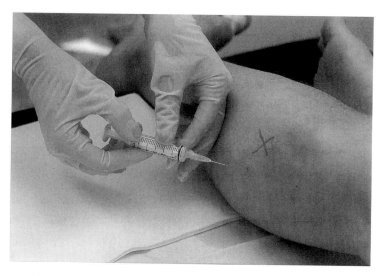

Fig. 4. Intramuscular gene therapy in chronic critical limb ischemia.

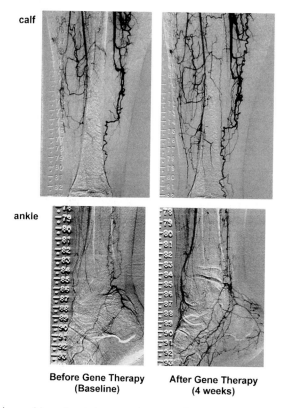

calf

ankle

Before Gene Therapy
(Baseline)

After Gene Therapy
(4 weeks)

Fig. 5. Serial angiographies after intramuscular gene therapy using phVEGF$_{165}$ showing small sized newly visible collateral networks at the ankle level.

rest pain resolved in 13 of 14 limbs and gangrene healed or showed considerable improvement in 26 of 41 limbs. Limb salvage occurred in 87% of patients with unreconstructable CLI (*unpublished data*). Despite below knee amputation in seven patients with intractable pain or infectious complications, results were promising compared to historic controls *(41)*. Complications were limited to transient lower extremity edema, consistent with VEGF-enhancement of vascular permeability; the edema was aggressively and successfully treated with diuretics *(42)*.

Although not found in any of the phVEGF$_{165}$-treated patients, all gene therapy designed to potentiate local angiogenesis carries the theoretical risk of potentiation of angiogenesis-driven diseases such as diabetic retinopathy *(43)* or tumor angiogenesis *(44)*. It should be noted, however, that previous laboratory studies have established that VEGF expression did not lead to malignant proliferation or metastasis, a finding in agreement with the notion that stimulation of angiogenesis is necessary but not sufficient for malignant growth *(45)*. There remains the question of whether atherosclerotic plaque neovascularization may be exacerbated by angiogenic therapy *(46)*.

It should be noted that at least three mechanisms can explain the angiogenic effect of VEGF seen in patients. Because VEGF is mitogenic in vitro, the most obvious explanation is that the angiogenic effect in vivo was achieved via a similar mechanism, that is, from proliferation and migration of endothelial cells followed by formation of new blood vessels. Another possibility is recruitment of preexisting collateral blood vessels rather than *de novo* vessel formation. The importance of this distinction is emphasized further by the different stimuli that may be involved in regulation of arteriogenesis and angiogenesis. Whereas proximal occlusion of a limb artery leads to ischemia distally, angiographically observed collaterals frequently develop or are visible around the site of occlusion in a territory that itself is not ischemic. Finally, VEGF improves vasomotor function of large and small arteries of animals with chronic ischemia.

FGF

Another open-labeled clinical phase I trial in chronic CLI using naked plasmid DNA encoding aFGF was finished in 2001 *(47)*. Based on the identical concept of intramuscular gene therapy as used for phVEGF$_{165}$, 51 patients with unreconstructable CLI were treated with intramuscular injection of plasmid DNA coding aFGF. Overall 75% of patients showed healing or considerable improvement of ischemic tissue lesions. According to the yet unpublished data, there were no safety concerns during short-term 1-yr follow-up. A randomized, double-blinded, placebo-controlled phase II trial is planned to be conducted in Europe and the United States.

The largest, randomized, double blind, placebo-controlled study comparing placebo and single or double dose (30 µg/kg) of recombinant bFGF in patients with moderate to severe intermittent claudication is the TRAFFIC trial *(48)*. Protein was given by intraarterial infusion at d 1, and according to the protocol at d 30. Primary efficacy analysis of peak walking time at 90 d gave a weak but statistically not significant change between groups. Repeat infusion at 30 d was not better than the single dose. There were no serious adverse events associated with the treatment, so that intraarterial infusion of recombinant bFGF appears to be safe, although there was a trend for more proteinuria >300 mg/d (placebo 3, single dose 9, double dose 11 mg%).

SUMMARY

The use of gene transfer or recombinant protein is a new developing field of basic and applied research for vascular insufficiency. An understanding of some of the basic concepts and mechanisms of vasculogenesis, arteriogenesis, and especially angiogenesis established the foundation for this rapidly growing specialty of therapeutic angiogenesis. Several growth factors have been identified, isolated, and characterized. In animal models of hind limb and myocardial ischemia, angiogenic growth factors have been shown to induce capillary growth and collateral development. VEGF, aFGF, and bFGF appear to have the most promise for clinical development. Early clinical trials with these three growth factors in patients with CLI show some evidence of therapeutic benefit. Bioavailability and angiogenic bioactivity by intamuscular gene transfer has been demonstrated in human studies. The best method of administration and transfection needs to be determined; for transfection, viral vectors or the plasmid-based approach needs further study. Intraarterial recombinant protein and intramuscular injection in the ischemic limb both appear of therapeutic benefit but dosing regimes, timing of injections, and the most potent therapeutic growth remain to be determined.

REFERENCES

1. Risau W, Sariola H, Zerwes H-G, Sasse J, Ekblom P, Kemler R. Vasculogenesis and angiogenesis in embryonic stem cell-derived embryoid bodies. Development 1988;102:471–478.
2. Ferrara N, Carver-Moore K, Chen H, Dowd M, LuL, O'Shea Ks. Heterozygous embryonic lethality induced by targeted inactivation of the VEGF gene. Nature 1996;380:439–442.
3. Schaper W, Brahander MD, Lewi P. DNA synthesis and mitoses in coronary collateral vessels of the dog. Circ Res 1971;28:671–679.
4. Klagsbrun M, D'Amore PA. Regulators of angiogenesis. Annu Rev Physiol 1991;53:217–239.
5. Suri C, Jones PF, Patan S. Requisite role of angiopoietin-1, a ligand for the TIE2 receptor, during embryonic angiogenesis. Cell 1996;87:1171–1180.
6. Maisonpierre PC, Suri C, Jones PF, Bartunkova S. Angiopoietin-2, a natural antagonist for Tie2 that disrupts in vivo angiogenesis. Science 1997;277:55–60.
7. Sato Y, Rifkin DB. Inhibition of endothelial cell movement by pericytes and smooth muscle cells: activation of latent tranforming growth factor-beta 1-like molecule by plasmin during co-culture. J Cell Biol 1989;109:309–315.
8. Schaper W. Molecular mechanisms of coronary collateral growth. Circ Res 1996;79:911–919.
9. Waltenberger J, Lange J, Kranz A. Vascular endothelial growth factor A-induced chemotaxis of monocytes is attenuated in patients with diabetes mellitus. Circulation 2000; 102:185–190
10. Baffour R, Berman J, Garb JL, Rhee SW, Kaufman J, Friedmann P. Enhanced angiogenesis and growth of collaterals by in vivo administration of recombinant basic fibroblast growth factor in a rabbit model of acute lower limb ischemia: dose–response effect of basic fibroblast growth factor. J Vasc Surg 1992; 16:181–191.
11. Pu LQ, Sniderman AD, Brassard R, Lachapelle KJ, Graham AM, Lisbona R. Enhanced revascularization of the ischemic limb by means of angiogenic therapy. Circulation 1993;88:208–215.
12. Banai S, Jaklitsch MT, Shou M, et al. Angiogenic-induced enhancement of collateral blood flow to ischemic myocardium by vascular endothelial growth factor in dogs. Circulation 1994;89:2183–2189.
13. Takeshita S, Zheng LP, Asahara T, et al. Therapeutic angiogenesis: a single intra-arterial bolus of vascular endothelial growth factor augments collateral vessel formation in a rabbit ischemic hindlimb. J Clin Invest 1994;93:662–670.
14. Dvorak HF, Brown LF, Detmar M, Dvorak AM. Vascular permeability factor/vascular endothelial growth factor, microvascular hyperpermeability, and angiogenesis. Am J Pathol 1995;146:1029–1039.

15. Thomas KA. Vascular endothelial growth factor, a potent and selective angiogenic agent. J Biol Chem 1996;271:603–606.
16. Klagsbrun M, D'Amore PA. Vascular endothelial growth factor and its receptors. Cytokine Growth Fact Rev 1996;7:2593-#270.
17. Ferrara N, Houck K, Jakeman L, Leung DW. Molecular and biological properties of the vascular endothelial growth factor family of proteins. Endocrinol Rev 1992;13:18–32.
18. Goldberg MA, Schneider TJ. Similarities between the oxygen-sensing mechanisms regulating the expression of vascular endothelial growth factor and erythropoietin. J Biol Chem 1994;269: 4355–4359.
19. Levy PL, Levy NS, Goldberg MA. Post-transcriptional regulation of vascular endothelial growth factor by hypoxia. J Biol Chem 1996;271:2746–2753.
20. Brogi E, Schatteman G, Wu T, et al. Hypoxia-induced paracrine regulation of vascular endothelial growth factor receptor expression. J Clin Invest 1996;97:469–476.
21. Waltenberger J, Mayr U, Pentz S, Hombach V. Functional upregulation of the vascular endothelial growth factor receptor KDR by hypoxia. Circulation 1996;94:1647–1654.
22. Bauters C, Asahara T, Zheng LP, et al. Physiologic assessment of augmented vascularity induced by VEGF in ischemic rabbit hindlimb. Am J Physiol 1994;267:H1263–H1271.
23. Bauters C, Asahara T, Zheng LP, et al. Recovery of disturbed endothelium-dependent flow in the collateral-perfused rabbit ischemic hindlimb after administration of vascular endothelial growth factor. Circulation 1995;91:2802–2809.
24. Takeshita S, Kearney M, Loushin C, et al. In vivo evidence that vascular endothelial growth factor stimulates collateral formation inducing arterial cell proliferation in a rabbit ischemic hindlimb. J Am Coll Cardiol 1994;23:294A. (Abstract)
25. Clauss M, Gerlach M, Gerlach H, et al. Vascular permeability factor: a tumor-derived polypeptide that induces endothelial cell and monocyte procoagulant activity, and promotes monocyte migration. J Exp Med 1990;172:1535–1545.
26. Wang H, Keiser A. Vascular endothelial growth factor upregulates the expression of matrix metalloproteinases in vascular smooth muscle cells. Circ Res 1998; 83:832–840.
27. Losordo DW, Pickering JG, Takeshita S, et al. Use of the rabbit ear artery to serially assess foreign protein secretion after site specific arterial gene transfer in vivo: evidence that anatomic identification of successful gene transfer may underestimate the potential magnitude of transgene expression. Circulation 1994;89:785–792.
28. Riessen R, Rahimizadeh H, Blessing E, Takeshita S, Barry JJ, Isner JM. Arterial gene transfer using pure DNA applied directly to a hydrogel-coated angioplasty balloon. Hum Gene Ther 1993;4:749–758.
29. Takeshita S, Tsurumi Y, Couffinhal T, et al. Gene transfer of naked DNA encoding for three isoforms of vascular endothelial growth factor stimulates collateral development in vivo. Lab Invest 1996;75: 487–501.
30. Wolff JA, Malone RW, Williams P, et al. Direct gene transfer into mouse muscle in vivo. Science 1990;247:1465–1468.
31. Tsurumi Y, Takeshita S, Chen D, et al. Direct intramuscular gene transfer of naked DNA encoding vascular endothelial growth factor augments collateral development and tissue perfusion. Circulation 1996;94:3281–3290.
32. Joukov V, Pajusola K, Kaipainen A, et al. A novel vascular endothelial growth factor, VEGF-C, is a ligand for the Flt4 (VEGFR-3) and KDR (VEGFR-2) receptor tyrosine kinases. EMBO J 1996;15: 290–298.
33. Witzenbichler B, Asahara T, Murohara T, et al. Vascular endothelial growth factor-C (VEGF-C/VEGF-2) promotes angiogenesis in the setting of tissue ischemia. Am J Pathol 1998;153:381–394.
34. Kielian M, Jungerwirth S. Mechanisms of enveloped virus entry into cells. Mol Biol Med 1990;7: 17–31.
35. Isner JM. Therapeutic angiogenesis: a new frontier for vascular therapy. Vasc Med 1996;1:79–87.
36. Isner JM, Walsh K, Symes J, et al. Arterial gene transfer for therapeutic angiogenesis in patients with peripheral artery disease. Hum Gene Ther 1996;7:959–988.
37. European Working Group on Critical Leg Ischemia . Second European consensus document on chronic critical leg ischemia. Circulation 1991;84(Suppl):IV, 26.
38. Isner JM. Arterial gene transfer of naked DNA for therapeutic angiogenesis: early clinical results. Adv Drug Deliv Rev 1998;30:185–197.

39. Isner JM, Pieczek A, Schainfeld R, et al. Clinical evidence of angiogenesis following arterial gene transfer of pnVEGF 165 in a patient with ischemic limb. Lancet 1996;348:370–374.

40. Baumgartner I, Pieczek A, Manor O, et al. Constitutive expression of phVEGF 165 following intramuscular gene transfer promotes collateral vessel development in patients with critical limb ischemia. Circulation 1998;97:1114–1123.

41. Lepantalo M, Matzke S. Outcome of unreconstructed chronic critical leg ischaemia. Eur J Vasc Endovasc Surg 1996;11:153.

42. Baumgartner I, Rauh G, Pieczek A, et al. Lower extremity edema associated with gene transfer of naked DNA encoding vascular endothelial growth factor. Ann Intern Med. 2000;132:880–884.

43. Aiello LP, Avery RL, Arrigg PG, et al. Vascular endothelial growth factor in ocular fluids of patients with diabetic retinopathy and other retinal disorders. N Engl J Med 1994;331:1480–1487.

44. Plate KH, Breier G, Weich HA, Risau W. Vascular endothelial growth factor is a potential tumour angiogenesis factor in human gliomas in vivo. Nature 1992;359:845–848.

45. Ferrara N, Winer J, Burton T, et al. Expression of vascular endothelial growth factor does not promote transformation but confers a growth advantage in vivo to Chinese hamster ovary cells. J Clin Invest 1993;91:160–170.

46. Pickering JG, Weir l, Jekanowski J, Kearney MA, Isner JM. Proliferative activity in peripheral and coronary atherosclerotic plaque among patients undergoing percutaneous revascularization. J Clin Invest 1993;91:1469–1480.

47. Comerota AJ, Throm RC, Strandness E, et al. A phase I clinical study to evaluate safety and biological activity of NV1FGF (human FGF1 expression plasmid) in patients with severe peripheral arterial occlusive disease. Molecular Therapy 2000; Abstracts of Scientific Presentations. The Third Annual Meeting of the American Society of Gene Therapy. Abstract 548.

48. Lederman RT. TRAFFIC (Therapeutic Angiogenesis with rFGF-2 for Intermittent Claudication). Presentation at the American College of Cardiology 50th Scientific Session. Progress in Clinical Trials. Clin Cardiol 2001;24:481.

49. Lazarous DF, Unger EF, Epstein SE, et al. Basic fibroblast growth factor in patients with intermittent claudication: results of a phase I trial. J Am Coll Cardiol 2000;36:1239–1244.

12 Endovascular Therapy

Christopher J. White, MD

CONTENTS

INTRODUCTION

The first report of "endovascular therapy" for peripheral arterial disease (PAD) was by Dr. Charles Dotter in 1964 *(1)*. In 1974, Dr. Andreas Gruentzig developed a balloon catheter for dilation of vascular lesions *(2)*. Currently, percutaneous transluminal angioplasty (PTA) employs a wide variety of devices ranging from metal stents to endovascular radiation devices for restenosis and is recognized as a safe and effective alternative to surgery for selected patients. Endovascular therapy offers several distinct advantages over surgical revascularization for selected peripheral vascular lesions *(3–5)*. It may be performed with local anesthesia, enabling the treatment of patients who are at high risk for general anesthesia. The morbidity and mortality from endovascular therapy is very low when compared to surgical revascularization. Problems secondary to angioplasty are generally related to vascular access. Following endovascular therapy patients are usually ambulatory on the day of treatment, and unlike the situation after vascular surgery can often return to normal activity within 24–48 h of an uncomplicated procedure. Finally, endovascular therapies may be repeated if necessary, generally without increased difficulty or increased patient risk compared to the first procedure, and prior angioplasty does not usually preclude surgery if required at a later date.

SUPRACLAVICULAR ENDOVASCULAR THERAPIES

Subclavian Artery Intervention

The treatment of subclavian or innominate artery stenosis is a major concern to the physician caring for patients with internal mammary artery coronary bypass grafts,

From: *Contemporary Cardiology: Peripheral Arterial Disease: Diagnosis and Treatment*
Edited by: J. D. Coffman and R. T. Eberhardt © Humana Press Inc., Totowa, NJ

which are jeopardized by proximal subclavian stenoses. Significant subclavian stenosis may cause a subclavian steal syndrome resulting in coronary ischemia in a patient with an internal mammary artery coronary bypass graft, symptoms of vertebrobasilar insufficiency, or upper extremity claudication.

The primary surgical treatment for symptomatic subclavian stenosis is carotid to subclavian artery bypass. Although the immediate clinical success with surgical revascularization is good, complication rates are significant, averaging 13% including stroke in 3% and death in 2% (6–8). Recent data suggest that endovascular therapy with stent placement is preferable to surgery in most patients with symptomatic subclavian and innominate stenosis (8,9).

Our multicenter trial of 245 patients undergoing subclavian artery intervention from six centers reported an overall success rate of 98.5%, with a major complication rate of 1% (10). The clinical symptoms are shown in Table 1. The pressure gradient across the stenoses was reduced from 52.5 mmHg to 3.1 mmHg ($p < 0.01$) (Fig. 1). After almost 2 yr of follow-up, the primary patency rate was 89% and the secondary patency rate was 98.5%.

Peripheral vascular stenting of aortic arch vessel disease is at least as efficacious as surgical procedures with less morbidity and mortality. The long-term patency and symptomatic improvement of subclavian lesions are excellent, which makes endovascular therapy with stent placement the treatment of choice in centers with experienced interventionalists.

Carotid Artery Intervention

Carotid artery stent placement is a promising technique for stroke prevention (Fig. 2). When compared to surgical endarterectomy, the "gold standard," percutaneous therapy has the potential to be safer, less traumatic, and more cost effective. In addition, percutaneous therapy has the advantage of treating patients at increased surgical risk of complications and is not limited to the cervical portion of the carotid artery. Target event rates for 30-d stroke and death rates are approx 6% for symptomatic patients and 3% for asymptomatic patients based on randomized surgical trials.

The largest single center series of carotid stents published to date is from Roubin and colleagues who recently reported the 5-yr results for 528 patients and 604 vessels treated with carotid stenting (11). They found an excellent outcome in both symptomatic and asymptomatic patients with an overall 30-d stroke and death rate of 7.4% (Table 2). Of interest the highest risk group of patients were those over 80 yr of age (Table 3).

Patients with extracranial carotid artery disease who require cardiac surgery are difficult management problems due to the increased risk of stroke complicating coronary bypass surgery. Waigand and colleagues treated 53 carotid arteries with ≥ 70% carotid stenoses in 50 patients who were scheduled for coronary bypass surgery or high-risk coronary angioplasty (12). The majority (72%) of the patients had asymptomatic carotid lesions. Periprocedural stroke and death occurred in one (2%) patient. None had a neurological event associated with coronary revascularization. At a mean follow-up of 10 mo, there have been no major strokes or neurological deaths. Recurrent stenosis was seen in 3 of 46 (6.5%) carotid arteries that were treated successfully with balloon angioplasty. One patient had asymptomatic compression of a balloon expandable stent. The authors concluded that carotid stenting was a reasonable and safe alternative to combined carotid and coronary surgery in patients with severe coronary disease.

Table 1
Frequency of Indications for Subclavian artery Stent Placement

Indications	Frequency
Arm claudication	42.6%
Subclavian steal	25.0%
Compromised LIMA graft	23.6%
Vascular access	15.0%
Other	6.7%

Data as obtained for 245 patients reported by Jain SP et al. JACC 1998;31:63A *(10)*.

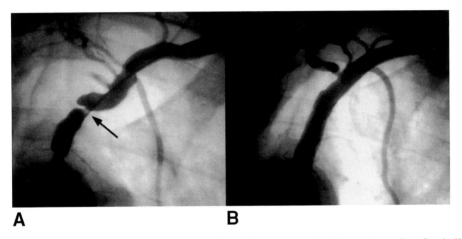

Fig. 1. (A) Baseline angiogram of proximal left subclavian stenosis. **(B)** Angiography after balloon expandable stent placement. Note the brisk antegrade filling of vertebral artery.

The results of CAVATAS (Carotid And Vertebral Artery Transluminal Angioplasty Study), a randomized trial of carotid intervention versus surgery, have reported favorable results *(13)*. A total of 504 patients were randomized to either carotid endarterectomy (*n* = 253) or carotid angioplasty (*n* = 251) between 1992 and 1997. The majority of the patients (96%) had recently symptomatic lesions. Only 26% of the angioplasty patients received a bailout carotid stent for a failed angioplasty result, the remainder were treated with balloon angioplasty alone. The 30-d endpoint of disabling stroke or death showed no difference between the angioplasty arm (10%) or the surgical arm (9.9%). The surgical event rate (9.9%, 95% CI 6.2–13.6%) overlapped with the results of the European Carotid Surgery Trial (7.0%, 95% CI 5.8–8.1%) and the North American Symptomatic Carotid Endarterectomy Trial (6.5%, 95% CI 5.2–7.8%).

Complications of cranial nerve injury and myocardial ischemia were reported only in the surgical group. Long-term follow-up has shown no difference in neurological events between the groups. The authors concluded that angioplasty and surgery were equivalent for safety and efficacy but the angioplasty group experienced less procedural morbidity.

Currently, in centers with experienced interventionalists, carotid stenting can be recommended as the treatment of choice for selected high-risk or unfavorable carotid endarterectomy candidates (Table 4). The target event (30-d stroke and death) rates should be below 6% for symptomatic patients and 3% for asymptomatic patients.

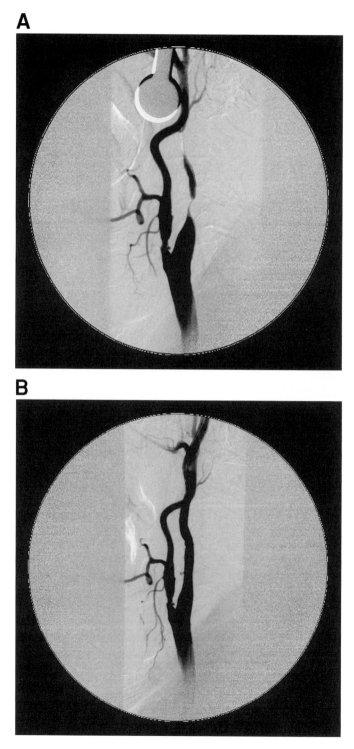

Fig. 2. (A) Baseline carotid angiogram with critical stenosis of the right internal carotid artery. **(B)** Angiogram demonstrating resolution of the stenosis following self-expanding stent placement.

Table 2
Complications at 30 d for Carotid Artery Stent Placement

Event	Rate
Stroke and death	7.4%
Major stroke	1.0%
Minor stroke	4.8%
Death	1.6%

Data from 604 vessels as reported by Roubin GS et al. Circulation 2001;103:532 *(11)*.

Table 3
Age-Dependent Risk of Stroke at 30 d in Elderly Patients with Carotid Artery Stent Placement

	< 80 yr old	≥ 80 yr old	p Value
Major stroke	0.4%	5.0%	< 0.001
Stroke and death	6.0%	16.0%	< 0.01

Data as reported by Roubin GS et al. Circulation 2001;103:532 *(11)*.

Table 4
Carotid Stent Indications

Increased surgical risk:
  Medical comorbidity
  Repeat endarterectomy
  Contralateral carotid occlusion
  Age ≥ 80 yr

Difficult surgical access:
  High cervical lesion
  Intrathoracic lesion
  Prior radiation therapy or radical neck surgery

Carotid stenting is contraindicated in patients with angiographic evidence of intravascular thrombi or filling defects, and in centers where neurovascular rescue is not available. Relative contraindications include severe aortic arch vessel tortuosity and inability to dilate the lesion due to calcification.

Devices to minimize the risk of distal embolization, presumably the major cause of procedure-related strokes, are currently undergoing clinical trials. The devices are designed to limit, or prevent, the number and size of particles that are released from carotid atherosclerotic disease during angioplasty and/or stenting. There are three classes of device including distal occlusion ballons, proximal occlusion balloons, and filters. Each device has theoretical benefits and limitations. At the present time, there is not enough clinical information to prefer one strategy or device over another. As data become available, operators will be able to risk stratify their patients to further enhance the safety of the procedure.

Vertebral Artery Intervention

It is well known that ligature of one of the two vertebral arteries is well tolerated in humans, making the clinical presentation of vertebrobasilar insufficiency a relatively infrequent occurrence *(14)*. Atherosclerotic occlusive disease of the origin of both vertebral arteries is the most common cause for vertebrobasilar insufficiency; however, other combinations of carotid, subclavian, and innominate stenoses can compromise the posterior circulation and precipitate symptoms of vertebrobasilar insufficiency requiring an assessment of the circle of Willis to define the anatomy in patients with symptomatic vertebrobasilar symptoms. Initial therapy of symptomatic patients consists of anticoagulation and platelet inhibitors, with aortic arch and four-vessel cerebrovascular angiography indicated if symptoms continue despite medical management *(15)*.

Sundt and colleagues *(16)* reported the first successful treatment of the vertebrobasilar system by intraoperative PTA in 1980. Since Sundt's initial report, multiple case reports and clinical series have described the successful use of PTA to treat posterior circulation atherosclerotic disease *(17–19)*. Several case reports describing percutaneous stent placement for the treatment of vertebral artery atherosclerotic occlusive disease have been published *(20,21)*. Most recently, Malek and colleagues reported a series of 21 patients with posterior circulation ischemia treated with balloon angioplasty and stent placement including 8 subclavian arteries and 13 vertebral arteries *(22)*.

We have studied the safety and efficacy of percutaneous primary vertebral artery stenting for the treatment of posterior circulation ischemia in 37 vertebral arteries of 32 patients *(23)*. Indications for vertebral stenting were diplopia ($n = 4$), blurred vision ($n = 4$), dizziness ($n = 23$), transient ischemic attacks ($n = 4$), drop attack ($n = 1$), gait disturbance ($n = 1$), headache ($n = 2$), and asymptomatic critical stenosis ($n = 1$). Nine patients exhibited more than one symptom and one patient without symptoms had a critical stenosis of a solitary vertebral artery treated with stenting prior to coronary artery bypass grafting. Unilateral vertebral artery stenting was performed in 26 (81%) patients and bilateral stenting in 6 (19%) patients. Of 38 lesions, 33 (87%) were located within 1 cm of the ostium, one (3%) lesion was located in the V_1 segment, and four (10%) lesions were located in the V_2 segment of the vertebral artery.

Procedural success was achieved in all 32 (100%) patients (Fig. 3). One patient (3%) experienced a TIA 1 hr after the procedure, which spontaneously resolved within 5 min. Repeat angiography revealed a patent stent without any focal spasm or occlusion of the intracranial arteries.

Follow-up was available in all 32 patients at a mean of 10.6 mo. All patients were alive. One (3%) patient had recurrent dizziness at 3.5 mo and was found to have in-stent stenosis, which was successfully treated with balloon angioplasty. The remaining 31 patients remain asymptomatic at the follow-up.

RENAL ARTERY ENDOVASCULAR THERAPY

Atherosclerotic renal artery stenosis, the most common cause of secondary hypertension, affects fewer than 5% of the general hypertensive population *(24)*. There are, however, several clinical "high-risk" subsets of patients in whom atherosclerotic renal artery stenosis is much more common, such as those with poorly controlled hypertension, elderly patients with renal insufficiency, and patients with severe hypertension associated with coronary or PAD (Table 5) *(25,26)*.

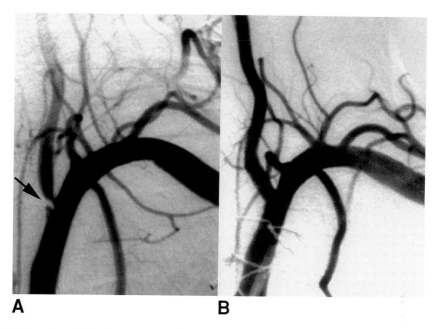

Fig. 3. (A) Baseline subclavian artery angiography demonstrating 80% narrowing at the ostium of the left vertebral artery. **(B)** Angiography after placement of a coronary self-expanding stent.

In patients undergoing coronary angiography for suspected coronary artery disease, the incidence of renal artery stenosis ranges from 15% to 18% *(27)*. In patients with known aneurysmal or occlusive PAD, associated renal artery stenosis is found in 28% *(28)*. In patients with renal insufficiency the incidence of renal artery stenosis is as high as 24% *(29)*.

The natural history of renal artery stenosis is to progress over time. The incidence of stenosis progression in angiographic studies ranges from 39% to 49% *(30,31)*. Many of these lesions progress to complete occlusion with loss of renal function. In a prospective study of patients with renal artery stenosis treated medically, progression occurred in 42% (11% progressed to occlusion) over a 2-yr period *(32)*. Of particular importance is the realization that progression of renal artery stenosis and loss of renal function are *independent* of the ability to medically control blood pressure *(33)*. Renal artery revascularization with stent placement has been demonstrated to improve or slow the progression of renal failure in these patients *(34,35)*.

Indications for Renal Intervention

The clinical indications for percutaneous renal artery revascularization are similar to those for surgical revascularization. Patients with ≥ 70 % diameter stenosis of the renal artery and poorly controlled hypertension are candidates for percutaneous intervention. For aortoostial lesions, restenosis lesions, or following a suboptimal balloon angioplasty (≥ 30% residual diameter stenosis or dissection), the use of endovascular stents is preferred (Fig. 4) *(36)*. For patients with fibromuscular dysplasia or renal branch artery lesions, we prefer balloon angioplasty with provisional stenting for unsatisfactory results *(37,38)*.

Table 5
Hypertensive Patients at Increased Risk of Renal Artery Stenosis

Abdominal bruit (systolic and diastolic)
Onset of hypertension < 20 yr or > 55 yr
Malignant hypertension
Refractory or difficult to control hypertension
Azotemia with ACE inhibitors
Atrophic kidney
Hypertension and associated atherosclerotic disease
Elderly with renal insufficiency

Patients with renal failure and associated renal artery stenosis may benefit from percutaneous revascularization, although this has not been demonstrated in any systematic study. Traditional teaching requires that both renal arteries be compromised to cause renal failure, but in the setting of patients with hypertensive renal insufficiency, a unilateral stenosis may serve to protect the affected kidney from hypertensive damage. This kidney might be expected to respond with improved function if the offending stenotic lesion is treated *(39)*.

Finally, treatment of isolated renal artery stenotic lesions, which do not cause uncontrolled hypertension or renal insufficiency, has been debated as a means to preserve renal function. Timely intervention and correction of these lesions may prevent progressive narrowing of the vessel and loss of renal function. Patients on hemodialysis whose parenchyma is supplied by stenotic renal arteries, and those with renal artery stenosis and refractory congestive heart failure or unstable angina, should also be considered candidates for angioplasty or stenting *(40)*.

Contraindications to Renal Intervention

Contraindications to renal angioplasty and stenting are relative and not absolute. The risk to benefit ratio of the procedure must be considered. Patients with atheroembolic disease or a "shaggy" aorta are at increased risk of cholesterol emboli with catheter manipulation in the aorta (*see* Chapter 17). Patients with renal artery aneurysms are at risk of rupture and surgical correction should be considered.

Clinical Outcomes of Renal Stent Placement

A randomized trial comparing balloon angioplasty to medical therapy in 106 patients with uncontrolled hypertension and renal artery stenosis ($\geq$ 50% diameter stenosis) demonstrated failure of medical therapy in 44% (22 of 50 patients) at 3 mo requiring crossover to angioplasty therapy *(41)*. At 3 mo, there was evidence of improved blood pressure control, a requirement for fewer medications, and improved renal function in the angioplasty group. At 1 yr follow-up, 16% ($n = 8$) of the medically treated patients experienced occlusion of the stenotic renal artery vs none in the angioplasty group.

Dorros and colleagues demonstrated that renal artery stent placement was more effective than balloon angioplasty alone in improving or abolishing pressure gradients across renal artery lesions treated *(42)*. In 76 patients (92 renal arteries) undergoing primary renal artery stent placement, the technical success rate was 100% and the angiographic restenosis rate at 6 mo was 25%. Clinical follow-up demonstrated that 78% of their

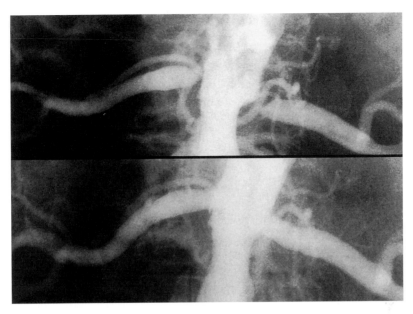

Fig. 4. (Top) Baseline aortogram with bilateral renal artery stenosis. **(Bottom)** Angiogram after balloon expandable stent placement.

patients had stable or improved renal function, with a significant decrease in blood pressure and number of antihypertensive medications for the entire group *(43)*.

A randomized trial comparing balloon angioplasty to stent placement in 85 patients with atherosclerotic renal artery stenosis and hypertension demonstrated a higher success rate and superior long-term patency rate with stent placement compared to balloon angioplasty *(44)*. At 6 mo the angiographic restenosis rate for the balloon angioplasty group was 48% compared to only 14% ($p < 0.01$) for the stent group.

Treatment of Unstable Angina and Congestive Heart Failure

We analyzed the results of renal artery stent placement in another group of 48 patients with unstable angina ($n = 23$) or congestive heart failure (CHF) ($n = 25$) who had hypertension refractory to medical therapy and $\geq 70\%$ stenosis of one ($n = 30$) or both ($n = 18$) renal arteries *(40)*. For the entire cohort of patients hypertension control was achieved within 24 h in 87% and a sustained benefit was seen in 74% at 6 mo.

Our experience with renal stenting in patients with renovascular hypertension and refractory unstable angina or CHF is very encouraging. These patients were unmanageable with medical therapy alone. The placement of renal stents successfully reduced their afterload and allowed these patients to be managed medically.

Preservation of Renal Function

Two reports have demonstrated that renal artery stent placement improved or slowed the progression of renal artery stenosis in a group of patients with impaired renal function and atherosclerotic renal artery stenosis *(34,35)*. The renal function of these patients was analyzed by plotting the slopes of the reciprocal serum creatinine values before and after successful stent placement. The authors found that the progression of renal failure was significantly slowed after stent placement.

ABDOMINAL AORTIC ENDOVASCULAR THERAPY
Aortic Occlusive Disease

Distal abdominal aortic disease has been conventionally treated with endarterectomy or bypass grafting. Frequently, distal aortic occlusive disease is associated with occlusive disease of the iliac arteries. The potential advantages of a percutaneous (nonsurgical) technique compared to an aortoiliac reconstruction are no requirement for general anesthesia or an abdominal incision, and percutaneous therapy is associated with a shorter hospital stay and lower morbidity *(45)*. Although axillofemoral extraanatomic bypass offers a lower risk surgical alternative for patients with terminal aorta occlusive disease and severe comorbidities, it has the disadvantages of a lower patency rate than direct surgical bypass of the lesions and requires that surgical intervention of a normal vessel be performed to achieve inflow.

Since 1980, balloon angioplasty has been used successfully, although not extensively, in the terminal aorta *(46)*. An extension of this strategy has been the use of endovascular stents in the treatment of infrarenal aortic stenoses. While balloon dilation of these lesions has been reported to be effective, the placement of stents offers a more definitive treatment with a larger acute gain in luminal diameter, scaffolding of the lumen to prevent embolization of debris, and, theortically, an enhanced long-term patency compared to balloon angioplasty alone *(47)*. Stents are an attractive therapeutic option for the management of large artery occlusive disease to maintain or improve the arterial luminal patency after balloon angioplasty. The utility of stents for infrarenal aortic stenoses has not been demonstrated in randomized trials; however, the clinical results are encouraging.

The use of covered stent grafts to treat long-segment aortoiliac occlusive disease has been reported by Marin and colleagues in 42 patients with limb-threatening ischemia (47). The stent grafts were handmade and were constructed using Palmaz stents and 6-mm polytetrafluoroethylene (PTFE) thin-walled grafts. Surgical exposure of the femoral access site was obtained and the lesion crossed with a guidewire. The stent was sewn to the proximal end of the graft and deployed with balloon inflation at the inflow site to the lesion. The distal end of the graft was surgically anastomosed at the outflow site. Procedural success was obtained in 91% (39 of 43 arteries). The 18-mo patency rate was 89% and the 2-yr limb salvage rate was 94%.

Abdominal Aortic Aneurysm Exclusion

It is estimated that more than 100,000 abdominal aortic aneurysms are diagnosed each year in the United States and approx 40,000 require surgical correction. It is generally accepted that there is clinical benefit in electively repairing aneurysms > 5.0 cm, and in patients with hypertension and chronic obstructive lung disease aneurysms > 3.0 cm should be repaired *(48)*. In low-risk subsets of patients, the operative mortality is 5% compared to 10% in higher risk patients. The experience with covered stent grafts to exclude abdominal aortic and aortoiliac aneurysms is still early in its clinical experience, and is performed with stent grafts that require surgical access to introduce these large-diameter devices.

In one large series, 331 aortoiliac aneurysms were referred for endovascular repair, but only 154 (47%) were found to be suitable candidates (Table 6) *(49)*. Successful aneurysm exclusion with the endograft was accomplished in 87% of the patients. Major

Table 6
Abdominal Aortic Aneurysm Classification

Type A: proximal and distal neck > 10 mm length and < 25 mm in diameter without involvement of the iliac arteries

Type B: proximal neck > 10 mm and < 25 mm diameter; involvement of aortic bifurcation, and iliac diameter < 12 mm

Type C: proximal neck > 10 mm and < 25 mm diameter; involvement of aortic bifurcation and common iliac arteries, and iliac diameter < 12 mm

Type D: Involvement of both internal iliac arteries

Type E: Proximal neck < 10 mm or diameter > 25 mm

complications included death (0.6%), limb amputation (0.6%), emergency surgery (0.6%), vessel occlusion (1.2%), need for dialysis (1.2%), distal embolization (3.3%), and access site complications (3.9%). A total of 17 "endoleaks" were observed, of which 2 fabric tears and 1 proximal leak closed spontaneously; 13 were sealed with the placement of an additional stent graft; and 2 patients refused further treatment. At a mean follow-up of 13 mo, the secondary patency (including endovascular repair of stent graft leaks) was 87% with an overall mortality rate of < 1%. Although the initial clinical experience with these devices is encouraging, longer term data will be necessary to determine what role this procedure will have in the management of aneurysmal disease.

Although no randomized trials comparing stent grafts to conventional surgery have been completed, Cohnert and colleagues reported the outcome of 37 matched pairs undergoing elective infrarenal abdominal aneurysm repair and stent-graft placement *(50)*. Interestingly, there was no difference in length of stay in the hospital, there were more deaths in the stent-graft group, and the 30-d mortality and morbidity was trending higher for the stent-graft group (Fig. 5).

LOWER EXTREMITY ENDOVASCULAR THERAPY
Iliac Artery Intervention

Traditional surgical therapies for iliac lesions include aortoiliac and aortofemoral bypass. These bypass procedures have a 74–95% 5-yr patency, which is comparable, but not superior, to percutaneous intervention *(51)*. Ameli and colleagues reported a series of 105 consecutive patients undergoing aortofemoral bypass *(52)*. The majority (58%) of their patients had mild to moderate clinical symptoms and were treated for claudication. The operative mortality was 5.7%, the early graft failure rate was 5.7%, and the 2-yr graft patency was 92.8%.

Iliac angioplasty is a well-accepted therapy for selected patients meeting defined clinical and anatomic criteria (Table 7). The availability of endovascular stents has significantly broadened the type of iliac lesions that may be treated percutaneously (Fig. 6) *(53)*. The overall clinical benefit of iliac stent placement has been demonstrated using a meta-analysis of more than 2000 patients from eight reported angioplasty (PTA) series and six stent series *(54)*. The patients who received iliac stents had a statistically higher procedural success rate and a 43% reduction in late (4-yr) failures in patients treated with stents compared to those treated with balloon angioplasty.

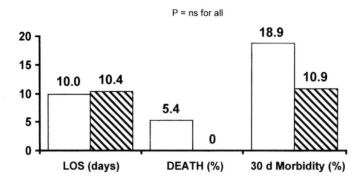

Fig. 5. Matched pairs comparison of aortic stent graft vs conventional aneurysm repair *(50).*

Table 7
Stratification of Lesion for Iliac Artery Balloon Angioplasty

Favorable	*Unfavorable*
Stenosis	Occlusion
Discrete lesions ($\leq$ 3 cm)	Long lesions ($\geq$ 5 cm)
Noncalcified	Aortoiliac aneurysm
Nondiabetic	Atheroembolic disease
Patent runoff ($\geq$ 2)	Extensive bilateral aortoiliac disease

Clinical results for provisional iliac stent placement with the Palmaz stent in 184 iliac lesions demonstrated a 91% procedural success rate and a 6-mo patency rate of 99% *(55).* Long-term follow-up of these iliac lesions demonstrated a 4-yr primary patency rate of 86% and a secondary patency rate of 95%. Results for provisional iliac stent placement with the self-expanding Wallstent have demonstrated patency rates at 1 yr of 95%, 2 yr of 88%, and 4 yr of 82% in 118 treated lesions *(56).*

The immmedate post-procedure results of a randomized trial of PTA with provisional stenting (stent placement for unsatisfactory balloon angioplasty results) vs *de novo* stenting in iliac arteries demonstrated that pressure gradients across the lesions after primary stent placement (5.8 ± 4.7 mmHg) were significantly lower after stent placement than after PTA alone (8.9 ± 6.8 mmHg) but not after provisional stenting (5.9 ± 3.6 mmHg) (57). The primary technical success rate, defined as a post-procedural gradient of < 10 mmHg, revealed no difference between the two treatment strategies (primary stent = 81% vs PTA plus provisional stenting = 89%). By using provisional stenting, the authors avoided stent placement in 63% of the lesions, and still achieved an equivalent acute hemodynamic result compared to primary stenting. Longer term follow-up will be necessary to evaluate the patency of these vessels.

Primary placement of Palmaz balloon expandable stents has been evaluated in a multicenter trial for iliac placement in 486 patients followed for up to 4 yr (mean 13.3 ± 11 mo) *(58).* Using life-table analysis, clinical benefit was present in 91% at 1 yr, 84% at 2 yr, and 69% of the patients at 43 mo of follow-up. The angiographic patency rate of the iliac stents was 92%. Complications occurred in 10% and were predominantly

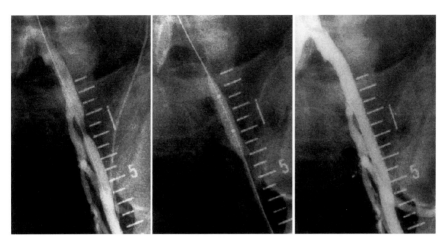

Fig. 6. (Left) Left external iliac stenosis. **(Middle)** Stent deployment. **(Right)** Post-stent result.

related to the arterial access site. Five patients suffered thrombosis of the stent, of which four were recanalized with thrombolysis and balloon angioplasty. A preliminary report from a European randomized trial of primary iliac (Palmaz) stent placement vs balloon angioplasty demonstrated a 4-yr patency of 92% for the stent group vs a 74% patency for the balloon angioplasty group (Table 8) *(59)*.

Iliac stent placement may also be used as an adjunctive procedure to surgical bypass procedures. Clinical results of using iliac angioplasty with or without stent placement to preserve inflow for a femorofemoral bypass over a 14-yr period in 70 consecutive patients have been very encouraging *(60)*. They found that the patients requiring treatment of the inflow iliac artery with angioplasty or stent placement did just as well as those without iliac artery disease at 7 yr after surgery. These results suggest that percutaneous intervention can provide adequate long-term inflow for femorofemoral bypass as an alternative to aortofemoral bypass in patients at increased risk for a major operation.

Femoropopliteal PTA

Percutaneous angioplasty has a primary success rate between 70% and 97% for femoropopliteal atherosclerotic lesions, with the success rate being higher for stenoses than for total occlusions with patency between 50% and 70% at 3–5 yr *(61,62)*. These results compare favorably with the results of infrainguinal surgical bypass. In patients with above-knee autogenous vein graft femoropopliteal bypass surgery, the 5-yr cumulative patency is 78%, whereas a 52% 5-yr patency for Gortex™ femoropopliteal grafts has been reported *(51)*. For below knee autogenous saphenous vein grafts, the patency rate is lower than for above-knee grafts, with one study reporting a 2-yr patency of 62% in those treated with ticlopidine compared to 55% in those without ticlopidine *(63)*.

A randomized trial comparing PTA to surgery for patients with femoropopliteal lesions showed no significant difference between the two modalities after 3 yr of follow-up for study related deaths, amputations, and late interventions (Fig. 7) *(64)*. PTA and surgery had equivalent outcomes for the hemodynamic results (ankle–brachial index) and that a successful angioplasty was as equally durable as a surgical bypass procedure (Fig. 8). Even in the case of a failed angioplasty, the patient could undergo successful surgical therapy without placing the patient at higher risk of limb loss or surgical

Table 8
Randomized Trial Comparing Iliac PTA vs Stent

Procedure	Technical success	Hemodynamic success	Clinical success	Complication rate	4-Yr Patency
Stent (n = 123)	98.4%	97.6%	97.6%	4.1%	91.6%
PTA (n = 124)	91.9%	91.9%	89.5%	6.5%	74.3%

Data reported by Perler BA, et al. J Vasc Surg 1996;24:363 *(60)*.

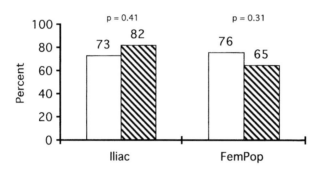

Fig. 7. Bar graph demonstrating the results of a randomized trial of PTA vs surgery *(64)*.

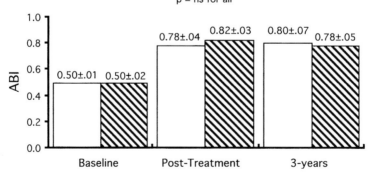

Fig. 8. Bar graph of hemodynamic results comparing PTA vs surgery *(64)*.

failure. In femoropopliteal lesions that are amenable to either angioplasty or surgery, angioplasty should be the first choice for its lower morbidity and cost and equivalent long-term results and durability.

The long-term patency of femoropopliteal angioplasty depends on clinical as well as anatomic variables *(65,66)*. Clinical factors that negatively impact long-term patency of PTA include female sex, diabetes, and the presence of rest pain or threatened limb loss.

Technical factors that correlate with long-term failure of angioplasty include longer lesion length, multiple vs single lesions, lesion eccentricity, and a poor angiographic appearance post-angioplasty.

The status of the distal runoff vessels in the tibial vessels also impacts the long-term success of PTA in the femoropopliteal vessels. In one study of 370 patients undergoing angioplasty for lower limb ischemia, patients with less than or equal to one-vessel runoff had a 3-yr patency of only 25%, compared with 78% in patients with two- or three-vessel runoff *(67)*. Minar and colleagues analyzed restenosis at 2 yr in 207 patients following successful femoropopliteal angioplasty and used a multivariate analysis to assess variables affecting restenosis (Table 9) (68).

Femoropopliteal Stents

There have been isolated reports of the application of endovascular stents in femoropopliteal vessels. A theoretic risk of stent compression or damage from external trauma exists for balloon-expandable stents in this location, making self-expanding more attractive in this extraskeletal location. Henry and colleagues reported their experience with balloon-expandable stents (Palmaz™) in 126 patients after suboptimal or failed balloon angioplasty (provisional stenting) *(55)*. They achieved technical success in 99% of the patients. The 4-yr patency rate for femoral stents was 66% and for popliteal stents it was 50%. Primary patency was more likely to be obtained in short ($\leq$ 3 cm) vs long ($>$ 3 cm) lesions, stenoses rather than occlusions, single stents vs multiple stents, and larger ($\geq$ 7 cm) rather than smaller ($<$ 7 cm) diameter vessels.

A smaller clinical experience has been reported for the self-expanding Wallstent in femoropopliteal arteries (Fig. 9). Zollikofer and colleagues reported the results of Wallstent placement after failed or suboptimal balloon angioplasty in 15 femoropopliteal vessels *(69)*. Twelve were occlusions and three were stenoses. Single stents were placed in three lesions and multiple (two to six) stents were placed in 12 lesions. At an average follow-up of 20 mo, the primary patency rate was 20% and the secondary patency rate was 54%. Stent thrombosis occurred in six lesions and in-stent restenosis occurred in six lesions.

Henry and Amor have reported their experience with self-expanding nitinol stents *(67)*. A more recent update of 433 patients (stenosis 292 and occlusion 141) showed the 4-yr primary patency rate of 79% for femoral lesions and 85% for popliteal lesions (*personal communication*). There was no reported difference in long-term patency between occlusions and stenoses. At present, pending randomized trials for femoropopliteal stent placement, stent placement should be reserved for failed PTA.

Tibioperoneal Angioplasty

Below-the-knee angioplasty has been generally reserved for cases of threatened limb loss because of the technical difficulty using conventional peripheral angioplasty equipment in these vessels, and the fear of potential limb loss should a complication occur. Surgical bypass below the knee also has an increased failure rate compared with iliofemoral or femoropopliteal revascularization. Although published experience is limited, the procedural success rates for tibioperoneal angioplasty are about 85% and 1–2 yr patency rates range between 40% and 85% *(70,71)*. Surgical saphenous vein bypass graft patency is 50–60% at 5 yr and is similar to long-term angioplasty results *(72)*. Recent reports using the *in situ* technique for distal vein graft bypass procedures sug-

Table 9
Variables Affecting Restenosis Following Femoropopliteal Angioplasty

	2-Yr patency (%)	p Value
Claudication	64%	0.06
Limb threat	50	
Two- to three-vessel runoff	68	0.02
Zero- to one-vessel runoff	49	
Stenosis (single)	74	0.06
Stenosis (multiple)	63	
Occlusion (< 10 cm)	59	0.06
Occlusion (≥ 10 cm)	47	
Diabetes (+)	68	0.05
Diabetes (−)	54	
Male	68	0.06
Female	56	

Data reported by Minar E, et al. Circulation 1995;91:2167 *(68)*.

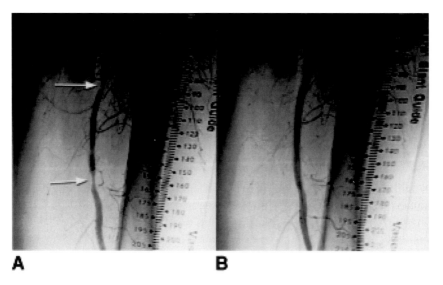

A   **B**

Fig. 9. (A) Baseline angiography of tandem superficial femoral artery stenoses. **(B)** Angiography after placement of a self-expanding stent to cover both lesions.

gests a superior patency to the conventional reversed saphenous vein graft technique *(73)*.

The development of smaller more flexible balloon catheters over steerable guidewires, based on the design of coronary balloon angioplasty systems, has improved the results of intervention (Fig. 10). In 111 patients with tibioperoneal angioplasty for claudication (47%), tissue loss (27%), or rest pain (26%), Dorros and colleagues had a primary success rate of 90% for all lesions, including 99% for stenoses and 65% for occlusions *(74)*. At the time of hospital discharge 95% of the patients were symptomatically improved.

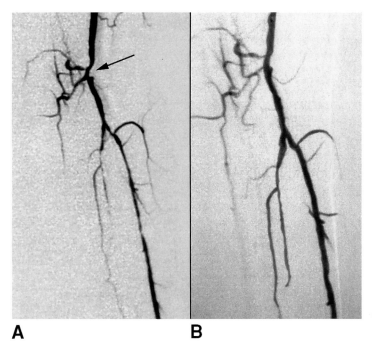

Fig. 10. (A) Baseline angiography of popliteal stenosis (*arrow*) and posterior tibioperoneal lesions. **(B)** Angiogram following balloon angioplasty of the popliteal and posterior tibial artery.

These excellent results, as well as our own experience, support the contention that angioplasty of the tibioperoneal vessels should not necessarily be reserved for limb-salvage situations, however, caution is still advised in patient selection because the surgical options are limited if angioplasty fails.

THROMBOLYSIS FOR ACUTE PERIPHERAL ARTERIAL OCCLUSIONS

Twenty-three years ago, Poliwoda and colleagues described the first use of peripheral intravenous infusions of streptokinase for chronic arterial occlusions *(75)* (*see* Chapter 7). A number of other reports followed, demonstrating that treatment of chronic arterial occlusions with intravenous streptokinase had a disappointingly low success rate and high complication rate.

More aggressive infusion techniques together with the use of newer thrombolytic agents such as urokinase and recombinant tissue plasminogen activator (rt-PA) have resulted in an improvement in the clinical results of intraarterial thrombolysis and decreased complication rate *(76)*. The technique of direct intraarterial infusion of thrombolytic agents has been used with increasing success in both chronic symptomatic occlusions and acute thrombosis with threatened limb loss. Thrombolysis is also a useful adjunct to percutaneous angioplasty for occlusions of peripheral bypass grafts in both the lower and upper extremities and native arteries in the upper extremities *(77,78)*.

Newer, "clot-specific," agents have been used in an attempt to improve efficacy and reduce complication rates. Success rates of 76–88% using rt-PA with bleeding complications in up to 20% of patients have been reported *(79)*. One randomized trial of thrombolysis in occluded bypass grafts comparing urokinase to tissue plasminogen activator failed to show any difference in successful thrombolysis or in clinical outcome; however, this study did note lower fibrinogen levels and increased speed of clot lysis in the patients given rt-PA *(76)*.

For patients presenting with acute thrombotic occlusion of the lower extremity (< 7 d), initial catheter-directed thrombolysis appears to be more efficacious than immediate surgical revascularization *(80)*. In a randomized trial (surgery vs urokinase) of 114 patients, the cumulative limb-salvage rate was similar among the two groups, but the cumulative survival rate at 12 mo was significantly improved in the thrombolysis group compared with the surgical group (84 vs 58%, $p = 0.01$). The benefit from thrombolysis was achieved without an increase in hospital days or cost compared to the surgical group.

A large multicenter randomized trial, STILE, was initiated to determine the benefits of catheter-directed thrombolysis (urokinase or rt-PA) compared to surgical revascularization in patients with symptomatic lower extremity native artery or bypass graft occlusions of less than 6 mo duration *(81)*. This trial was stopped prematurely after enrolling 393 patients because of a high incidence of failure to deliver the thrombolytic agent to the target lesion in the thrombolysis group. The angiographer was unable to place the treatment catheter into the occluded bypass graft in 41% of patients and into the target native artery in 22% of patients. In a subgroup analysis, there was an advantage for the catheter-directed thrombolysis in patients with acute presentations (< 14 d). Patients treated with catheter-directed thrombolysis had an 11% risk of amputation vs 30% in the surgical group ($p = 0.02$). Mortality in the thrombolysis group (5.6%) was lower when compared to the surgery group (10%). The authors concluded that catheter-directed thrombolysis was most appropriate for those patients presenting with acute ischemia rather than chronic ischemia of the extremities. Although debate continues regarding the optimal agent and dosage regimen, it is clear that intraarterial, catheter-directed thrombolysis is the treatment of choice in acute thrombotic and embolic peripheral arterial occlusions.

SUMMARY

The paradigm for peripheral vascular revascularization is changing as percutaneous intervention replaces some open surgical procedures. Endovascular stents have been the most prominent factor behind this transformation. Stents have succeeded by providing predictable outcomes with excellent durability. In general, percutaneous revascularization with stents offers the same or better durability than bypass grafts with far less morbidity and mortality. Strong patient preferences and physician interest ensure continued growth and support for device development and further technical evolution.

REFERENCES

1. Dotter CI, Judkins MP. Transluminal treatment of arteriosclerotic obstruction: description of a new technique and a preliminary report of its application. Circulation 1964;30:654–670.
2. Gruntzig A, Hopff H. Perkutane rekanalisation chronischer arterieller verschlusse mit einem neuen dilatationskatehetr modifikation der Dotter-Technik. Dtsch Med Wochenschr 1974;99:2502–2507.
3. O'Keeffe ST, Woods BO, Beckmann CF. Percutaneous transluminal angioplasty of the peripheral arteries. Cardiol Clin 1991;9:519–521.
4. Health and Public Policy Committee, American College of Physicians. Percutaneous transluminal angioplasty. Ann Intern Med 1983;99:864–869.
5. Isner JM, Rosenfeld K. Redefining the treatment of peripheral artery disease: role of percutaneous revascularization. Circulation 1993;88:1534–1557.

6. Beebe HG, Stark R, Johnson ML, Jolly PC, Hill LD. Choices of operation for subclavian vertebral arterial disease. Am J Surg 1980;139:616–623.
7. Dorros G, Lewin RF, Jamnadas P, Mathiak LM. Peripheral transluminal angioplasty of the subclavian and innominate arteries utilizing the brachial approach: acute outcome and follow-up. Cathet Cardiovasc Diagn 1990;19:71–76.
8. Gershony G, Basta L, Hagan AD. Correction of subclavian artery stenosis by percutaneous angioplasty. Cathet Cardiovasc Diagn 1990;21:165–169.
9. Hadjipetrou P, Cox S, Piemonte T, Eisenhauer A. Percutaneous revascularization of atheroclerotic obstruction of aortic arch vessels. J Am Coll Cardiol 1999;33:1238–1245.
10. Jain SP, Zhang SY, Khosla S, et al. Subclavian and innominate arteries stenting: acute and long term results (abstract). J Am Coll Cardiol 1998;31:63A.
11. Roubin GS, New G, Iyer SS, et al. Immediate and late clinical outcomes of carotid artery stenting in patients with symptomatic and asymptomatic carotid artery stenosis. Circulation 2001;103:532–537.
12. Waigand J, Gross CM, Uhlich F, et al. Elective stenting of carotid artery stenosis in patients with severe coronary artery disease. Eur Heart J 1998;19:1365–1370.
13. CAVATAS investigators. Endovascular versus surgical treatment in patients with carotid stenosis in the carotid and vertebral artery transluminal angioplasty study (CAVATAS): a randomized study. Lancet 2001;357:1729–1737.
14. Alexander W. The treatment of epilepsy by ligature of the vertebral artery. Brain 1942;5:170–180.
15. Smith RB III. The surgical treatment of peripheral vascular disease. In: Hurst JW, Schlant RC, Rackley CZ, Sonnenblick EH, Wenger NK, eds. The Heart, 7th edit. New York: McGraw-Hill, 1992; pp.2235–2236.
16. Sundt TM Jr, Smith HC, Campbell JK, Vietstra RE, Cucchiara RF, Stanson AW. Transluminal angioplasty for basilar artery stenosis. Mayo Clin Proc 1980;55:673–680.
17. Higashida RT, Tsai FY, Halbach VV, Dowd CF, Hiemima GB. Cerebral percutaneous transluminal angioplasty. Heart Dis Stroke 1993;2:497–502.
18. Higashida RT, Tsai FY, Halbach VV, et al. Transluminal angioplasty for atherosclerotic disease of the vertebral and basilar arteries. J Neurosurg 1993;78:192–198.
19. Terada T, Higashida RT, Halbach VV, et al. Transluminal angioplasty for atherosclerotic disease of the distal vertebral and basilar arteries. J Neurol Neurosurg Psychiatry 1996;60:377–381.
20. Storey GS, Marks MP, Dake M, Norbash AM, Steinberg GK. Vertebral artery stenting following percutaneous transluminal angiography. J Neurosurg 1996;84:883–887.
21. Feldman RL, Rubin JJ, Kuykendall RC. Use of coronary Palmaz-Schatz stent in the percutaneous treatment of vertebral artery stenoses. Cathet Cardiovasc Diagn 1996;38:312–315.
22. Malek AM, Higashida RT, Phatouros CC, et al. Treatment of posterior circulation ischemia with extracranial percutaneous balloon angioplasty and stent placement. Stroke 1999;30:2073–2085.
23. Jenkins JS, White CJ, Ramee SR, et al. Vertebral artery stenting. Cathet Cardiovasc Intervent 2001; 54:1–5.
24. Simon N, Franklin SS, Bleifer KH, Maxwell MH. Clinical characteristics of renovascular hypertension. JAMA 1972;220:1209–1218.
25. Olin JW, Melia M, Young JR, Graor RA, Risius B. Prevalence of atherosclerosis renal artery stenosis in patients with atherosclerosis elsewhere. Am J Med 1990;88:46N–51N.
26. Harding MB, Smith LR, Himmelstein SI, et al. Renal artery stenosis: prevalence and associated risk factors in patients undergoing routine cardiac catheterization. J Am Soc Nephrol 1992;2: 1608–1616.
27. Jean WJ, Al-Bitar I, Zwicke DL, Port SC, Schmidt DH, Bajwa TK. High incidence of renal artery stenosis in patients with coronary artery disease. Cathet Cardiovasc Diagn 1994;32:8–10.
28. Valentine RJ, Clagett GP, Miller GL, Myers SI, Martin JD, Cherm A. The coronary risk of unsuspected renal artery stenosis. J Vasc Surg 1993;18:433–440.
29. O'Neil EA, Hansen KJ, Canzanello VJ, Pennell TC, Dean RH. Prevalence of ischemic nephropathy in patients with renal insufficiency. Am Surg 1992;58:485–490.
30. Greco BA, Breyer JA. The natural history of renal artery stenosis: who should be evaluated for suspected ischemic nephropathy? Semin Nephrol 1996;16:2–11.
31. Schreiber MJ, Pohl MA, Novick AC. The natural history of atherosclerotic and fibrous renal artery disease. Urol Clin N Am 1984;11:383–392.
32. Zierler RE, Bergelin RO, Isaacson JA, Strandness DE. Natural history of atherosclerotic renal artery stenosis: a prospective study with duplex ultrasonography. J Vasc Surg 1994;19:250–258.

33. Dean RH, Kieffer RW, Smith BM, et al. Renovascular hypertension: anatomic and renal function changes during drug therapy. Arch Surg 1981;116:1408–1415.

34. Harden PN, MacLeod MJ, Rodger RS, et al. Effect of renal artery stenting on progression of renovascular renal failure. Lancet 1997;349:1133–1136.

35. Watson PS, Hadjipetrou P, Cox SV, Piemonte TC, Eisenhauer AC. Effect of renal artery stenting on renal function and size in patients with atherosclerotic renovascular disease. Circulation 2000;102:1671–1677.

36. White CJ, Ramee SR, Collins TJ, Jenkins JS, Escobar A, Shaw D. Renal artery stent placement: utility in difficult lesions for balloon angioplasty. J Am Coll Cardiol 1997;30:1445–1450.

37. Archibald GR, Beckmann CF, Libertino JA. Focal renal artery stenosis caused by fibromuscular dysplasia: treatment by percutaneous transluminal angioplasty. Am J Radiol 1988;151:593–596.

38. Cluzel P, Raynaud A, Beyssen B, Pagny SY, Gaux JC. Stenosis of renal branch arteries in fibromuscular dysplasia: results of percutaneous transluminal angioplasty. Radiology 1994;193:227–232.

39. Kaylor WM, Novick AC, Ziegelbaum M, Vidt DG. Reversal of end stage renal failure with surgical revascularization in patients with atherosclerotic renal artery occlusion. J Urol 1989;141:486–488.

40. Khosla S, White CJ, Collins TJ, Jenkins JS, Shaw D, Ramee SR. Effects of renal artery stent implantation in patients with renovascular hypertension presenting with unstable angina or congestive heart failure. Am J Cardiol 1997;80:363–366.

41. van Jaarsveld BC Krijnen P, Pieterman H, et al. The effect of balloon angioplasty on hypertension in atherosclerotic renal artery stenosis. N Engl J Med 2000;342:1007–1014.

42. Dorros G, Prince C, Mathiak L. Stenting of a renal artery stenosis achieves better relief of the obstructive lesion than balloon angioplasty. Cathet Cardiovasc Diagn 1993;29:191–198.

43. Dorros G, Jaff M, Jain A, Dufek C, Mathiak. Follow-up of primary Palmaz–Schatz stent placement for atherosclerotic renal artery stenosis. Am J Cardiol 1995;75:1051–1055.

44. van de Ven PJ, Kaatee R, Beutler JJ, et al. Arterial stenting and balloon angioplasty in ostial atherosclerotic renovascular disease: a randomised trial. Lancet 1999;353:282–286.

45. Tegtmyer CG, Hartwell GD, Selby GB, Robertson R Jr, Kron IL, Tribble CG. Results and complications of angioplasty in aortoiliac diseases. Circulation 1991;83:153–160.

46. Diethrich EB. Endovascular treatment of abdominal aortic occlusive disease: the impact of stents and intravascular ultrasound imaging. Eur J Vasc Surg 1993;7:228–236.

47. Marin ML, Vieth FJ, Sanchez LA, et al. Endovascular repair of aortoiliac occlusive disease. World J Surg 1996;20:679–686.

48. Cronenwett JL. Infrainguinal occlusive disease. Semin Vasc Surg 1995;8:284–288.

49. Blum U, Voshage G, Lammer J, et al. Endoluminal stent grafts for infrarenal abdominal aortic aneurysms. N Engl J Med 1997;336:13–20.

50. Cohnert TU, Oelert F, Wahlers T, et al. Matched pair analysis of conventional versus endoluminal AAA treatment outcomes during the intitial phase of an aortic endografting program. J Endovasc Ther 2000;7:94–100.

51. Johnston KW. Balloon angioplasty: predictive factors for long-term success. Semin Vasc Surg 1989;3: 117–122.

52. Ameli FM, Stein M, Provan JL, Aro L, Prosser R. Predictors of surgical outcome in patients undergoing aortobifemoral bypass reconstruction. J Cardiovasc Surg 1990;30:333–339.

53. Sullivan TM, Childs MB, Bacharach JM, Gray BH, Piedmonte MR. Percutaneous transluminal angioplasty and primary stenting of the iliac arteries in 288 patients. J Vasc Surg 1997;25:829–839.

54. Bosch JL, Hunink MGM. Meta-analysis of the results of percutaneous transluminal angioplasty and stent placement for aortoiliac occlusive disease. Radiology 1997;204:87–96.

55. Henry M, Amor M, Thevenot G, et al. Palmaz stent placement in iliac and femoropopliteal arteries: primary and secondary patency in 310 patients with 2–4 year follow up. Radiology 1995;197:167–174.

56. Vorwerk D, Gunther RW, Schurmann K, Wendt G. Aortic and iliac stenosis: follow-up results of stent placement after insufficient balloon angioplasty in 118 cases. Radiology 1996;198:45–48.

57. Tetteroo E, Haaring C, van der Graaf Y, van Schaik JP, van Engelen AD, Mali WP. Intraarterial pressure gradients after randomized angioplasty or stenting of iliac artery lesions. Dutch Iliac Stent Trial Study Group. Cardiovasc Intervent Radiol 1996;19:411–417.

58. Palmaz JC, Laborde JC, Rivera FJ, Encamacion CE, Lutz JD, Moss JG. Stenting of the iliac arteries with the Palmaz stent: experience from a multicenter trial. Cardiovasc Intervent Radiol 1992;15: 291–297.

59. Richter GM, Noeldge G, Roeren T, et al First long-term results of a randomized multicenter trial: iliac balloon-expandable stent placement versus regular percutaneous transluminal angioplasty. In: Lierman D, ed. State of the Art and Future Developments. Morin Heights, Canada: Polyscience, 1995; pp. 30–35.

60. Perler BA, Williams GM. Does donor iliac artery percutaneous transluminal angioplasty or stent placement influence the results of femorofemoral bypass? Analysis of 70 consecutive cases with long-term follow up. J Vasc Surg 1996;24:363–370.

61. Capek P, McLean GK, Berkowitz HD. Femoropopliteal angioplasty: factors influencing long-term success. Circulation 1991; 83(Suppl I):70–80.

62. Hewes RC, White RI Jr, Murray RR, et al. Long term results of superficial femoral artery angioplasty. Am J Radiol 1986;146:1025–1029.

63. Becquemin J. Effect of ticlopidine on the long-term patency of saphenous vein grafts in the legs. N Engl J Med 1997;337:1726–1731.

64. Wilson SE, Wolf GL, Cross AP. Percutaneous transluminal angioplasty versus operation for peripheral arteriosclerosis: report of a prospective randomized trial in a selected group of patients. J Vasc Surg 1989;9:1–9.

65. Jeans WD, Armstrong S, Cole SE, Horrocks M, Baird RN. Fate of patients undergoing transluminal angioplasty for lower-limb ischemia. Radiology 1990;177:559–564.

66. Stokes KR, Strunk HM, Campbell DR, Gibbons GW, Wheeler HG, Clouse ME. Five-year results of iliac and femoropopliteal angioplasty in diabetic patients. Radiology 1990;174:977–982.

67. Henry M, Amor M, Byer R, et al. Clinical experience with a new nitrol self-expanding stent in peripheral arteries. J Endovasc Surg 1996;3:369–379.

68. Minar E, Ahmadi A, Koppensteiner R, et al. Comparison of effects of high-dose and low-dose aspirin on restenosis after femoropopliteal percutaneous transluminal angioplasty. Circulation 1995;91: 2167–2173.

69. Zollikofer C, Antonucci F, Pfyffer M, et al. Arterial stent placement with use of the Wallstent: midterm results of clinical experience. Radiology 1991;179:449–456.

70. Schwarten DE, Cutliff WB. Arterial occlusive disease below the knee: treatment with percutaneous transluminal angioplasty performed with low-profile catheters and steerable guide wires. Radiology 1988;169:71–74.

71. Matsi PJ, Manninen HI, Suhonen MT, Pirinen AE, Soimakallio S. Chronic critical lower-limb ischemia: prospective trial of angioplasty with 1–36 months of follow-up. Radiology 1993;188: 381–387.

72. Davis RK, Bosher EP, Brown PW. Critical elements in successful tibial artery reconstruction based on a 10-year experience with reversed vein grafts. In: Veith FJ, ed. Critical Problems in Vascular Surgery. St. Louis: Quality Medical Publishing, 1989; pp. 47–51.

73. Bergmark C, Johansson G, Olofsson P, Swedenborg J. Femoro-popliteal and femoro-distal bypass: a comparison between in situ and reversed technique. J Cardiovasc Surg 1991;32:117–120.

74. Dorros G, Lewin RF, Jamnadas P, Mathiak LM. Below-the-knee angioplasty: tibioperoneal vessels, the acute outcome. Cathet Cardiovasc Diagn 1990; 19:170–178.

75. Poliwoda H, Alexander K, Buhl V, Holsten D, Wagner HH. Treatment of chronic arterial occlusions with streptokinase. N Engl J Med 1969;280:689–692.

76. Meyerovitz MF, Goldhaber SZ, Reagan K, et al. Recombinant tissue-type plasminogen activator versus urokinase in peripheral arterial graft occlusions: a randomized trial. Radiology 1990;175:75–78.

77. Sullivan KL, Gardiner GA, Kandarpa K, et al. Efficacy of thrombolysis in infrainguinal bypass grafts. Circulation1991;83(Suppl I):99–105.

78. Widlus DM, Venbrux AC, Benenati JF, et al. Fibrinolytic therapy for upper-extremity arterial occlusions. Radiology 1990;175:393–399.

79. Graor RA, Risius B, Lucas V, et al. Thrombolysis with recombinant human tissue-type plasminogen activator in patients with peripheral artery and bypass graft occlusions. Circulation 1986;74(Suppl 1): 15–20.

80. Ouriel K Shortell CK, DeWeese JA, et al. A comparison of thrombolytic therapy with operative revascularization in the initial treatment of acute peripheral arterial ischemia. J Vasc Surg 1994;19: 1021–1030.

81. Stile Investigators. Results of a prospective randomized trial evaluating surgery versus thrombolysis of ischemia of the lower extremity. Ann Surg 1994;220:251–268.

13

Surgical Revascularization

James O. Menzoian, MD and
Joseph D. Raffetto, MD

INTRODUCTION

Indications for vascular surgical reconstruction for peripheral arterial disease (PAD) generally include two clinical presentations: intermittent claudication (IC) and critical limb ischemia (CLI), which includes rest pain, nonhealing ulcers, and gangrene. Prior to any consideration of intervention for IC, lifestyle modification including an exercise program, smoking cessation, weight loss, correction of hyperlipidemia, and a trial of pharmacologic agents is essential. Recent studies have demonstrated that abnormal levels of homocysteine and antiphospholipid antibodies not only can contribute to PAD, but also affect graft function and patency, thereby warranting medical treatment *(1–5)*. Patients with CLI, however, without a lumen-opening intervention and/or surgical revascularization will almost certainly be faced with a major limb amputation.

Revascularization procedures are divided into two anatomic types: inflow procedures and outflow procedures (infrainguinal disease) with the femoral artery acting as the reference point. Patients with a diminished or absent femoral artery pulse are considered to have an inflow problem, while those with a strong femoral artery pulse and no distal pulses have an outflow problem. The level of the anatomic obstruction does not necessarily correlate with the clinical presentation of IC or CLI. Patients with inflow or outflow disease can present with either IC or CLI; however, many patients with CLI have multilevel obstructive disease.

From: *Contemporary Cardiology: Peripheral Arterial Disease: Diagnosis and Treatment*
Edited by: J. D. Coffman and R. T. Eberhardt © Humana Press Inc., Totowa, NJ

INFLOW DISEASE

We now review a variety of surgical options for patients who present with either IC or CLI and have anatomic obstructive disease at the aortoiliac level.

Aortoiliac Occlusive Disease

AORTOFEMORAL BYPASS

Patients with aortoiliac occlusive disease presenting with either IC or CLI have diminished to absent femoral pulses. The best intervention for these patients is aortobifemoral bypass using a synthetic graft. The results with this procedure are some of the most successful in vascular surgery with excellent clinical improvement and excellent long-term graft patency. There are numerous reports of graft patency rates of 85–90% at 5 and 10 yr (Table 1). The results in patients with IC are generally better that those in patients with CLI. A meta-analysis of 23 studies shows that there is a fairly constant excellent patency rate for this procedure from a variety of centers over the study period of 1970–1996 (Fig. 1). In addition, this procedure can be carried out with an acceptable operative morbidity and mortality *(6)*. Modern series report an operative mortality of 1–2%.

Numerous considerations are essential in making the decision to proceed with this type of bypass. Because this procedure involves cross-clamping the abdominal aorta, the hemodynamic effects on the heart must be considered due to the afterload changes associated with cross-clamping and subsequent release of the aortic clamp. An appropriate evaluation of cardiac function prior to offering this type of surgery is critical. The type and extent of this cardiac evaluation depends on the individual patient. Clinical features to be considered include a history of coronary heart disease, previous myocardial infarction, or congestive heart failure, and any electrocardiographic abnormalities. A more extensive discussion of the preoperative evaluation of these patients can be found in Chapter 14.

There are important technical issues that must be taken into consideration to ensure optimal success of an aortobifemoral bypass graft. These include the patency of the inferior mesenteric artery (IMA) and maintenance of blood flow in the external and internal iliac arteries. In those patients with an occlusion of the IMA, the aortic anastomosis with the new bypass graft can be done in either an end-to-end or end-to-side manner. However, if the IMA is patent, it is important to maintain flow into the IMA. An end-to-end anastomosis with sewing off the distal aorta will result in a loss of prograde blood flow into the IMA. In addition, if there is associated iliac artery disease preventing retrograde flow from the femoral anastomosis, there will be a loss of flow into the IMA, which could result in intestinal ischemia. Similarly, an end-to-end anastomosis at the aorta will not allow retrograde flow into the internal iliac arteries if the external iliac arteries are occluded and thus could result in pelvic ischemia causing impotence or colon ischemia *(7)*.

Another consideration of aortofemoral surgery is the impact on sexual function with efforts to avoid causing sexual dysfunction. An injury to the sympathetic nerves at the aortic bifurcation can result in retrograde ejaculation. This is best prevented by avoiding extensive surgical dissection at the aortic bifurcation. In addition, embolization into the internal iliac arteries can result in vasculogenic impotence. On the other hand,

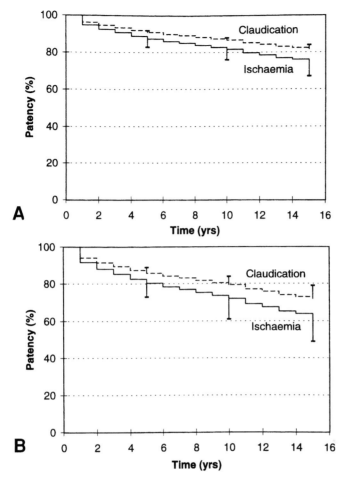

Fig 1. Pooled patency curves, adjusted for symptomatic status (critical ischemia vs intermittent claudicaiton) for both limb-based **(A)** and patient-based reporting **(B)** Error bars represent 95% confidence intervals. (Reprinted with permission from DeVries et al., J Vasc Surg 1997;26:558–561.)

sexual function in men can be improved by aortic surgery, which increases blood flow to the internal iliac arteries *(8)*.

The operative approach to aortofemoral surgery can be either the standard transabdominal or a retroperitoneal approach. Advocates of the retroperitoneal approach report decreased morbidity with less pulmonary complications, shorter intensive care unit stays, decreased length of hospitalizations, and early toleration of an enteral diet. There are enthusiasts of both methods but a review of all reported series does not show a clear benefit to either, although there does appear to be slightly less morbidity with the retroperitoneal approach *(9,10)*.

Reported results with aortofemoral surgery show that there is no benefit of any one available graft material over another. The available grafts for use at the aortic level include Dacron, either woven or knitted, polytetrafluoroethylene (PTFE); and cryopreserved allografts. The latter graft is generally reserved for use when aortic infections are present.

AXILLOFEMORAL BYPASS

Axillofemoral bypass is an extraanatomic approach to aortoiliac occlusive disease. Its major advantages are an avoidance of a large abdominal incision and aortic cross clamping. This procedure can be carried out under local anesthesia if necessary. Its major disadvantage is poorer long-term graft patency (Table 1). Although there are some recent publications suggesting patency rates nearly equivalent to aortofemoral bypass, this opinion is not generally held. Passman and colleagues have reported a 5-yr graft patency rate of 74% and suggest that in appropriate circumstances this operation can be considered as a reasonable option *(11)*.

Comparison of the results of axillofemoral bypass to aortofemoral bypass is problematic because there are no randomized trials evaluating the two procedures in comparable patients. There are large discrepancies in patency results in reported series, which may be due to a variety of factors. The patency of axillofemoral bypass seems to depend on the quality of the outflow from the femoral artery. In patients with an occluded superficial femoral artery, long-term patencies of axillofemoral bypass are inferior *(12)*. Some surgeons feel that the poor quality of the inflow axillary artery in a large percentage of patients is often unappreciated. Calligaro and colleagues found that 25% of their patients had a stenosis of 50% or greater in the donor axillary artery even without a blood pressure differential in the two arms, which is the usual guideline used to judge the quality of the donor axillary artery *(13)*. It has also been suggested that axillounilateral bypass should not be done because of poor long-term patency when compared with axillobifemoral bypass. Many surgeons feel that improved patencies in some modern series are the result of the use of externally supported large-diameter grafts (8 mm vs 6 mm), but again in the absence of a randomized trial this conclusion is not clear *(14)*.

A variety of options are available for treating the patient with inflow disease. The "gold standard" to which these must be compared is the aortofemoral bypass. This operation has the best long-term patency and clinical improvement for aortoiliac occlusive disease. There appears to be a tradeoff between aortofemoral and axillofemoral bypass procedures, which includes long-term patency and operative morbidity and mortality. Although recent series do report improved results with extraanatomic axillofemoral bypass surgery, the results are not comparable to the results with aortofemoral bypass. It is our opinion that in those patients with no significant cardiac or medical risk factors, aortofemoral bypass is the procedure of choice.

Unilateral Inflow Disease

Patients presenting with unilateral iliac occlusive disease pose an interesting challenge because of the number of options available for treatment. In those patients with stenotic lesions amenable to angioplasty and/or stent placement this is a very reasonable option with excellent results from the point of view of clinical improvement and long-term patency (see Chapter 12). However, in patients with total occlusion, there are a variety of alternative approaches including aortobifemoral bypass, aortounilateral bypass, iliofemoral bypass, iliac endarterectomy, and femoral–femoral bypass.

AORTOUNILATERAL FEMORAL BYPASS

This operation can be performed using either a transabdominal or a retroperitoneal approach. It has not gained widespread acceptance. The reported patencies are variable and, in addition, the commonly held belief that these patients will progress to develop bilateral disease makes this approach unpopular.

ILIOFEMORAL BYPASS

This procedure is usually limited to occlusive disease that involves the external iliac artery. The common iliac artery must be relatively disease free to serve as the donor artery for the bypass. The retroperitoneal approach to the common iliac artery is favorable and has the added advantage of a smaller, less painful incision than the standard incision used for abdominal aortic surgery. Again, reported results are variable, probably related to many issues such as the quality of the donor common iliac artery and the femoral artery and its runoff vessels *(15)*. These authors are pleased with their experience with this operative procedure.

ILIAC ENDARTERECTOMY

This procedure is included for completeness; however, it has not gained widespread acceptance. The results of iliac endarterectomy depend greatly on the technique used to ensure the adequacy of a complete endarterectomy not only in length, but also in depth and an assurance of a good endpoint into a relatively normal artery *(16)*.

FEMORAL–FEMORAL BYPASS

Under the circumstances of unilateral iliac artery occlusive disease, this operation is probably the most popular. Again, there are conflicting reports regarding clinical improvement and long-term graft patency. The major advantage of this operative approach is its low operative morbidity and mortality. It also can be done under local anesthesia in the appropriate patient. There are, however, many considerations prior to undertaking this operative approach, which include the following:

1. What is the status of the donor iliac and femoral artery?
2. What is the status of the recipient femoral artery and its outflow arteries?
3. Is the superficial femoral artery patent?
4. What is the quality of the deep femoral artery?
5. Is the operation being done for IC or CLI?
6. Is the operation being done for native ipsilateral occlusive disease or following an occlusion of one limb of a previous aortobifemoral bypass?

Femoral–femoral bypass is an operative procedure that can be accomplished with a low operative morbidity and mortality but the tradeoff is a compromised long-term graft patency compared to iliofemoral bypass. It can give excellent relief of symptoms from IC when both the superficial femoral artery and the deep femoral arteries are patent. It should not be performed in patients with IC and superficial femoral artery occlusion *(17)*. In patients with CLI who present a poor risk due to medical comorbidities, a femoral–femoral bypass can be accomplished with concomitant profundaplasty if there is minimal tissue loss of the limb *(18)*. It should probably be combined with an outflow procedure when the superficial femoral artery is occluded in patients with significant tissue loss and gangrene. It is also an acceptable procedure in patients with unilateral limb occlusion of a previous aortobifemoral bypass *(12)*.

There is often a discussion of steal phenomenon in association with femoral–femoral bypass surgery. Decreased pressure in the donor limb can be demonstrated in a large number of patients undergoing this type of bypass, but it is rarely clinically significant

(18). Even though clinical steal phenomenon is uncommon, Flanagan and colleagues demonstrated that when there is either a significant degree of inflow stenoses in the donor iliac artery or significant outflow occlusive disease in the recipient artery, patency rates of the bypass grafts are decreased.

A femoral–femoral bypass is an operative procedure that can be accomplished with low morbidity and with respectably good patency rates when there is good runoff and no hemodynamically significant stenoses in the donor iliac artery. The tradeoff for this lower operative morbidity is a decreased long-term patency when compared with aortofemoral bypass procedures.

INFRAINGUINAL DISEASE

The majority of patients undergoing revascularization of the lower extremity are those with CLI. A minority (approx 5%) of patients with IC will require lower extremity bypass, as > 75% will have relief (or stabilization) of their symptoms by lifestyle modification and/or pharmacologic therapy. As previously stated, the indications for surgery in patients with CLI are rest pain, nonhealing ulcers, and gangrene. Without surgical revascularization or in nonreconstructable limbs, the amputation rate is exceedingly high, ranging between 40% and 50% *(19,20)*. It is well established that patients with lower extremity arterial disease have significant cardiopulmonary disease and have decreased life expectancy compared to age- and gender-matched population without PAD *(12,21,22)*.

This section reviews surgical procedures and interventions of the lower extremity involving either a single or multisegment obstruction of a named artery, with specific attention to the profunda femoris or femoral–popliteal arterial system and the tibial–peroneal arterial branches. Technical issues regarding conduit type, orientation of the vein (reversed, *in situ*, nonreversed), adjunctive surgical procedures (arteriovenous fistulas, vein cuffs), complications, and outcomes are also reviewed.

The femoral artery is subdivided anatomically into the common femoral, profunda femoris, and the superficial femoral arteries. Extending from the superficial femoral artery is the popliteal artery, which begins at the hiatus in the adductor magnus muscle, passing through the knee joint, and ending at the origin of the anterior tibial artery. There is a rich collateral blood supply between the descending branch of the profunda femoris artery to the superior and inferior genicular branches to the popliteal artery *(23)*. The femoral artery demonstrates a propensity for atherosclerotic disease within the confluence of the common femoral and profunda femoris arteries, and in the superficial femoral artery, especially at the adductor hiatus. Although atherosclerosis more commonly affects the superficial femoral artery, the profunda has been found to have significant disease at its orifice and branches in up to 75% of limbs, mandating surgical reconstruction.

Profundaplasty

Profundaplasty should be considered only if the inflow is adequate or inflow revascularization is performed and the target outflow is the profunda femoris artery. Profundaplasty is most commonly performed in conjunction with an inflow procedure such as aortofemoral, iliofemoral, femoral–femoral, or axillofemoral bypass. Profundaplasty implies opening the profunda and common femoral arteries and anastomosing the inflow graft or placing a patch on the confluence of the two arteries. Endarterectomy of the profunda femoris or common femoral artery is rarely performed due to difficulty in obtaining clear surgical endpoints, leading to intimal flaps, and because of the ease of simply patching the artery. Various studies have documented the profunda femoris artery as an adequate outflow artery in conjunction with profundaplasty, when the superficial femoral artery is occluded (24,25). Cumulative patency and limb salvage rates are > 90% at 5 yr. Patients with CLI undergoing profundaplasty with a concomitant inflow procedure have acceptable results; however, compared to patients with claudication, long-term patency and limb salvage rates are inferior (26). Isolated profundaplasty is rarely performed for CLI given the availability of more effective distal revascularization options. Patients undergoing profundaplasty that only have proximal profunda femoris artery disease fare better with respect to limb salvage compared to those with diffuse disease extending into its first-, second-, and third-order branches (27). Because the profunda femoris artery provides important collateral vessels to the knee region, profundaplasty may be an important adjunct to knee salvage following amputation (28). Specific complications of profundaplasty are related to the groin dissection and include lymphatic disruption with lymphocele or impaired lymph drainage, hematoma, groin infection, and femoral nerve injury. Meticulous surgical technique is imperative to keep these local operative complications below 5%. Systemic complications are those related to underlying cardiopulmonary disease and medical comorbidities.

Femoral Popliteal Bypass

Femoral popliteal bypass can be performed for both IC and CLI. Most commonly patients with claudication have obstruction of the superficial femoral artery necessitating a bypass to the popliteal artery. In a study evaluating 4468 infrainguinal revascularizations over a 10-yr period, 9% (or 409 reconstructions) were for claudication and 91% for CLI (29). Of the 409 revascularizations for IC, 77% had the distal target artery to the popliteal (above knee in 40%, and below knee in 37%), while the remaining 23% were to the tibial vessels (29). Thus a significant group of patients with claudication may require tibial bypass because of an unsuitable popliteal target, even though tibial bypass in claudicants represented only 2.1% of the total (4468) infrainguinal revascularizations performed (29). When looking at risk factors for infrainguinal disease and in particular smoking and diabetes, smoking is strongly associated with claudication and generally one sees a sparing of tibial vessel disease, while diabetes has a predilection for tibial vessel disease (30). Based on the aforementioned it appears that claudication is more commonly associated with superficial femoral artery disease, and that femoral popliteal bypass is the usual treatment for this lesion. In contrast, most bypasses performed for CLI are to tibial vessels and the objective is to achieve restoration of pulsatile flow into the foot. As in claudication, a significant subgroup of patients (30–40%) with CLI can be successfully treated with femoral popliteal bypass (31,32). In a series by Shah and colleagues evaluating 2058 bypasses using *in situ* saphenous vein, 69% of all revascularizations terminated into the infrapopliteal arteries of which 91% had limb threatening ischemia as the indication for surgery. Therefore, approx 30% of patients with CLI had a femoral popliteal bypass (31).

In planning the femoral popliteal bypass an important consideration is the type of conduit chosen. A number of grafts have been utilized in revascularization. Equally important is the performance of the graft measured in long-term patency and the outcome of either limb salvage or amputation. Commonly used grafts in the above-knee position are autogenous vein (most commonly greater saphenous), umbilical vein, PTFE, and Dacron (knitted polyester), and less commonly venous and arterial homografts, which require additional studies to confirm their role in infrainguinal arterial reconstructions. The Veterans Cooperative study prospectively randomized 752 patients undergoing femoral popliteal bypasses above the knee, to either saphenous vein (SV), human umbilical vein (HUV), or PTFE. At 2 yr the assisted primary patency rates were similar (SV 81%, HUV 70%, PTFE 69%). However, at 5 yr the assisted primary patency rates were superior for saphenous vein (73%) compared to HUV (53%) or PTFE (39%) *(32)*. Major amputation rates were 8.4% with saphenous vein, 9.6% with HUV, and 12.5% with PTFE. Other studies comparing vein to PTFE have found primary graft patencies at 2 yr of 83% and 67%, respectively, indicating acceptable short-term graft function when PTFE above the knee is used as an alternative conduit *(33)*. When considering prosthetic grafts for above knee bypass, both PTFE and Dacron have similar primary patencies at 3 (61% vs 64%) and 5 yr (45% vs 43%), respectively, and limb salvage rates of > 90% can be expected *(34,35)*. Furthermore, to reduce the risk of graft thrombosis, a prosthetic graft diameter of at least 7 mm should be used and preferably the patient's age should be > 65 yr *(35)*.

When revascularization is performed to the below-knee popliteal artery, the autogenous vein has superior patencies compared to other graft materials. Representative 5-yr primary patency rates in patients treated for both claudication and CLI range between 68% and 77%. There is little difference whether the saphenous vein is reversed (77%) or *in situ* (68%) *(see* Table 1). When the indication for femoral to below knee popliteal bypass is CLI and autogenous arm vein is used, 5-yr primary patency rates of up to 70% are approached, with limb salvage rates of 78%. HUV at the below-knee popliteal level has acceptable 5-yr primary patency of 60%, whereas PTFE yields only 40% patency at 5 yr *(36)*. It is clear that vein grafts with a diameter of at least 3.5–4 mm should be considered the conduit of choice, and that other conduits should be considered only in the absence of autogenous vein.

In circumstances of CLI where rest pain and gangrene or ulcer exist, and no suitable autogenous conduit is available, and/or no tibial or pedal vessel can be revascularized, it is acceptable to bypass to an isolated popliteal segment (no direct connection between popliteal artery and tibial vessels) if present. For an isolated popliteal bypass to remain patent and have clinical effect, adequate collaterals need to be present and reach the foot. In a study evaluating previously failed tibial bypass and limited tissue gangrene, isolated popliteal bypass had a primary patency and limb salvage rate at three years of 73% and 86%, respectively *(37)*.

Complications of femoral popliteal bypass surgery can be categorized as systemic, local wound, and graft-related. Systemic complications include cardiopulmonary events and death. It is well known that high-risk patients with perioperative myocardial ischemia undergoing noncardiac surgery have an 18% risk of cardiac events including death *(38)*. Specifically, myocardial infarction, unstable angina, arrhythmias, and congestive heart failure are a significant risk in patients undergoing major vascular surgery, with perioperative event rates of 11% and mortality of 2% *(39)*. Major wound complications range from 6% to 12% *(32,40)*, and the 30-d graft thrombosis rates for femoral popliteal bypass are 4.9% for saphenous vein, 12.3% for HUV, and 2.3% for PTFE.

Endovascular Therapies

Endovascular therapies have gained widespread application in aortoiliac disease, renal artery stenosis, and the arch vessels. The role for endovascular therapy in the vasculature of the lower extremities remains to be defined.

Short single (< 3 cm) stenoses of the femoropopliteal artery are ideal for percutaneous transluminal angioplasty (PTA). Favorable predictive factors are nondiabetic, proximal location, stenosis instead of occlusion, good runoff, no residual stenosis following PTA, and normal renal function *(41)*. A retrospective study evaluating femoropopliteal PTA had a technical success rate of 94.6%. The clinical success (free from progession of disease, amputation, nonhealing wounds) and anatomic patency at 4 yr were 40% and 52%, respectively *(42)*. Others have found PTA of the femoropopliteal artery in patients treated for claudication and CLI inferior to bypass grafting, reporting primary success rates of only 27% at 5 yr *(43)*. A study evaluating 307 PTAs of the femoral, popliteal, and tibial vessels for both stenoses and occlusive disease in patients with CLI demonstrate a 1-yr patency of < 15% *(44)*. Although PTA does not preclude future bypass grafting, the durability of the procedure and costs must be factored into overall patient care. Careful patient selection in those with a high risk for surgery, limited life expectancy, limited or no CLI, and having favorable predictive factors should be considered for PTA as a therapeutic option for focal lesions (< 5 cm) of the femoropopliteal artery. Placement of stents in the femoropopliteal artery as a primary therapeutic intervention is not indicated with either IC or CLI. Stents may have a role in salvaging a PTA procedure that has resulted in arterial dissection, elastic recoil, or thrombosis *(45)*.

The role of endovascular endarterectomy of the superficial artery has recently been evaluated. The endarterectomy system consisted of a ring cutter and primary stenting. The 1-yr primary patency in 17 patients presenting both with claudication and CLI was only 26%, and 59% of these patients required surgical revascularization *(46)*. The number of patients entered in the study was small; endarterctomy with stent placement cannot be recommended, especially when surgical bypass offers greater patency and reliability.

Tibial Bypass

The tibial vessels refer to the anterior tibial artery and the tibioperoneal trunk, which divides into the posterior tibial and peroneal arteries. The anterior tibial artery continues into the ankle and foot as the dorsalis pedis artery, which gives off its main two branches, the lateral tarsal and arcuate arteries. The posterior tibial artery also continues in the foot branching into the medial and lateral plantar arteries, the latter forming the deep plantar artery giving off digital branches and forming the plantar arch with the dorsalis pedal artery. The peroneal artery terminates at the ankle with collaterals to the anterior tibial and posterior tibial arteries via anterior and posterior communicating branches, respectively *(23)*. The inframalleolar arteries include the dorsalis pedis, tarsal branches, posterior tibial, and its lateral and medial branches and are often referred as pedal vessels. Patients with diabetes have a predilection for developing atherosclerosis in the tibial and pedal arteries *(30)*. However, the majority of patients presenting with CLI have multilevel disease involving not only the tibial arteries but also the femoropopliteal segments and inflow aortoiliac vessels *(45)*. The majority of revascularizations to the tibial vessels are for CLI, although approx 23% are performed for severe claudication *(29,31)*.

Revascularization to tibial vessels includes the anterior tibial, posterior tibial, and peroneal arteries. Basic principles to ensure graft patency and favorable outcome include:

1. The inflow artery may be at any level (common femoral, profunda, superficial femoral, popliteal, and tibial) provided that there is noncompromised flow.
2. The distal outflow artery should have the best continuous runoff that will provide perfusion to the foot.
3. Greater saphenous and autogenous veins are the conduits of choice.
4. The best quality target artery should be selected and no attempt should be made to decrease the length of the vein so that a less suitable more proximal artery can be chosen.

The most common inflow artery in a tibial bypass is the common femoral artery. In instances in which the superficial femoral and popliteal arteries are patent, these arterial sites may be considered as the inflow vessel to revascularize the distal tibial or pedal arteries. This is especially useful when sufficient vein length is limited. The majority of bypasses using the distal superficial femoral and popliteal arteries as inflow sites are for CLI, especially in the diabetic patient, because of the predilection for tibial disease with sparing of the superficial femoral–popliteal artery *(47)*. Acceptable 5-yr primary patency of 41% and limb salvage of 69% at 6 yr have been reported; however, even the presence of a 20% or greater stenosis in the inflow artery can lead to early failure *(48)*. The application of PTA of the inflow artery during concomitant revascularization may be of benefit *(47)*. The profunda femoris artery can also serve as an inflow vessel for infrainguinal bypass, and is especially useful when there is inadequate vein graft length, a need to avoid the groin due to scarring from previous operations or infections, and when concomitant profundaplasty is required. Primary patency rates of 78% at 3 yr have been reported and yield similar results to grafts originating from the common femoral, superficial femoral, and popliteal arteries *(49)*.

When the saphenous vein is inadequate or unavailable, arm vein is an excellent conduit bypass. Both the cephalic and basilic veins are suitable and can be reversed or nonreversed with valve lysis applied in the latter case. Faries and colleagues reported on 520 revascularizations with 98% having CLI as the indication and with the majority of the bypasses targeting the distal artery at the tibial and pedal sites. The overall 5-yr primary patency and limb salvage rates were 54.5% and 71.5%, respectively. Interestingly, the authors found that composite arm vein grafts (spliced vein requiring venovenostomy) had patency similar to a single-vein conduit, and that the probability of using the contralateral greater saphenous vein for subsequent infrainguinal bypass (97%) or cardiac bypass (3%) was 26.4% at 2 yr *(50)*.

A number of factors affect reported results of primary patency and limb salvage, leading to wide variability and discrepancies among various studies. Of importance are adherence to reporting standards, clearly defined indications for surgery, patient population and comorbid factors, technical issues, follow-up strategies (noninvasive test vs physical exam), and adjuvant measures applied (vein cuffs, arteriovenous fistulas, anti-

Table 1
Primary Patency and Limb Salvage Rates After Surgical Revascularization

Bypass/conduit	Indication	5-Yr patency	5-Yr LS
Aortofemoral	IC/CLI	85%	n.a.
Axillofemoral	IC/CLI	71%	92%
AK Femoropopliteal/			
RSV	IC	69%	n.a.
AV	IC	60%	n.a.
HUV	IC	70%	n.a.
PTFE	IC	60%	n.a.
BK Femoropopliteal/			
RSV	IC/CLI	77%	75%
ISV	IC/CLI	68%	78%
AV	CLI	70%	78%
HUV	IC/CLI	60%	n.a.
PTFE	IC/CLI	40%	n.a.
Femorotibial/			
RSV	CLI	62%	82%
ISV	CLI	68%	83%
AV	CLI	58%	82%
HUV	CLI	37%	n.a.
PTFE	CLI	21%	48%

LS, limb salvage; IC, intermittent claudication; CLI, critical limb ischemia; AK, above knee; BK, below knee; RSV, reverse saphenous vein; ISV, *in situ* saphenous vein; AV, arm vein; HUV, human umbilical vein; PTFE, polytetrafluoroethylene; n.a., not available.
Adapted with permission of the publisher from Weitz JI, et al. Circulation 1996;94:3026–3049.

coagulation, etc.). The American Heart Association Scientific Council evaluated multiple studies and reported 5-yr primary patency results for femorotibial bypass for CLI with reverse saphenous vein, *in situ* vein, arm vein, HUV, and PTFE of 62%, 68%, 58%, 37%, and 21%, respectively *(36)*. There was a reported 5-yr limb salvage for reverse saphenous vein, *in situ* vein, arm vein, and PTFE of 82%, 83%, 82%, and 48%, respectively *(36)*. These reports are consistent with those published by the Trans Atlantic Intersociety Consensus evaluating a large body of studies with similar categories including indication, conduit, reverse or nonreversed vein, and distal artery anastomosis *(45)*. Table 1 summarizes the 5-yr primary patency and limb salvage results with respect to conduit, bypass performed, and surgical indication for both infrainguinal revascularizations and inflow bypass procedures, as many patients may undergo both procedures either simultaneously or more commonly staged. For infrainguinal revascularizations, particularly to the below-knee popliteal and tibial pedal vessels, the superiority of autogenous vein is evident. Autogenous vein is the conduit of choice and should be used in all instances if available to ensure improved patency and limb salvage.

In instances in which the tibial vessels are not continuous into the foot and patent vessels are present in the foot, inframalleolar bypass is warranted for limb salvage. Plantar artery revascularization has been reported by various authors mainly to salvage limbs with CLI *(51,52)*. These bypasses should be undertaken only with vein. Although a complete pedal arch is favorable for graft function, an incomplete pedal arch does not preclude proceeding with revascularization. Primary patency rates at 2 yr range between 67% and 74%, and limb salvage is about 78%.

In circumstances in which the pedal arteries preclude revascularization for CLI, and a patent peroneal artery is available, bypass to the peroneal is acceptable. The peroneal artery collateralizes to the pedal arteries via the anterior and posterior branches, providing adequate flow to the foot to allow for wound healing. In a study comparing graft function at either the dorsalis pedis or peroneal artery in patients with CLI having similar demographics and risk factors, secondary patency and limb salvage rates at 5-yr for the dorsalis pedis and peroneal were grafts 68% vs 76%, and 87% vs 93%, respectively *(53)*. The authors found no statistical differences and concluded that the artery chosen should be based on limitations of graft length and site of adjacent wounds *(53)*.

In constructing venous bypasses of the lower extremity the saphenous vein can be *in situ*, nonreversed, or reversed. Advantages of the *in situ* technique include limiting wound size and reducing wound site complications. It also allows for better size match between the vein and artery at the proximal and distal anastomoses. A theoretical consideration is that leaving the vein *in situ* could reduce trauma to surrounding tissues and the vasa vasorum possibly improving patencies. An *in situ* or nonreversed vein requires the valves to be lysed with a valvulotome to allow for inline arterial blood flow. Disadvantages of *in situ* and nonreversed vein is damage to the vein during valve leaflet valvulotomy, inadequate visualization of the entire vein for assessment of size, sclerosis and duplication of the vein, and inadequate disconnection of arteriovenous fistulas once the vein has been arterialized. Most of these potential problems can be resolved by preoperative interrogation of the vein by duplex ultrasound, careful handling of the vein during valvulotomy, and intraoperative completion arteriography or duplex evaluation. Reversing the greater saphenous vein requires removing the vein from its anatomic subcutaneous bed. This allows for direct visualization of the vein and does not require manipulation of the endoluminal surface with valve cutters, thereby removing the possibility of intimal injuries and tears, and incomplete valve lysis. Despite the pros and cons for either technique, there are no statistical differences in patency of the grafts or limb salvage, and either method for infrainguinal revascularization is considered equivalent *(45,54–56)*.

The complications of femoral tibial bypass are essentially those of femoral popliteal bypass with similar rates of complications as previously described. The majority of patients having revascularization to the tibial and pedal vessels have underlying cardiopulmonary disease, and comorbid risk factors. Special attention to preoperative evaluation and medical management of hypertension, angina, congestive heart failure, diabetes, dyslipidemia, and tobacco use is imperative for a favorable result.

Endovascular Approach

Endovascular PTA of the tibial and peroneal vessels has a high rate of failure, particularly in patients with diabetes (44). As many as 60–90% of patients with tibial disease have diabetes. A problem with PTA of the tibioperoneal artery is that very few patients present with focal disease, therefore making PTA less likely to restore flow when diffuse disease is present with poor runoff. In selected patients with focal tibial disease, PTA is feasible with acceptable limb salvage rates; however, diligent follow-up is mandatory *(45)*.

ADJUNCTIVE SURGICAL PROCEDURES

In an effort to provide improved graft patencies especially when autogenous vein is unavailable, a multitude of surgical adjunctive procedures have been developed. These include distal vein patches and cuffs, arteriovenous fistulas, and composite grafts.

Vein Patches and Cuffs

Commonly applied vein patches and cuffs are the Miller patch/cuff, Taylor patch, and Linton patch. All patches and cuffs conform a small segment of vein to the distal anastomosis where the prosthetic graft comes into direct contact or adjacent to the target artery. Taylor and colleagues described an anastomotic vein patch in popliteal and infrapopliteal bypasses using PTFE. The principle is that the vein patch is autogenous tissue and, in theory, should have better compliance and reduced progression of myointimal hyperplasia, which is a major factor in late graft failure. The authors reported 5-yr primary patency rates for popliteal anastomoses of 71% and tibioperoneal anastomoses of 54%. Of interest, all patients were given perioperative aspirin and prostaglandin E_1, and no anticoagulation postoperatively *(57)*. Reports of interposition vein cuffs (Miller cuff) in patients with CLI and claudication have been published. Vein cuffs placed in above-knee PTFE bypass offer no advantage to PTFE alone; however, vein cuffs in below-knee bypasses have a primary patency rate at 2 yr of 52% vs 29% with no cuff, and limb salvage rates were 20% greater when vein cuffs were applied *(58)*. Vein cuffs have also been used in tibial vessels for CLI. Primary patency rates of PTFE plus vein cuff vs PTFE alone at 2 yr were reported as 54% and 12%, respectively, and limb salvage rates of 61% and 22% at 42 mo, respectively *(59)*. Distal vein patches have also been advocated to prolong graft patency. The principle of a distal vein patch is to anastomose a 2- to 3-cm segment of vein to a tibial artery, and then anastomose the PTFE graft to the vein patch via a venotomy extending two thirds of the longitudinal distance of the vein patch. Neville and colleagues reported 80 distal vein patch PTFE bypasses to tibial vessels in 79 patients with CLI. The 4-yr primary patency and limb salvage rates were 63% and 79%, respectively *(60)*. Results with adjuvant vein cuffs and patches are encouraging, especially when applied to the below-knee popliteal and tibial arteries. Further randomized studies will be required to establish their role; however, vein cuffs and patches appear as an acceptable alternative when a paucity of autogenous vein exists.

Arteriovenous Fistulas

Arteriovenous fistula creation at the distal anastomosis has been advocated to improve below knee and tibial bypasses when PTFE is used. The principle is to decrease vascular resistance and increase flow in the graft without causing a steal phenomenon. The arteriovenous fistula can be constructed through a common ostia by suturing the artery and vein together at the distal anastomosis, or making a separate fistula distal to the anastomosis *(45)*. A study comparing arteriovenous fistula to vein cuffs in patients with CLI found primary patency at 3 yr of 48% vs 38%, respectively *(61)*. The limb salvage during that same time period was 76% and 92%, respectively *(61)*. An interesting study comparing infrapopliteal PTFE bypass with or without adjuvant arteriovenous fistula (AVF) concluded that no advantage was afforded by the fistula *(62)*. The 1-yr primary patency and limb salvage rates with an adjuvant AVF were 55% and 54%, respectively, compared with 53% and 43% without an AVF *(62)*. However, in this study all patients, regardless if the fistula was placed or not, had an interposition vein cuff performed *(62)*. If an arteriovenous fistula is performed, it is probably best reserved for tibioperoneal reconstructions.

Composite Grafts

A composite graft consists of a conduit that is composed of prosthetic material proximally that is sewn end to end to vein, which is placed at the distal anastomosis. A composite graft can be considered when patients have only a limited length of vein, therefore necessitating an additional conduit to increase the length of the graft to reach the distal target artery. Theoretical advantages are distal vein crossing the knee joint, prosthetic conduit at the inflow vessel, and using only enough synthetic material to complete the conduit. A study evaluating 96 PTFE–vein composite grafts for CLI, with target arteries to the below knee popliteal and tibioperoneal arteries reported 5-yr primary patency rates of 58%, and limb salvage of 80% *(63)*. Others have found that composite grafts have inferior patencies compared to arm vein in patients operated on for CLI, with > 90% of revascularizations being performed to the tibioperoneal and pedal vessels. The 5-yr primary patency and limb salvage for arm vein was reported at 54% and 76%, respectively *(64)*. For composite graft both graft patency and limb salvage were 0% at 5 yr *(64)*.

When considering the use of adjunctive procedures, patient selection is important. Specific indications for vein cuffs and patches, arteriovenous fistulas, and composite grafts will require further randomized studies to define their role in infrainguinal revascularization. Based on the current literature, in the presence of available autogenous vein, adjuvant surgical procedures to extend graft length should be limited.

END-STAGE RENAL DISEASE AND INFRAINGUINAL REVASCULARIZATION

Patients with end-stage renal disease (ESRD) on dialysis are at increased risk for development of infrainguinal arterial disease. The mortality rate is increased with an adjusted 5-yr survival rate of only 28% in patients on dialysis. A significant proportion of dialysis patients have diabetes mellitus and cardiovascular disease, and 54% of deaths in dialysis dependent patients are attributed to cardiac and cerebrovascular events *(65)*. In the United States the rate of patients progressing to ESRD requiring dialysis is increasing, in particular, in patients between the ages of 60 and 80 yr *(65–67)*. Many dialysis patients have significant cardiovascular disease including lower extremity arterial disease, and of those dialysis patients having infrainguinal arterial occlusions > 90% present with CLI requiring surgical therapy. The literature is controversial with regards to revascularization vs primary amputation in this high-risk group of patients, with reported operative mortality rates of 5–13%, and morbidity as high as 47% for revascularization *(68)*. Most studies evaluating ESRD patients on dialysis undergoing revascularization conclude that primary patency rates are lower than similar operations performed in patients without ESRD. Despite the lower patency rates, the limb salvage rate in patients with ESRD appears to be comparable to those patients without renal disease. Specific studies evaluating bypass procedures in patients with ESRD report primary patency rates at 2 yr of 68% and limb salvage of 84% *(69)*. In a study comparing patients with diabetes and ESRD on dialysis versus patients with only diabetes, the patients on dialysis had markedly worse primary patency at 1 yr of 53% vs 82% in diabetic nondialysis patients *(68)*. Of significance is the low survival rate of only 52% at 1 yr and 39% at 3 yr in patients on dialysis undergoing infrainguinal revascularization. Because of the limited life expectancy of patients on dialysis having CLI and lower short-term graft patency, some authors advocate primary amputation *(70)*. Patients with ESRD on dialysis with CLI present a formidable challenge. The surgeon must weigh the risks and benefits as well as the quality of life following infrainguinal reconstructions. Further studies are required to establish guidelines for revascularization in patients with ESRD, and at this time individualization of care is essential.

SUMMARY

Patients with CLI or IC requiring surgical reconstruction are generally complex because of other comorbid conditions. For this reason, any consideration of the possibility of surgical reconstruction should be well thought out and planned. Once nonoperative therapeutic interventions have been initiated and are found to be unsuccessful, it is appropriate to proceed with surgical reconstruction. A complete history and physical exam along with supporting noninvasive laboratory and confirming radiographic evaluation should be undertaken. If the problem is an inflow problem, then operative risk assessment for the type of surgical inflow procedure is essential. An important consideration is whether the patient can safely undergo an aortobifemoral bypass procedure or whether an extraanatomic procedure is a better option. If the patient requires an outflow procedure because of evidence of a compromised circulation distal to the femoral artery, again an appropriate preoperative evaluation to assess those risk factors that might influence the outcome of the surgical reconstruction should be undertaken.

REFERENCES

1. Boushey CJ, Beresford SA, Omenn GS, Motulsky AG. A quantitative assessment of plasma homocysteine as a risk factor for vascular disease: probable benefits of increasing folic acid intakes. JAMA 1995;274:1049–1057.
2. Criqui MH, Denenberg JO, Langer RD, Fronek A. The epidemiology of peripheral arterial disease: importance of identifying the population at risk. Vasc Med 1997;2:221–226.
3. Ridker PM, Stampfer MJ, Rifai N. Novel risk factors for systemic atherosclerosis: a comparison of C-reactive protein, fibrinogen, homocysteine, lipoprotein(a), and standard cholesterol screening as predictors of peripheral arterial disease. JAMA 2001;285:2481–2485.
4. Taylor LM, Moneta GL, Sexton GJ, Schuff RA, Porter JM. Prospective blinded study of the relationship between plasma homocysteine and progression of symptomatic peripheral arterial disease. J Vasc Surg 1999;29:8–19.
5. Lam EY, Taylor LM, Landry GJ, Porter JM, Moneta GL. Relationship between antiphospholipid antibodies and progression of lower extremity arterial occlusive disease after lower extremity bypass operations. J Vasc Surg 2001;33:976–982.
6. DeVries SO, Hunink MGM. Results of aortic bifurcation grafts for aortoiliac occlusive disease: a meta-analysis. J Vasc Surg 1997;26:558–569.
7. Amwli FM, Stein M, Aro L, Provan JL, Gray R, Grossman H. End-to-end vs end-to-side proximal anastomosis in aortobifemoral bypass surgery: does it matter? Can J Surg 1991;34:243–246.
8. Cormio L, Edgren J, Lepantalo M, et al. Aortofemoral surgery and sexual function. Eur J Vasc Endovasc Surg 1996;11:453–457.
9. Sicard GA, Reilly JM, Rubin BG, et al. Transabdominal versus retroperitoneal incision for abdominal aortic surgery: report of a prospective randomized trial. J Vasc Surg1995;21:174–183.

10. Cambria RP, Brewster DC, Abbott WM, et al. Transperitoneal versus retroperitoneal approach for aortic reconstruction J Vasc Surg 2000;11:314–325.

11. Passman MA, Taylor LM, Moneta GL et al. Comparison of axillofemoral and aortofemoral bypass for aortoiliac occlusive disease. J Vasc Surg 1996;23:263–271.

12. Rutherford RB, Patt A, Pearce WH. Extraanatomic bypass: a closer look. J Vasc Surg 1987;6:437–446.

13. Calligaro KD, Ascer E, Veith FJ, et al. Unsuspected inflow disease in candidates for axillofemoral bypass operations: a prospective study. J Vasc Surg 1990;11:832–837.

14. Harris JE, Taylor LM, McConnell DB, Moneta GL, Yeager RA, Porter JM. Clinical results of axillofemoral bypass using externally supported polytetrafluoroethylene. J Vasc Surg 1990;12: 416–421.

15. Darling RC, Leather RP, Chang BB, Lloyd WE, Shah DM. Is the iliac artery a suitable inflow conduit for iliofemoral occlusive disease? An analysis of 514 aortoiliac reconstructions. J Vasc Surg 1990;12: 409–415.

16. van den Dungen JJAN, Boontje JA, Kriveld A. Unilateral iliofemoral occlusive disease: long-term results of the semiclosed endarterectomy with the ring stripper. J Vasc Surg 1991;14:673–677.

17. Kalmar PG, Hoserg M, Johnston KW. The current role for femorofemoral bypass. J Vasc Surg 1987;6: 71–76.

18. Flanagan P, Pratt DG, Goodrean JJ. Hemodynamic and angiographic guidelines in selection of patients for femorofemoral bypass. J Vasc Surg1987;6:71–76.

19. Griffith CDM, Callum KG. Limb salvage surgery in a district general hospital: factors affecting outcome. Ann Coll Surg (Engl) 1988;70:95–98.

20. Norgen L, Alwmark A, Angqvist KA, et al. A stable prostacyclin analogue (Iloprost) in the treatment of ischemic ulcers of the lower limb: a Scandinavian–Polish placebo-controlled randomized multicenter study. Eur J Vasc Surg 1991;4:463–467.

21. Muluk SC, Muluk VS, Kelley ME, et al. Outcome events in patients with claudication: a 15-year study in 2777 patients. J Vasc Surg 2001;33:251–258.

22. Newman AB, Shemanski L, Manolio TA, et al. Ankle-arm index as a predictor of cardiovascular disease and mortality in the cardiovascular health study. Arterioscler Thromb Vasc Biol 1999;19:538–545.

23. Moore KL. The lower limb. In: Moore KL, ed. Clinically Oriented Anatomy, 2nd edit. Baltimore: Williams & Wilkins, 1985; pp.396–564.

24. Madiba TE, Mars M, Robbs JV. Aortobifemoral bypass in the presence of superficial femoral artery occlusion: does the profunda femoris artery provide adequate runoff? J R Coll Surg (Edinb) 1998;43: 310–313.

25. Prendiville EJ, Burke PE, Colgan MP, Wee BL, Moore DJ, Shanik DG. The profunda femoris: a durable outflow vessel in aortofemoral surgery. J Vasc Surg 1992;16:23–29.

26. Bastounis E, Felekouras E, Pikoulis E, Hadjinikolaou L, Georgopoulos S, Balas P. The role of profunda femoris revascularization in aortofemoral surgery: an analysis of factors affecting graft patency. Int Angiol 1997;16:107–113.

27. van der Plas JP, Dijk J, Tordoir JH, Jacobs MJ, Kitslaar PJ. Isolated profundaplasty in critical limb ischemia: still of any use? Eur J Vasc Surg 1993;7:54–58.

28. Panayiotopoulos YP, Reidy JF, Taylor PR. The concept of knee salvage: why does a failed femorocrural/pedal arterial bypass not affect the amputation level? Eur J Vasc Endovasc Surg 1997;14: 417–418.

29. Byrne J, Darling C, Chang BB, et al. Infrainguinal arterial reconstructions for claudication: is it worth the risk? An analysis of 409 procedures. J Vasc Surg 1999;29:259–269.

30. Menzoian JO, LaMorte WW, Paniszyn CC, et al. Symptomatology and anatomic patterns of peripheral vascular disease: differing impact of smoking and diabetes. Ann Vasc Surg 1989;3:224–228.

31. Shah DM, Darling RC, Chang BB, Fitzgerald KM, Paty PS, Leather RP. Long-term results of *in situ* saphenous vein bypass: analysis of 2058 cases. Ann Surg 1995;222:438–446.

32. Johnson WC, Lee KK. A comparative evaluation of polytetrafluoroethylene, umbilical vein, and saphenous vein bypass grafts for femoral–popliteal above-knee revascularizations: a prospective randomized Department of Veterans Affairs Cooperative Study. J Vasc Surg 2000;32:268–277.

33. Burger DHC, Kappetein AP, van Bockel H, Breslau PJ. A prospective randomized trial comparing vein with polytetrafluoroethylene in above-knee femoropopliteal bypass grafting. J Vasc Surg 2000;32: 278–283.

34. Post S, Kraus T, Muller-Reinartz U, et al. Dacron vs. polytetrafluoroethylene grafts for femoropopliteal bypass: a prospective randomized multicenter trial. Eur J Vasc Endovasc Surg 2001;22:226–231.

35. Green RM, Abbott WM, Matsumoto T, et al. Prosthetic above-knee femoropopliteal bypass grafting: five year results of a randomized trial. J Vasc Surg 2000;31:417–425.

36. Weitz JI, Byrne J, Clagett GP, et al. Diagnosis and treatment of chronic arterial insufficiency of the lower extremities: a critical review. Circulation 1996;94:3026–3049.

37. Samson RH, Showalter DP, Yunis JP. Isolated femoropopliteal bypass graft for limb salvage after failed tibial reconstruction: a viable alternative to amputation. J Vasc Surg 1999;29:409–412.

38. Mangano DT, Browner WS, Hollenberg M, London MJ, Tubau JF, Tateo IM. Association of perioperative myocardial ischemia with cardiac morbidity and mortality in men undergoing noncardiac surgery: the Study of Perioperative Ischemia Research Group. N Engl J Med 1990;323: 1781–1788.

39. de Virgilio C, Toosie K, Ephraim L, et al. Dipyridamole-thallium/sestamibi before vascular surgery: a prospective blinded study in moderate-risk patients. J Vasc Surg 2000;32:77–89.

40. Schwartz ME, Harrington EB, Schanzer H. Wound complications after *in situ* bypass. J Vasc Surg 1988;7:802–807.

41. Clark TW, Groffsky JL, Soulen MC. Predictors of long-term patency after femoropopliteal angioplasty: results from the STAR registry. J Vasc Interv Radiol 2001;12:923–933.

42. Karch LA, Mattos MA, Henretta PJ, McLafferty RB, Ramsey DE, Hodgson KJ. Clinical failure after percutaneous transluminal angioplasty of the superficial femoral and popliteal arteries. J Vasc Surg 2000;31:880–887.

43. Lofberg AM, Karacagil S, Ljungman C, et al. Percutaneous transluminal angioplasty of the femoropopliteal arteries in limbs with chronic critical lower limb ischemia. J Vasc Surg 2001;34: 114–121.

44. Parsons RE, Suggs WD, Lee JJ, Sanchez LA, Lyon RT, Veith FJ. Percutaneous transluminal angioplasty for the treatment of limb threatening ischemia: do the results justify an attempt before bypass grafting? J Vasc Surg 1998;28:1066-1071.

45. TASC Working Group. Management of peripheral arterial disease (PAD). J Vasc Surg 2000;31: S1–S296.

46. Nelson PR, Powell RJ, Proia RR, et al. Results of endovascular superficial femoral endarterectomy. J Vasc Surg 2001;34:526–531.

47. Verhelst R, Bruneau M, Nicolas AL, et al. Popliteal-to-distal bypass grafts for limb salvage. Ann Vasc Surg 1997;11:505–509.

48. Rosenbloom MS, Walsh JJ, Shuler JJ, et al. Long-term results of infragenicular bypasses with autogenous vein originating from the distal superficial femoral and popliteal arteries. J Vasc Surg 1988;7: 691–696.

49. Mills JL, Taylor SM, Fujitani RM. The role of the deep femoral artery as an inflow site for infrainguinal revascularization. J Vasc Surg 1993;18:416–423.

50. Faries PL, Arora S, Pomposelli FB, et al. The use of arm vein in lower-extremity revascularization: results of 520 procedures performed in eight years. J Vasc Surg 2000;31:50–59.

51. Ascer E, Veith FJ, Gupta SK. Bypasses to plantar arteries and other tibial branches: an extended approach to limb salvage. J Vasc Surg 1988;8:434–441.

52. Roddy SP, Darling RC, Chang BB, et al. Outcomes with plantar bypass for limb-threatening ischemia. Ann Vasc Surg 2001;15:79–83.

53. Darling RC, Chang BB, Shah DM, Leather RP. Choice of peroneal or dorsalis pedis artery bypass for limb salvage. Semin Vasc Surg 1997;10:17–22.

54. Belkin M, Knox J, Donoldson MC, Mannick JA, Whittemore AD. Infrainguinal arterial reconstruction with nonreversed greater saphenous vein. J Vasc Surg 1996;24:957–962.

55. Eugster T, Stierli P, Aeberhard P. Infrainguinal arterial reconstructions with autologous vein grafts: are the results for the *in situ* technique better than those of non-reversed bypass? A long-term follow-up study. J Cardiovasc Surg (Torino) 2001;42:221–226.

56. Watelet J, Soury P, Menard JF, Plissonnier D, Peillon C, Lestrat JP. Femoropopliteal bypass: *in situ* or reversed vein grafts? Ten-year results of a randomized prospective study. Ann Vasc Surg 1997;11: 510–519.

57. Taylor RS, Loh A, McFarland RJ, Cox M, Chester JF. Improved technique for polytetrafluoroethylene bypass grafting: long-term results using anastomotic vein patches. Br J Surg 1992;79:348–354.

58. Stonebridge PA, Prescott RJ, Ruckley CV. Randomized trial comparing infrainguinal polytetrafluoroethylene bypass grafting with and without vein interposition cuff at the distal anastomosis: the joint vascular research group. J Vasc Surg 1997;26:543–550.

59. Kansal N, Pappas PJ, Gwertzman GA, et al. Patency and limb salvage for polytetrafluoroethylene bypasses with vein interposition cuffs. Ann Vasc Surg 1999;13:386–392.
60. Neville RF, Tempesta B, Sidawy AN. Tibial bypass for limb salvage using polytetrafluoroethylene and a distal vein patch. J Vasc Surg 2001;33:266–272.
61. Kreienberg PB, Darling RC, Chang BB, Paty PS, Lloyd WE, Shah DM. Adjunctive techniques to improve patency of distal prosthetic bypass grafts: polytetrafluoroethylene with remote arteriovenous fistulae versus vein cuffs. J Vasc Surg 2000;31:696–701.
62. Hamsho A, Nott D, Harris PL. Prospective randomized trial of distal arteriovenous fistula as an adjunct to femoro-infrapopliteal PTFE grafts. Eur J Vasc Endovasc Surg 1999;17:197–201.
63. Bastounis E, Georgopoulos S, Maltezos C, Alexiou D, Chiotopoulos D, Bramis J. PTFE-vein composite grafts for critical limb ischemia: a valuable alternative to all-autogenous infrageniculate reconstructions. Eur J Vasc Endovasc Surg 1999;18:127–132.
64. Faries PL, LoGerfo FW, Arora S, et al. Arm vein conduit is superior to composite prosthetic-autogenous grafts in lower extremity revascularization. J Vasc Surg 2000;31:1119–1127.
65. Owen WF, Madore F, Brenner BM. An observational study of cardiovascular characteristics of long-term end-stage renal disease survivors. Am J Kidney Dis 1996;28:931–936.
66. Peri UN, Fenvez AZ, Middleton JP. Improving survival of octogenarian patients selected for hemodialysis. Nephrol Dial Transplant 2001;16:2201–2206.
67. Baek MY, Kwon TH, Kim YL, Cho DK. CAPD, an acceptable form of therapy in elderly ESRD patients: a comparative study. Adv Perit Dial 1997;13:158–161.
68. Hakaim AG, Gordon JK, Scott TE. Early outcome of *in situ* femorotibial reconstruction among patients with diabetes alone versus diabetes and end-stage renal failure: analysis of 83 limbs. J Vasc Surg 1998;27:1049–1055.
69. Harrington EB, Harrington ME, Schanzer H, Haimov M. End-stage renal disease: is infrainguinal limb revascularization justified? J Vasc Surg 1990;12:691–696.
70. Edwards JM, Taylor LM, Porter JM. Limb salvage in end-stage renal disease (ESRD): comparison of modern results in patients with and without ESRD. Arch Surg 1988;123:1164–1168.

14 Perioperative Cardiac Evaluation and Management for Vascular Surgery

Robert T. Eberhardt, MD and
April Nedeau, BS

CONTENTS

INTRODUCTION

Cardiovascular complications are the leading cause of morbidity and mortality following major vascular surgery, with rates estimated as high as 30% *(1)*. These complications include acute coronary syndromes, unstable angina or myocardial infarction (MI), pulmonary edema, and cardiac death. The ominous feature of a perioperative MI is that as many as 30–50% are fatal *(2)*. In patients with peripheral artery disease (PAD), rates of perioperative cardiac death are twice that of the general surgical population *(3,4)*. This is not surprising given the systemic nature of atherosclerosis and the increased prevalence of coexistent coronary artery disease (CAD), reported in as many as 70% of patients with PAD *(5)*.

In addition to the role of CAD, the physiologic response to surgery and anesthesia contributes to an environment that is conducive to these cardiovascular events. During the perioperative period, cardiovascular homeostasis is altered with depressed myocardial function, heightened vascular tone, increased coronary artery sheer stress, and enhanced platelet aggregation. Other physiologic stressors include fluctuation in intravascular volume, body temperature, autonomic nervous system activity, and serum catecholamines. The combination of these factors provides the basis for the development of the cardiovascular complications and leads to the characteristic timing of events. Acute MI has a bimodal distribution with an important peak occurring 48–72 h after surgery. Similarly, pulmonary edema may occur early in recovery or later with fluid

From: *Contemporary Cardiology: Peripheral Arterial Disease: Diagnosis and Treatment*
Edited by: J. D. Coffman and R. T. Eberhardt © Humana Press Inc., Totowa, NJ

mobilization about 72 h following surgery. Thus the second and third postoperative days are an important time from the cardiac standpoint owing to the development of these cardiac events.

It should be emphasized that the presence of PAD selects a population that carries high cardiovascular risk and requires special preoperative consideration. A preoperative assessment is designed to identify individuals at high risk, thus permitting attempts to reduce risk and minimize morbidity and mortality. This chapter provides an overview of the issues involved in the preoperative cardiac evaluation and perioperative management of the patient undergoing vascular surgery.

CORONARY ARTERY DISEASE AND ITS IMPACT

It is well established that PAD is associated with coexistent CAD—the prevalence of which depends on the methods utilized to establish the diagnosis. In patients undergoing vascular surgery, clinically evident "CAD" is present in 30–50% of cases *(6)*. The prevalence is greatly increased with the use of invasive methodology, such as coronary angiography. Coronary angiograms performed in 1000 consecutive patients undergoing elective vascular surgery at the Cleveland Clinic revealed "significant" CAD (defined by at least a 50% stenosis involving one or more coronary vessels) in 60% of patients *(5)*. Employing the criteria of a 70% or greater stenosis, "significant" CAD was found to involve one coronary vessel in 27% of patients, two coronary vessels in 19% of patients, and three coronary vessels in 11% of patients. Furthermore, about 25% of patients undergoing elective vascular surgery had "severe correctable" CAD *(5)*.

The presence of CAD accounts for most of the adverse outcomes of vascular surgery contributing to the increased development of acute MI and coronary death. Ischemic heart disease with MI accounted for 40–60% of deaths in those undergoing vascular reconstructive surgery *(7)*. The presence of "suspected" CAD increases postoperative mortality following vascular surgery approximately fourfold compared with no "overt" CAD *(6)*. The perioperative cardiac event rate in patients with clinical evidence of CAD was 11% compared to 1.7% in those without evidence of CAD.

In addition to the periprocedural concerns, the presence of CAD detrimentally influences late survival in patients undergoing elective vascular surgery. The presence of "suspected" CAD is associated with a twofold increase in the 5-yr mortality compared to those without "overt" disease *(6)*. The survival rates were poor in 1112 patients undergoing abdominal aortic aneurysm repair with a 5-yr survival of 67.5% and 10-yr survival of 40.7% *(8)*. In this group afflicted with vascular disease, reduced survival correlated strongly with evidence of ischemic heart disease.

CORONARY REVASCULARIZATION

The detrimental impact that CAD has on outcomes in patients with PAD undergoing vascular surgery encourages a strategy favoring coronary revascularization. Despite the intuitive appeal of this approach, there is scant evidence demonstrating that this improves clinical outcomes during vascular surgery. All the studies reported to date have been retrospective in nature, as there have been no prospectively conducted trials. Advocates of this approach point to the effects of coronary revascularization in patients with PAD on short-term (or perioperative) outcomes as well as long-term survival.

Coronary Artery Bypass Graft Surgery

Several retrospective studies have suggested that there is a "protective" effect of coronary artery bypass graft surgery (CABG) during subsequent vascular surgery *(9)*. In patients with CAD and angina pectoris, CABG performed either prior to or simultaneously with carotid endarterectomy was associated with a lower mortality during carotid endarterectomy, from 18% to 3% *(10)*. Similarly, in patients found to have "severe correctable" CAD during preoperative coronary angiography, mortality was low (0.8%) if the vascular surgery was preceded by CABG *(9)*. In the CASS (Coronary Artery Surgery Study) registry, prior CABG was associated with a reduced mortality during noncardiac surgery, from 2.4% to 0.9% *(11)*. Prior CABG in patients undergoing high-risk surgery was associated with fewer operative deaths (1.7% vs 3.3%, $p = 0.03$) and myocardial infarction (0.8% vs 2.7%, $p = 0.002$) compared with medical management *(12)*.

Looking beyond the perioperative impact, CABG may influence long-term survival. In patients undergoing vascular surgery, prior CABG was associated with half the 5-yr mortality compared with those with suspected CAD without CABG *(6)*. The European Coronary Surgery study compared CABG to medical therapy in 768 men with angina and at least two-vessel CAD *(13)*. The outcomes were not dramatically different in these two groups at 5 yr. However, if the presence or absence of PAD was considered, there was a marked difference between medical therapy and CABG. In patients with PAD, 8-yr survival was 85% in the CABG group compared with 52% in the medical therapy group. These data support a possible long-term beneficial effect of coronary revascularization in patients with PAD.

Percutaneous Revascularization

Given the appropriate coronary anatomy, it seems logical that percutaneous coronary revascularization may reduce the risk of major perioperative cardiac complications. However, as with CABG, there are no prospectively conducted randomized trials to support percutaneous revascularization prior to vascular surgery. The reported outcomes from retrospective analysis have varied by centers and with the techniques utilized.

BALLOON ANGIOPLASTY

Several studies have reported on the impact of percutaneous coronary revascularization, using balloon angioplasty, on the perioperative outcomes from noncardiac surgery. In a study from the Mayo Clinic, 50 patients with symptomatic CAD and abnormal stress tests underwent percutaneous transluminal coronary angioplasty (PTCA) prior to noncardiac surgery *(14)*. The majority of these patients had advanced symptoms with Canadian Heart Association Class III or IV angina or unstable angina. PTCA was performed at a median of 9 d prior to noncardiac surgery. The frequency of major cardiac complications with noncardiac surgery was 5.6% for MI and 1.9% for death. This may be compared with an anticipated rate as high as 30% in this high-risk group. Another study from the Cleveland Clinic reported outcomes in 194 patients who underwent PTCA within 3 mo prior to vascular surgery *(15)*. Over half of these patients had a previous MI. During the elective vascular surgery in this high-risk group only one patient died and one suffered a myocardial infarction, although the cardiac morbidity was 13.4% primarily due to postoperative congestive heart failure.

In contrast, the practice of routine coronary angiography and revascularization has been questioned. A review of 297 patients with an ischemic response on persantine thallium prior to vascular surgery found that 70 patients had undergone coronary angiography with 25 having subsequent coronary revascularization *(16)*. Although no coronary events were reported in those having coronary angiography, the complications of the coronary evaluation and intervention may offset any potential benefit. Comparing the 70 patients who underwent angiography to 70 matched patients without coronary imaging, there was no reduction in perioperative events including nonfatal and fatal MI with angiographic-guided therapy. Furthermore, there was no benefit in terms of long-term survival rates with up to 4 yr of follow-up.

CORONARY STENTING

Since their introduction in the 1990s, coronary stents have become the mainstay of interventional cardiology, accounting for the majority of the procedures. The use of these devices during coronary revascularization prior to vascular surgery has appeal. Contrary to this belief, "catastrophic outcomes" have been reported when surgery was performed soon after coronary stenting *(17)*. Analysis of 40 consecutive patients who underwent coronary stenting within 6 wk prior to noncardiac surgery found a high rate of MI, bleeding, and death. In this study, perioperative coronary stenting, performed on an average of 13 d before surgery, was associated with 7 MI, 11 major bleeds, and 8 deaths. All the MI and deaths and most of the bleeding episodes (8 of 11) occurred in patients who underwent stenting within 2 wk of surgery. The mortality rate among the 25 operated within 2 wk was 32%.

The periprocedural use of antiplatelet therapy, primarily aspirin and ticlopidine, was often interrupted and may have contributed to the adverse outcomes. Of the eight deceased patients, five patients had both aspirin and ticlopidine stopped 0–2 d before surgery. In contrast, the continued use of aggressive antiplatelet therapy was also not felt to be safe, as three of five patients in whom both agents were continued had a major bleeding episode and died.

Retrospective analysis of the effect of coronary revascularization on perioperative events often overlooks the risk associated with both procedures. This is especially important if the rationale for coronary revascularization is for "protection" rather than used as a symptom-driven therapy. The complication rate of coronary revascularization, both surgical and percutaneous, is much greater in those with PAD, with a nearly twofold increased risk *(18)*. As a general rule coronary revascularization prior to noncardiac surgery should be considered only if it would be appropriate if no surgery were anticipated *(19)*. Performing "prophylactic" coronary revascularization either surgically or percutaneously has not been shown to be beneficial. It is advocated that selective revascularization be performed based on clinical manifestations.

PREOPERATIVE EVALUATION

The concern for coexistent occult CAD in patients with PAD undergoing vascular surgery has led to various suggestions regarding the aggressiveness of the preoperative evaluation. This has ranged from simply a clinical evaluation to routine angiography with coronary revascularization. The goal of the preoperative evaluation prior to vascular surgery is the same as that prior to any surgery—to identify and attempt to attenuate risk associated with increased perioperative cardiovascular morbidity and mortality.

Clinical Evaluation

Factors contributing to the perioperative risk arise from patient-specific issues, as well as issues specific to the surgical procedure being performed. Patient-specific features include clinical predictors, based on the medical history, examination, electro-cardiogram (EKG), laboratory findings, and functional capacity. The sum of these patient-specific features is often used to estimate the risk inherent to individual patients. This must be placed in to the context of the risk inherent to the surgery and the need for surgery itself.

CLINICAL PREDICTORS

Identification of clinical predictors has been an ongoing challenge over several decades. In the 1960s, preoperative predictors adversely impacting perioperative cardiac morbidity were recognized from routine history and physical examination, including a recent MI and decompensated congestive heart failure (CHF). In landmark work in the 1970s, Goldman and colleagues published a multifactorial cardiac risk index, assigning relative values to various clinical features and using the sum of the scores to predict operative risk *(20)*. Clinical attributes included age, history of a recent MI, physical examination findings of heart failure or aortic stenosis, EKG alterations, and laboratory abnormalities. This risk index was subsequently modified by Detsky and colleagues to include additional criteria, such as unstable angina, a history of CHF, or remote MI *(21)*. Over the next couple of decades, cardiac indices served as a resource to estimate peri-operative risk. However, many physicians consider this method inconvenient, as it requires assigning and calculating weighted values for each patient. In addition, the predictive value of such cardiac indices has been found to be poor in patients undergoing vascular surgery *(22)*.

In an effort to simplify risk assessment, the American College of Cardiology and the American Heart Association (ACC/AHA) task force created guidelines for the perioperative cardiovascular evaluation *(19)*. A useful approach is to segregate the clinical predictors as major, intermediate, and minor based on the relative risk. Major clinical predictors are associated with a marked increased risk and include unstable coronary syndromes, decompensated CHF, significant arrhythmias, and severe valvular heart disease. Patients with conditions in this category require intense management, and delay or cancellation of surgery may be obligatory. Intermediate clinical predictors are associated with increased risk as supported by the literature and merit a thorough preoperative assessment. This includes mild angina, remote MI, compensated CHF, and diabetes mellitus. Minor clinical predictors, although widely accepted as cardiovascular disease markers, have not been sufficiently validated as independent risk factors. These include advanced age, abnormal EKG, nonsinus rhythm, low functional capacity, history of stroke, and uncontrolled hypertension.

Several other features may be included in the classification of perioperative clinical predictors (Table 1). Severe valvular heart diseases present different degrees of risk. Severe aortic or mitral stenosis carries high risk and both are major clinical predictors, while severe aortic or mitral regurgitation carries moderate risk and both are intermediate predictors. While multiple other medical issues may influence the operative risk,

Table 1
Clinical Predictors of Perioperative Cardiovascular Risk

MAJOR PREDICTORS
    Unstable coronary syndrome
        Recent myocardial infarction (within 1 mo)
        Unstable or severe angina
    Decompensated congestive heart failure
    Significant arrhythmia
        Uncontrolled SVT or VT
        High-grade AV Block
    Severe valvular heart disease
        Critical aortic stenosis
        Severe mitral stenosis

INTERMEDIATE PREDICTORS
    Mild angina pectoris
    Prior myocardial infarction
    Compensated or prior congestive heart failure
    Diabetes mellitus
    Moderate valvular heart disease
        Severe aortic or mitral regurgitation
    Chronic renal insufficiency

MINOR PREDICTORS
    Advanced age
    Abnormal electrocardiogram
    Rhythm other than sinus
    Low functional capacity
    Uncontrolled systemic hypertension
    Prior stroke

SVT, supraventricular tachycardia; VT, ventricular tachycardia; AV, atrioventricular. Modified from Eagle KA, et al., J Am Coll Cardiol 1996;27:910–948.

chronic renal insufficiency stands out as a strong predictor (23,24). A recent report found that in patients undergoing abdominal aortic aneurysm repair preoperative chronic renal insufficiency was associated with a greater than ninefold increased risk ($p < 0.0001$) (25).

FUNCTIONAL CAPACITY

Functional capacity is another important determinant of perioperative and long-term cardiovascular risk. It is the maximal aerobic demand or energy expenditure performing physical activities and expressed as the metabolic equivalent (MET). An activity scale index, such as the Duke Activity Status Index, provides clinicians with a series of questions to estimate the MET level achieved during routine daily physical activities. The energy demand performing simple activities, such as personal hygiene activities, daily household chores, and walking distances on level ground, is in the range of 1–4 METs. With more strenuous events, such as stair climbing, heavy housework, and moderate recreational activities, the energy utilized is in the range of 4–10 METs. Functional capacity and MET level achieved are strongly associated with perioperative risk. The risk is increased threefold with poor functional capacity (< 4 METs) and reduced with high functional capacity (> 7 METs). Thus, the finding of a poor functional capacity often warrants a more thorough evaluation.

SURGICAL-SPECIFIC RISK

Surgery carries a risk of cardiovascular complications specific to the type of operation and condition under which it is being performed. A major contributor to the surgical-specific risk is the magnitude and duration of the hemodynamic stress. Wide deviations in heart rate, blood pressure, oxygenation, and vascular volume, as well as alterations in the coagulation cascade and platelet activity, are inherent to certain operations. The surgery-specific risk is directly related to the alteration of these variables during the procedure. The procedure may also select a population of patients with elevated risk, such as in the case of vascular surgery. Operations being performed under emergent conditions carry higher risk.

Surgical procedures may be divided into high, intermediate, and low risk based on the observed cardiovascular event rates (19). The categorization by the ACC/AHA task force places all peripheral vascular surgeries, other than carotid surgery, as high-risk (19). These high-risk procedures have a perioperative MI and death rate of above 5%. Intermediate risk procedures, includes carotid endarterectomy, have an event rate of 1–5%.

Further delineation or stratification of the risk of individual peripheral vascular operations is often performed by clinicians, as it seems intuitive that certain procedures carry higher risk. There is greater hemodynamic stress associated with aortic level procedures due to cross-clamping and declamping of the aorta. Similarly, distal peripheral bypass grafting to the pedal level involves a longer time to perform the operation. While it is well established that carotid surgeries are associated with a lower event rate, the risk attributed to other vascular surgeries is less clear. Although the assumption is that aortic operations have greater event rates than peripheral procedures, contradictory evidence is available. L'Italien and colleagues reported on the outcomes of 547 vascular surgeries, finding that the complication rate was similar (or greater) following the 177 infrainguinal surgeries compared with the 321 abdominal aortic surgery (death or MI rate of 16% vs 11%) (26). While such analysis is retrospective and is greatly influenced by patient selection, it emphasizes that the risk with vascular surgery is high and requires careful perioperative assessment and management to reduce this risk.

Risk Stratification Testing

Various modalities have been utilized to stratify the risk of cardiac complications with vascular surgery, given the inconsistent predictive value of clinical predictors in this group of patients. Testing has been useful in patients at intermediate risk by clinical predictors and those with poor functional capacity. The methods evaluate for the presence of coronary ischemia and/or left ventricular dysfunction, both of which are predictive of increased perioperative risk (19).

TREADMILL STRESS TESTING

Exercise stress testing is useful to diagnose coronary artery disease, clarify functional status, and predict long-term outcomes. The reported sensitivity and specificity for detecting obstructive CAD is 68% and 77%, provided an adequate level of stress is achieved *(27)*. In addition, information about functional capacity provides insight into mortality *(28)*. Poor functional capacity is associated with high mortality, while a good functional capacity is associated with lower mortality. In the medical treatment group of the CASS study, the inability to exercise for at least 3 min on a standard Bruce protocol treadmill test was associated with a > 5% annual mortality (29). In contrast, the ability to exercise for more than 9 min on a standard Bruce protocol treadmill test was associated with < 1% annual mortality.

Treadmill exercise testing is also used to predict perioperative outcomes. Two features of the stress test that are important are the presence of coronary ischemia and the functional capacity, or exercise duration. Carliner and colleagues reported 16% of 32 patients with an abnormal exercise response prior to elective surgery died or had a MI *(30)*. In contrast, 93% of 168 patients with a normal exercise response had no cardiac events. The diagnostic and prognostic value of exercise treadmill testing requires individuals reach an adequate level of stress (85% of the age-adjusted, maximally predicted heart rate). Unfortunately only about 30% of vascular surgery patients are able to achieve adequate workloads as a consequence of their disease *(1)*. The use of preoperative treadmill testing with supplemental arm ergometry was performed in 100 patients undergoing vascular surgery. The event rate was low (6%) in the 30 patients able to achieve the target heart rate, but much higher (24%) in the 70 patients unable to achieve target heart rate. The greatest perioperative risk appears to be in those with an ischemic EKG response to exercise that occurs at a low workload.

Pharmacologic Stress Testing

Pharmacologic stress testing is often used in patients who are unable to exercise or have limited ambulatory ability to assess for CAD and coronary ischemia. Patients undergoing vascular surgery often have limited exercise capacity favoring the use of pharmacologic stress testing to evaluate for CAD and predict operative risk. In general, an abnormal stress test has been found to increase the perioperative risk.

Myocardial Perfusion Imaging. Myocardial perfusion imaging, most commonly with dipyridamole thallium imaging, has been used to predict cardiac risk (death or MI) with vascular surgery. The positive predictive value of a test revealing thallium redistribution has ranged from 5% to 50% with a mean of about 15% (Table 2) *(31–41)*. The negative predictive value of a normal scan is generally quite high, about 95%. Although the risk is greatest in those with ischemia as demonstrated by thallium redistribution, the risk may also be elevated in those with fixed thallium defects owing to prior MI.

The use of such testing remains fairly controversial because of the relatively low positive predictive value. In a review of 457 patients undergoing elective abdominal aortic surgery, Baron and colleagues found perfusion imaging had a poor predictive value *(42)*. Clinical features including the presence of definite CAD and age above 65 were better predictors. Other investigators have sought to quantify the scan abnormalities concluding that the "ischemic burden" or number of reversible defects improves the predictive value *(38)*.

Dobutamine Stress Echocardiogram. Dobutamine echocardiography, which utilizes the ability of a catecholamine stimulus to increase myocardial oxygen demand and induce wall motion abnormalities in regions of ischemic myocardium, has been evaluated as a method to predict operative risk. Although less extensively studied than dipyridamole thallium, it seems to provide an even greater predictive value both positive and

Table 2
Dipyridamole–Thallium Imaging and Cardiac Events with Vascular Surgery

Authors	N	Event rate	Positive predictive value		Negative predictive value	
			%	N	%	N
Eagle et al. 1989 (31)	200	8	16	13/82	98	116/118
Lane et al. 1989 (32)	101	11	12	10/81	95	19/20
Younis et al. 1990 (40)	111	7	15	6/40	97	69/71
Hendel et al. 1992 (33)	327	9	14	24/167	99	97/98
Lette et al. 1992 (34)	355	8	17	28/161	98	160/162
Brown et al. 1993 (35)	231	5	13	10/77	99	192/194
Baron et al. 1994 (36)	457	19	21	54/254	84	171/203
Bry et al. 1994 (37)	237	7	11	12/110	96	122/127
Stratmann et al. 1996 (41)	197	5	5	6/110	97	84/87
Vanzetto et al. 1996 (38)	134	22	50	24/48	93	80/86
de Virgilio et al. 2000 (39)	80	11	14	4/29	90	46/51
TOTAL	2620	10	15	194/1284	95	1271/133

negative. The criteria for an abnormal test have varied in the past, but the criterion now accepted is new or worsening wall motion abnormalities. The positive predictive value has ranged from about 15% to 40%, while the negative predictive value has ranged from 95% to 100% (Table 3) (43–49). Investigators have evaluated the value of the ischemic threshold to predict risk. Ischemia that occurs below 60% of the maximally predicted heart rate appears to have much greater risk than that which occurs above the 60% maximally predicted heart rate (50,51).

AMBULATORY ELECTROCARDIOGRAPHIC MONITORING

Postoperative myocardial ischemia is well known to predict a high risk of subsequent MI and death (52,53). This has led investigators to evaluate the use of preoperative ambulatory EKG monitoring to predict the presence of CAD and estimate the risk of perioperative events in patients undergoing noncardiac surgery (52,54). The predictive value of ischemic ECG changes (ST segment depressions 1–2 mm) is comparable to dipyridamole thallium testing (55). This test, however, has limitations, including the need for an interpretable baseline EKG to demonstrate ischemia and the need to wear a monitor for 24–48 hr. This test has not gained general acceptance in clinical practice.

ECHOCARDIOGRAM

Perioperative assessment of left ventricular function has been evaluated using radionucleotide or contrast ventriculography and echocardiography. The risk of a cardiac complication is increased in patients with an ejection fraction below 35% (19,56,57). Depressed left ventricular function has been shown to be predictive of postoperative CHF, but was an inconsistent predictor of MI (19,56,57). Current clinical practice favors the use of echocardiography, which also provides information regarding diastolic and valvular function. The utility of echocardiograph to predict perioperative risk has not

Table 3
Dobutamine Echocardiography and Cardiac Events with Vascular Surgery

Authors	N	Event rate	Positive predictive value		Negative predictive value	
			%	N	%	N
Lalka et al. 1992 (44)	60	22	29	11/38	95	21/22
Eichelberger et al. 1993 (45)	75	7	19	5/27	100	48/48
Langan et al. 1993 (46)	74	4	17	3/18	100	56/56
Davila-Roman et al. 1993 (47)	91	9	17	4/23	100	68/68
Poldermans et al. 1995 (48)	300	9	38	27/71	100	229/229
Pellikka et al. 1996 (49)	80	10	29	7/24	98	55/56
TOTAL	699	9	28	58/208	99	488/491

been without controversy. Echocardiography did not significantly alter the predictive value when it was added to a predictive model that contained clinical risk factors (58). In contrast, echocardiography added predictive value to pharmacologic nuclear stress testing when both tests were abnormal (from 22% to 52%) (59). The current indication, as advised by the ACC/AHA task force, for the use of perioperative echocardiography is in patients with current or poorly controlled CHF (class I indication) and in patients with previous CHF or unexplained dyspnea (class II indication) (19).

Combining Clinical Risk and Testing

The optimal approach to the preoperative evaluation utilizes information from both the clinical features and the risk-stratification testing. Eagle and colleagues reported on the value of combining clinical variables and thallium dipyridamole testing in 200 patients undergoing vascular surgery (3). The risk of a cardiac event was low (3%) if there were no clinical variables and high (50%) if three or more variables were present. Thallium imaging was useful to stratify the risk in the intermediate risk group with one or two variables. While controversial, these findings have led to an approach to selectively utilize preoperative testing based on the clinical predictors.

We favor an approach to the preoperative vascular surgical evaluation that is modified from the AHA/ACC task force. This stepwise approach considers the clinical predictors, and functional capacity, as well as the need for surgery (Fig. 1). The approach places emphasis on the need for lower extremity revascularization when considering if risk-stratification testing is necessary. The preoperative evaluation prior to elective procedures, such as those for intermittent claudication, is more critical. Risk stratification testing is advocated for these elective vascular procedures in patients with intermediate-risk clinical predictors or poor functional capacity. In contrast, the preoperative evaluation prior to mandatory procedure, such as those for critical limb ischemia, is a "minimalist" approach that favors pursuing surgery with aggressive medical therapy. Risk stratification testing is advocated with mandatory procedures in patients with both intermediate-risk clinical predictors (particularly active coronary disease) and poor functional capacity. We prefer the use of dobutamine echocardiography for noninvasive

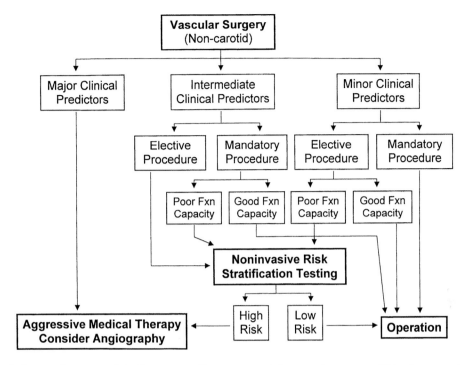

Fig. 1. A stepwise approach to the preoperative assessment for vascular surgery. This places emphasis on the need for surgery when considering if further risk stratification testing is required. Fxn, functional.

stress testing because it can assess for ischemia, including the ischemic threshold and burden, as well as left ventricular function.

Complications of the Cardiac Evaluation

Although designed to reduce the operative risk, the cardiac evaluation may adversely affect the outcome of the vascular surgery, owing to its effects on the timing of surgery. Since many cardiac evaluations require diagnostic testing to be scheduled, there is often an inevitable delay in the proposed vascular procedure. The effect of this delay might be significant and influence the feasibility and outcome of the vascular surgery.

A review of the experience in 161 patients undergoing vascular surgery at the VA Medical Center in Denver found that 42 patients had a "extended" cardiac evaluation with some risk stratification testing. The cardiac workup required a mean of 30 d to complete and the time from initial workup to surgery required a mean of 79 d *(60)*. Although debatable, adverse events related to the workup were reported in 16 patients (38%). Eight patients refused subsequent surgery after the cardiac workup, seven of whom had abdominal aortic aneurysms. Two patients with salvageable limbs at the onset required amputation on completion of the cardiac workup. Other complications attributed to cardiac catheterization, PTCA, or CABG included prosthetic graft infection, pseudoaneurysm formation, sternal wound infection, renal failure, and brain anoxia.

Thus it is possible for an extended cardiac evaluation prior to noncardiac surgery to result in unnecessary delays that may adversely impact on the surgical outcome as well as the patient's willingness to have surgery. This emphasizes the importance of an expedited, coordinated approach to the preoperative preparation for vascular surgery.

Long-Term Prognostic Value

Preoperative cardiac testing has the potential utility of predicting long-term risk and may select a group of patients that requires more aggressive therapy. There is support for the role of stress testing, including pharmacologic stress testing, to provide prognostic information regarding late cardiac complications in the surgical patient.

Late cardiac complications were evaluated in 172 patients who underwent vascular surgery with a preoperative myocardial imaging evaluation. During a mean follow-up of 21 mo, late cardiac complications occurred with greater frequency in those with an abnormal imaging evaluation compared to those with a normal scan (26% vs 4%, $p <$ 0.0001) *(41)*. The rate of late events was 32% in patients with a reversible defect (p < 0.001) and 22% in those with fixed defects ($p < 0.03$). The extent of ischemia may also predict risk as the higher the number of reversible defects the poorer the event-free survival *(61)*.

As with myocardial perfusion imaging, dobutamine echocardiography has been used to predict long-term outcomes. Late cardiac complications were evaluated in 316 patients with a dobutamine echocardiogram prior to noncardiac surgery with a mean follow-up of 19 mo *(62)*. Extensive and limited stress-induced wall motion abnormalities were independent predictors of late cardiac events with a relative risk of 6.5 and 2.9. The larger the "ischemic burden" on preoperative stress testing, the more likely it is that a cardiac complication will occur in the long term.

PERIOPERATIVE MANAGEMENT ISSUES

Perioperative Medical Management

Perioperative medical management is strategically aimed at factors that increase the risk of perioperative cardiovascular complications. In this way, medical conditions can be maximally treated with the hope of reducing the risk of cardiac complications during the preioperative period.

ISCHEMIC HEART DISEASE

Two important issues to consider in patients with known or suspected CAD undergoing vascular surgery are antiischemic management and the timing of coronary revascularization, if performed prior to surgery. Medical management for known or suspected ischemic heart disease in the vascular surgical patient includes aggressive β-blockade. Several studies have found a benefit of perioperative β-blocker use in reducing cardiac complications. Stone and colleagues gave a single oral dose of β-blocker to 89 patients with mild hypertension prior to surgery—58% of which was vascular surgery *(63)*. The incidence of perioperative ST-segment depression was 28% in the control group vs 2% in the treatment group *(63)*. Poldermans and colleagues evaluated the effect of preoperative β-blockade on cardiac outcomes in a group of 112 high-risk patients, identified with ischemia on dobutamine echocardiography, undergoing vascular surgery *(64)*. Patients were randomized to receive standard care or aggressive β-blockade with bisoprolol to keep the heart rate below 80 beats per minute. The rate of death from cardiac causes and nonfatal MI was lower in the bisoprolol group compared with the control group (3.4% vs 34%, $p < 0.001$) *(64)*. Thus there is accumulating evidence supporting the use of preoperative β-blockers in patients with PAD to reduce the risk of cardiovascular complications, even in those with inducible coronary ischemia. We advocate titration of β-blockers during the week prior to surgery, if possible, for a target heart rate of 60 beats per minute and close monitoring perioperatively to maintain a heart rate below 70 beats per minutes. Other classes of antiischemic agents, such as calcium channel blockers and nitrates, have not been shown to have this benefit but have not been adequately studied *(19)*. The appropriate use of antiplatelet therapy during the perioperative period for vascular surgery is uncertain. Although some surgeons are concerned about bleeding complications, most are willing to use aspirin. There is potential benefit of aspirin use on graft survival and perhaps on reducing cardiac events, although this has not been proven.

As previously discussed, although the rationale for considering coronary revascularization prior to vascular surgery is that restoring myocardial perfusion may enhance the safety of the vascular procedure and prolong life expectancy, this concept has not been proven by any prospectively conducted studies. There is an ongoing clinical trial that is evaluating the role of perioperative coronary revascularization or medical therapy in patients requiring elective vascular surgery *(65)*. The current practice favors performing coronary revascularization based on clinical indications rather than as a "prophylactic" measure. Even with this approach there is concern regarding an adverse effect of coronary revascularization that is performed in too close proximity to the vascular procedure. Although the operative risks for subsequent surgery were low in patients with prior CABG, the risk of death and medical complications were much higher if the operation was performed within 30 d *(66)*. Mortality was lower in 1093 patients who underwent both CABG and vascular surgery if there was a delay of 1 mo between the operations (0.2% with a delay compared with 4% without delay) *(67)*. Timing considerations are even more important with percutaneous coronary intervention. As previously described, the cardiac complication rate was exceedingly high if surgery was performed soon after intracoronary stent placement *(17)*. Following coronary stenting noncardiac surgery should be delayed at least 2 wk and preferably 4 wk to allow completion of antiplatelet therapy. If percutaneous revascularization is required within this time frame, "plain-old" balloon angioplasty should be considered.

HYPERTENSION

Although moderate hypertension is not considered an independent risk factor for cardiovascular complications, it is a useful marker of CAD *(19)*. Preoperative hypertension increases the likelihood of severe intraoperative blood pressure fluctuations and is associated with myocardial ischemia *(68,69)*. Several investigators have shown a reduction in the rate and duration of perioperative ischemia with preoperative blood pressure control and β-blockade *(63,70)*. Therefore, it is imperative to continue antihypertensive medications and avoid withdrawal of those agents that can cause rebound tachycardia and hypertension, such as β-blockers and clonidine.

HEART FAILURE AND CARDIOMYOPATHY

Heart failure, even if compensated, with depressed left ventricular function increases the risk of perioperative cardiac complications. Decompensated congestive heart failure dramatically increases the risk, including cardiac death, with noncardiac surgery *(20,21)*. Treatment of heart failure to restore a compensated state decreases the risk to an intermediate level *(19)*. Modification of the medical regimen is designed to optimize cardiovascular homeostasis by establishing euvolemia, reducing afterload, and regulating heart rate. Treatment of patients with heart failure focuses first on the presence of fluid overload, for which diuretic agents are used. After restoration of the volume status, or in the absence of fluid retention, the focus of treatment is on the use of angiotensin-converting enzyme inhibitors followed by β-blockers.

Cardiomyopathies, restrictive and hypertrophic, as well as the noncompliant or hyperdynamic left ventricle, increase the risk of perioperative cardiac complications. The presence of a cardiomyopathy warrants a careful evaluation with close monitoring of the fluid and hemodynamic status in the perioperative period. Hypertrophic cardiomyopathies have an increased tendency to develop outflow obstruction, particularly with a reduction in ventricular filling pressure with volume contraction. With restrictive cardiomyopathies volume contraction may decrease ventricular compliance and result in a significant drop in stroke volume. Avoiding volume depletion or the use of drugs that augment contraction, such as catecholamines, is imperative.

VALVULAR HEART DISEASE

Valvular heart disease may adversely affect the outcome of vascular surgery and warrants a careful evaluation to guide management. There are minimal data to support specific interventions, including valve replacement, to treat valvular heart disease prior to noncardiac surgery. Valve replacement is reserved for severe disease with clinical indications independent of the noncardiac surgery *(71)*. There are some data to support the feasibility of balloon valvuloplasty for aortic and mitral stenosis prior to noncardiac surgery as a palliative measure *(72)*. Aortic stenosis is the most feared of the valvular heart lesions as it carries the greatest perioperative risk and there is no effective medical therapy *(20)*. "Critical" aortic stenosis warrants careful consideration of the need for the noncardiac surgery and therapeutic interventions including valve replacement surgery or valvuloplasty, particularly for poor surgical candidates. Mitral stenosis is also associated with increased perioperative risk. Operative management of mild to moderate mitral stenosis is aimed at avoiding tachycardia, as this may lead to a decrease in diastolic filling and increase pulmonary congestion. Severe mitral stenosis may require either valve repair or replacement or valvuloplasty before noncardiac surgery. In general, regurgitant lesions are tolerated better than stenotic lesions during the perioperative period, given the response to medical therapy. Mitral and aortic regurgitation are treated with afterload reducing agents, such as angiotensin-converting enzyme inhibitors, and diuretics to optimize cardiac function. Another issue for patients with valvular heart disease, which is often overlooked, is the need for perioperative prophylactic antibiotics for endocarditis.

ARRHYTHMIAS AND CONDUCTION SYSTEM DISEASE

While there is evidence to support arrhythmias as risk factors for perioperative coronary events *(20)*, their significance is probably related to underlying cardiopulmonary disease *(73)*. Preoperative identification of an arrhythmia should prompt a thorough evaluation to search for cardiopulmonary disease, drug toxicity, or metabolic derangement. Several studies have suggested that in the absence of underlying disease most arrhythmias usually carry a benign prognosis *(74)*. Arrhythmias that are symptomatic or compromise hemodynamics necessitate further evaluation and treatment designed to suppress recurrence. Supraventricular arrhythmias can be treated with pharmacological or electrical cardioversion; however, when cardioversion is not an option, then rate control with digitalis, β-blockers, or calcium channel blockers may be employed. Anticoagulation in chronic atrial fibrillation can be safely withheld for 24–48 h postoperatively. Intravenous heparin is usually used postoperatively while reinitiating long-term anticoagulation with coumadin. Ventricular ectopy and nonsustained ventricular tachycardia usually do not require therapy except if contributing to myocardial ischemia or left ventricular dysfunction *(73)*. Sustained ventricular arrhythmias should be suppressed with an antiarrhythmic agent, such as lidocaine, procainamide, or amiodarone; however, initiating therapy immediately prior to surgery is discouraged.

Intraventricular conduction distrubances, in the absence of syncope or advanced heart block, are generally well tolerated perioperatively and do not require pacemaker placement *(75)*. The indications for temporary pacemaker placement are nearly identical to the indications for permanent pacemaker placement *(76)*. Most disturbances, including bifasicular block (right bundle branch block with left anterior or posterior fasicular block), or left bundle branch block with or without first degree atrioventricular block, do not need pacemaker placement in the absence of symptoms. However, given these conduction disturbances, medications that slow atrioventricular conduction should be avoided, if possible. Complete heart block and high-grade atrioventricular block may require preoperative and long-term pacing. Patients with a left bundle branch block who are to be monitored with a pulmonary artery (PA) catheter may require temporary pacing. Preexisting pacemakers should be interrogated and converted to an uninhibited mode.

Intraoperative Management

Surgery and anesthesia exert stress on the cardiovascular system. The cardiovascular response to these variables depends on baseline cardiac function and cardiac reserve. Investigators have attempted to individualize anesthetic management and intraoperative monitoring by determining the conditions that influence morbidity and mortality. The goal is to eliminate unnecessary procedural risk and attune intraoperative monitoring to enable rapid intervention, designed to produce better long-term outcomes.

ANESTHETIC MANAGEMENT

The mode of anesthesia and the choice of agents are two important variables to consider with anesthetic management. Studies comparing anesthetic techniques have found equivalent cardiac complication rates *(42,77)*. Although local anesthesia has the lowest risk, other anesthetic techniques are comparable. The various methods have different effects upon physiologic systems and may provide different relative risks and benefits.

Opioid anesthetics are valued for their relative hemodynamic stability; however, their use with respiratory depression predisposes to the need for postoperative mechanical ventilation often requiring weaning. Ventilator weaning, in the intensive care setting, has been associated with myocardial ischemia and MI.

Inhalation agents have similar effects on the cardiovascular system with depression of myocardial contractility and reduction in afterload. In a randomized study comparing primary anesthetic agents and outcomes of CABG, there was no significant difference between agents, including halothane, enflurane, and isoflurane *(78)*. The impact of newer agents, such as desflurane and sevoflurane, on cardiovascular outcomes has not been well investigated.

Spinal or epidural anesthesia is feasible with procedures at low dermatomal levels, such as infrainguinal bypass surgery. Its local distribution minimizes hemodynamic alterations; however, hypotension and reflex tachycardia may ensue if higher levels are involved. This method also does not prevent neurohumoral activation with increased serum catecholamines with stress. Although one study found a lower incidence of cardiac morbidity and clotting dysfunction with epidural anesthesia, several subsequent investigations have contradicted this finding *(2)*.

INTRAOPERATIVE MONITORING

Intraoperative monitoring is intended to detect hemodynamic instability or coronary ischemia to enable rapid intervention to reverse the problem. Acute elevation in the left ventricular diastolic pressure and pulmonary capillary wedge pressure is a sensitive indicator of myocardial ischemia *(79)*. The increase in the pulmonary capillary wedge pressure can be measured with a PA catheter to monitor for intraoperative ischemia. However, PA pressure monitoring had no benefit over central venous pressure monitoring, in patients undergoing major vascular surgery *(80)*. Although PA pressure monitoring may minimize intraoperative hemodynamic instability, several studies have indicated that it does not improve postoperative cardiac morbidity or mortality *(80,81)*. A recent case-controlled study found no benefit of PA catheterization prior to noncardiac surgery *(82)*. In fact, there was a higher rate of cardiovascular complications in patients having had a PA catheter even after adjustment for confounding factors. Similarly, a meta-analysis found no benefit of routine PA catheterization in moderate-risk patients undergoing vascular surgery *(83)*. It is known that patients with signs and symptoms of heart failure preoperatively have a 30–50% risk of developing postoperative heart failure; thus, careful monitoring of fluid balance is critical. The use of intraoperative PA catheters, even during major vascular surgery, is not recommended on a routine basis, but selectively in patients with known left ventricular dysfunction *(19)*.

An additional technique for intraoperative monitoring during surgery is transesophageal echocardiography (TEE). TEE may be used to detect intraoperative ischemia as demonstrated by the acute onset of new myocardial wall abnormalities. However, intraoperative TEE has a poor predictor value for postoperative cardiac morbidity *(84,85)*. TEE should not be used routinely during vascular surgery but may be considered selectively in high-risk patients.

The use of EKG monitoring has been used to evaluate for perioperative ischemia. Prolonged postoperative ST-segment changes are a strong independent predictor of myocardial events in high-risk noncardiac surgery patients *(53)*. Intraoperative ST-segment changes may be indicative of ischemia, but are dependent on subjective interpretation and their predictive value has not been well investigated. The specificity of ST-segment monitoring has been questioned; Mathew and colleagues observed ST-segment changes in low-risk, healthy women undergoing cesarean section without subsequent cardiac morbidity *(86)*. In contrast, computerized ST-segment trending limits subjectivity and may be superior to visual interpretation *(19)*. With this in mind, perioperative computerized ST-segment monitoring may be considered in high-risk patients.

Postoperative Surveillance

Postoperative myocardial ischemia is a harbinger of cardiac morbidity and mortality, especially in patients undergoing vascular surgery. However, it is challenging to identify postoperative myocardial ischemia and infarction due to its often painless nature. It has been estimated that 60% of postoperative MIs are "silent" as compared to 10–15% with nonsurgical MIs. This may be explained by residual anesthesia and analgesia or competing sensory stimulation, such as incision pain *(2)*. As a result, external instruments must be relied on to supply early indication of impending or evolving cardiac events.

The use of serial electrocardiograms and cardiac-specific enzymes has been evaluated for the detection of postoperative ischemia and MI. The predictive value of serial EKGs has been difficult to assess due to various diagnostic criteria used by investigators. Nonspecific ST and T wave changes are common in the postoperative period and do not necessarily predict increased cardiac morbidity. The role for monitoring creatine kinase isoenzymes (CK-MB) and newer myocardial-specific enzymes, such as troponin-I and troponin-T, is unclear owing to the poor predictive value of these tests. CK-MB can be released from noncardiac sources under peripheral ischemic conditions. Yeager and colleagues found in 1561 patients undergoing vascular surgery that the incidence of subsequent MI or coronary artery revascularization was significantly higher in patients with a perioperative MI *(87)*. However, the risk was not increased in patients with a "pure biochemical" MI defined by elevated cardiac enzymes in the absence of EKG changes or cardiovascular symptoms *(87)*. Therefore, it is reasonable to restrict surveillance for MI to patients with symptoms or EKG changes in the postoperative period.

The use of serial postoperative EKGs is recommended until the second or third postoperative day in patients with known or suspected CAD undergoing major vascular surgery. Postoperative cardiac enzyme monitoring should be reserved for high-risk patients in the presence of EKG abnormalities, symptoms, or cardiac dysfunction *(19)*.

SUMMARY

There is a high risk of major cardiovascular complications from vascular surgery attributed to the increased prevalence of CAD. The focus of the cardiac consultant and the preoperative cardiac evaluation is to identify features that increase the risk and attempt to reduce this risk. Patient-specific issues include clinical predictors and functional status assessment, which is often limited in the vascular surgical patients, prompting widespread use of risk-stratification testing. The most commonly used testing modalities are the pharmacologic stress tests to evaluate for ischemia. However, it is uncertain how to proceed with the information obtained, as the role of coronary revascularization prior to noncardiac surgery remains controversial. All the data regarding coronary revascularization, including CABG, PTCA, and coronary stenting, are retrospective. As a general guide, coronary revascularization should be performed only if it is appropriate independent of the surgery. There is also concern if coronary revascularization is performed immediately prior to noncardiac surgery. In contrast, medical therapy with β-blockade has been shown to reduce the risk of perioperative cardiac events, even in those with inducible ischemia. Given these uncertainties, a "minimalist" approach to preoperative testing is suggested in patients with "mandatory" indications for vascular surgery. A more critical, but selective, approach to preoperative testing is suggested in patients with "relative" indications for surgery. All patients should receive maximal perioperative medical therapy that focuses on the treatment of cardiac disorders to optimize cardiac function and hemodynamics. Intraoperative monitoring and postoperative surveillance is designed to detect hemodynamic instability or coronary ischemia to enable rapid intervention to reduce further complications.

REFERENCES

1. McPhail N, Calvin JE, Shariatmadar A, Barber GG, Scobie TK. The use of preoperative exercise testing to predict cardiac complications after arterial reconstruction. J Vasc Surg 1988;7:60–68.
2. Mangano DT. Perioperative cardiac morbidity. Anesthesiology 1990;72:153–184.
3. Eagle KA, Coley CM, Newell JB, et al. Combining clinical and thallium data optimizes preoperative assessment of cardiac risk before major vascular surgery. Ann Intern Med 1989;110:859–866.
4. McFalls EO, Doliszny KM, Grund F, Chute E, Chesler E. Angina and persistent exercise thallium defects: independent risk factors in elective vascular surgery. J Am Coll Cardiol 1993;21:1347–1352.
5. Hertzer NR, Beven EG, Young JR, et al. Coronary artery disease in peripheral vascular patients: a classification of 1000 coronary angiograms and results of surgical management. Ann Surg 1984;199:223–233.
6. Hertzer NR. Basic data concerning associated coronary disease in peripheral vascular patients. Ann Vasc Surg 1987;1:616–620.
7. Jamieson WR, Janusz MT, Miyagishima RT, Gerein AN. Influence of ischemic heart disease on early and late mortality after surgery for peripheral occlusive vascular disease. Circulation 1982;66:I92–I97.
8. Hollier LH, Plate G, O'Brien PC, et al. Late survival after abdominal aortic aneurysm repair: influence of coronary artery disease. J Vasc Surg 1984;1:290–299.
9. Hertzer NR, Young JR, Beven EG, et al. Late results of coronary bypass in patients presenting with lower extremity ischemia: the Cleveland Clinic Study. Ann Vasc Surg 1987;1:411–419.
10. Ennix CL, Lawrie GM, Morris GC, et al. Improved results of carotid endarterectomy in patients with symptomatic coronary disease: an analysis of 1,546 consecutive carotid operations. Stroke 1979;10: 122–125.
11. Foster ED, Davis KB, Carpenter JA, Abele S, Fray D. Risk of noncardiac operation in patients with defined coronary disease: the Coronary Artery Surgery Study (CASS) registry experience. Ann Thorac Surg 1986;41:42–50.
12. Eagle KA, Rihal CS, Mickel MC, Holmes DR, Foster ED, Gersh BJ. Cardiac risk of noncardiac surgery: influence of coronary disease and type of surgery in 3368 operations. CASS Investigators and University of Michigan Heart Care Program. Coronary Artery Surgery Study. Circulation 1997;96: 1882–1887.
13. European Coronary Surgery Study Group. Prospective randomised study of coronary artery bypass surgery in stable angina pectoris: second interim report. Lancet 1980;2:491–495.
14. Huber KC, Evans MA, Bresnahan JF, Gibbons RJ, Holmes DR. Outcome of noncardiac operations in patients with severe coronary artery disease successfully treated preoperatively with coronary angioplasty. Mayo Clinic Proc 1992;67:15–21.
15. Gottlieb A, Banoub M, Sprung J, Levy PJ, Beven M, Mascha EJ. Perioperative cardiovascular morbidity in patients with coronary artery disease undergoing vascular surgery after percutaneous transluminal coronary angioplasty. J Cardio Vasc Surg 1998;12:501–506.
16. Massie MT, Rohrer MJ, Leppo JA, Cutler BS. Is coronary angiography necessary for vascular surgery patients who have positive results of dipyridamole thallium scans? J Vasc Surg 1997;25:975–982.
17. Kaluza GL, Joseph J, Lee JR, Raizner ME, Raizner AE. Catastrophic outcomes of noncardiac surgery soon after coronary stenting. J Am Coll Cardiol 2000;35:1288–1294.
18. Rihal CS, Sutton-Tyrrell K, Guo P, et al. Increased incidence of periprocedural complications among patients with peripheral vascular disease undergoing myocardial revascularization in the Bypass Angioplasty Revascularization Investigation. Circulation 1999;100:171–177.

19. Eagle KA, Brundage BH, Chaitman BR, et al. Guidelines for perioperative cardiovascular evaluation for noncardiac surgery. Report of the American College of Cardiology/American Heart Association Task Force on Practice Guidelines (Committee on Perioperative Cardiovascular Evaluation for Noncardiac Surgery). J Am Coll Cardiol 1996;27:910–948.

20. Goldman L, Caldera DL, Nussbaum SR, et al. Multifactorial index of cardiac risk in noncardiac surgical procedures. N Engl J Med 1977;297:845–850.

21. Detsky AS, Abrams HB, McLaughlin JR, et al. Predicting cardiac complications in patients undergoing non-cardiac surgery. J Gen Intern Med 1986;1:211–219.

22. Lette J, Waters D, Lassonde J, et al. Multivariate clinical models and quantitative dipyridamole-thallium imaging to predict cardiac morbidity and death after vascular reconstruction. J Vasc Surg 1991;14:160–169.

23. Johnston KW, Scobie TK. Multicenter prospective study of nonruptured abdominal aortic aneurysms. I. Population and operative management. J Vasc Surg 1988;7:69–81.

24. Katz DJ, Stanley JC, Zelenock GB. Operative mortality rates for intact and ruptured abdominal aortic aneurysms in Michigan: an eleven-year statewide experience. J Vasc Surg 1994;19:804–815.

25. Huber TS, Wang JG, Derrow AE, et al. Experience in the United States with intact abdominal aortic aneurysm repair. J Vasc Surg 2001;33:304–310.

26. L'Italien GJ, Cambria RP, Cutler BS, et al. Comparative early and late cardiac morbidity among patients requiring different vascular surgery procedures. J Vasc Surg 1995;21:935–944.

27. Detrano R, Gianrossi R, Froelicher V. The diagnostic accuracy of the exercise electrocardiogram: a meta-analysis of 22 years of research. Prog Cardiovasc Dis 1989;32:173–206.

28. Morris CK, Ueshima K, Kawaguchi T, Hideg A, Froelicher VF. The prognostic value of exercise capacity: a review of the literature. Am Heart J 1991;122:1423–1431.

29. Weiner DA, Ryan TJ, McCabe CH, Chaitman BR, Sheffield LT, Ferguson et al. The value of preoperative exercise testing in predicting long-term survival in patients undergoing aortocoronary bypass surgery. Circulation 1984;70:I226–I231.

30. Carliner NH, Fisher ML, Plotnick GD, et al. Routine preoperative exercise testing in patients undergoing major noncardiac surgery. Am J Cardiol 1985;56:51–58.

31. Eagle KA, Coley CM, Newell JB, et al. Combining clinical and thallium data optimizes preoperative assessment of cardiac risk before major vascular surgery. Ann Intern Med 1989;110:859–866.

32. Lane SE, Lewis SM, Pippin JJ, et al. Predictive value of quantitative dipyridamole-thallium scintigraphy in assessing cardiovascular risk after vascular surgery in diabetes mellitus. Am J Cardiol 1989;64:1275–1279.

33. Hendel RC, Whitfield SS, Villegas BJ, Cutler BS, Leppo JA. Prediction of late cardiac events by dipyridamole thallium imaging in patients undergoing elective vascular surgery. Am J Cardiol 1992;70:1243–1249.

34. Lette J, Waters D, Cerino M, Picard M, Champagne P, Lapointe J. Preoperative coronary artery disease risk stratification based on dipyridamole imaging and a simple three-step, three-segment model for patients undergoing noncardiac vascular surgery or major general surgery. Am J Cardiol 1992;69:1553–1558.

35. Brown KA, Rowen M. Extent of jeopardized viable myocardium determined by myocardial perfusion imaging best predicts perioperative cardiac events in patients undergoing noncardiac surgery. J Am Coll Cardiol 1993;21:325–330.

36. Baron JF, Mundler O, Bertrand M, et al. Dipyridamole-thallium scintigraphy and gated radionuclide angiography to assess cardiac risk before abdominal aortic surgery. N Engl J Med 1994;330:663–669.

37. Bry JD, Belkin M, O'Donnell TF, et al. An assessment of the positive predictive value and cost-effectiveness of dipyridamole myocardial scintigraphy in patients undergoing vascular surgery. J Vasc Surg 1994;19:112–121.

38. Vanzetto G, Machecourt J, Blendea D, et al. Additive value of thallium single-photon emission computed tomography myocardial imaging for prediction of perioperative events in clinically selected high cardiac risk patients having abdominal aortic surgery. Am J Cardiol 1996;77:143–148.

39. de Virgilio C, Toosie K, Elbassir M, et al. Dipyridamole-thallium/sestamibi before vascular surgery: a prospective blinded study in moderate-risk patients. J Vasc Surg 2000;32:77–89.

40. Younis LT, Aguirre F, Byers S, et al. Perioperative and long-term prognostic value of intravenous dipyridamole thallium scintigraphy in patients with peripheral vascular disease. Am Heart J 1990;119:1287–1292.

41. Stratmann HG, Younis LT, Wittry MD, Amato M, Miller DD. Dipyridamole technetium-99m sestamibi myocardial tomography in patients evaluated for elective vascular surgery: prognostic value for perioperative and late cardiac events. Am Heart J 1996;131:923–929.

42. Baron JF, Bertrand M, Barre E, et al. Combined epidural and general anesthesia versus general anesthesia for abdominal aortic surgery. Anesthesiology 1991;75:611–618.

43. Lane RT, Sawada SG, Segar DS, et al. Dobutamine stress echocardiography for assessment of cardiac risk before noncardiac surgery. Am J Cardiol 1991;68:976–977.

44. Lalka SG, Sawada SG, Dalsing MC, et al. Dobutamine stress echocardiography as a predictor of cardiac events associated with aortic surgery. J Vasc Surg 1992;15:831–840.

45. Eichelberger JP, Schwarz KQ, Black ER, Green RM, Ouriel K. Predictive value of dobutamine echocardiography just before noncardiac vascular surgery. Am J Cardiol 1993;72:602–607.

46. Langan EM, Youkey JR, Franklin DP, Elmore JR, Costello JM, Nassef LA. Dobutamine stress echocardiography for cardiac risk assessment before aortic surgery. J Vasc Surg 1993;18:905–911.

47. Davila-Roman VG, Waggoner AD, Sicard GA, Geltman EM, Schechtman KB, Perez JE. Dobutamine stress echocardiography predicts surgical outcome in patients with an aortic aneurysm and peripheral vascular disease. J Am Coll Cardiol 1993;21:957–963.

48. Poldermans D, Arnese M, Fioretti PM, et al. Improved cardiac risk stratification in major vascular surgery with dobutamine-atropine stress echocardiography. J Am Coll Cardiol 1995;26:648–653.

49. Pellikka PA, Roger VL, Oh JK, Seward JB, Tajik AJ. Safety of performing dobutamine stress echocardiography in patients with abdominal aortic aneurysm > or = 4 cm in diameter. Am J Cardiol 1996;77: 413–416.

50. Poldermans D, Arnese M, Fioretti PM, et al. Improved cardiac risk stratification in major vascular surgery with dobutamine-atropine stress echocardiography. J Am Coll Cardiol 1995;26:648–653.

51. Das MK, Pellikka PA, Mahoney DW, et al. Assessment of cardiac risk before nonvascular surgery: dobutamine stress echocardiography in 530 patients. J Am Coll Cardiol 2000;35:1647–1653.

52. Mangano DT, Browner WS, Hollenberg M, London MJ, Tubau JF, Tateo IM. Association of perioperative myocardial ischemia with cardiac morbidity and mortality in men undergoing noncardiac surgery: the Study of Perioperative Ischemia Research Group. N Engl J Med 1990;323:1781–1788.

53. Landesberg G, Luria MH, Cotev S, et al. Importance of long-duration postoperative ST-segment depression in cardiac morbidity after vascular surgery. Lancet 1993;341:715–719.

54. Raby KE, Goldman L, Creager MA, et al. Correlation between preoperative ischemia and major cardiac events after peripheral vascular surgery. N Engl J Med 1989;321:1296–1300.

55. McPhail NV, Ruddy TD, Barber GG, Cole CW, Marois LJ, Gulenchyn KY. Cardiac risk stratification using dipyridamole myocardial perfusion imaging and ambulatory ECG monitoring prior to vascular surgery. Eur J Vasc Surg 1993;7:151–155.

56. Mosley JG, Clarke JM, Ell PJ, Marston A. Assessment of myocardial function before aortic surgery by radionuclide angiocardiography. Br J Surg 1985;72:886–887.

57. Pedersen T, Kelbaek H, Munck O. Cardiopulmonary complications in high-risk surgical patients: the value of preoperative radionuclide cardiography. Acta Anaesthesiologica Scandinavica 1990;34: 183–189.

58. Halm EA, Browner WS, Tubau JF, Tateo IM, Mangano DT. Echocardiography for assessing cardiac risk in patients having noncardiac surgery. Study of Perioperative Ischemia Research Group. Ann Intern Med 1996;125:433–441.

59. Kontos MC, Brath LK, Akosah KO, Mohanty PK. Cardiac complications in noncardiac surgery: relative value of resting two-dimensional echocardiography and dipyridamole thallium imaging. Am Heart J 1996;132:559–566.

60. Krupski WC, Nehler MR, Whitehill TA, et al. Negative impact of cardiac evaluation before vascular surgery. Vasc Med 2000;5:3–9.

61. Cohen MC, Curran PJ, L'Italien GJ, Mittleman MA, Zarich SW. Long-term prognostic value of preoperative dipyridamole thallium imaging and clinical indexes in patients with diabetes mellitus undergoing peripheral vascular surgery. Am J Cardiol 1999;83:1038–1042.

62. Poldermans D, Rambaldi R, Fioretti PM, et al. Prognostic value of dobutamine-atropine stress echocardiography for peri-operative and late cardiac events in patients scheduled for vascular surgery. Eur Heart J 1997;18(Suppl D):D86–D96.

63. Stone JG, Foex P, Sear JW, Johnson LL, Khambatta HJ, Triner L. Myocardial ischemia in untreated hypertensive patients: effect of a single small oral dose of a beta-adrenergic blocking agent. Anesthesiology 1988; 68:495–500.

64. Poldermans D, Boersma E, Bax JJ, et al. The effect of bisoprolol on perioperative mortality and myocardial infarction in high-risk patients undergoing vascular surgery. Dutch Echocardiographic Cardiac Risk Evaluation Applying Stress Echocardiography Study Group. N Engl J Med 1999;341: 1789–1794.

65. McFalls EO, Ward HB, Krupski WC, et al. Prophylactic coronary artery revascularization for elective vascular surgery: study design. Veterans Affairs Cooperative Study Group on Coronary Artery Revascularization Prophylaxis for Elective Vascular Surgery. Controll Clin Trials 1999;20:297–308.

66. Crawford ES, Morris GC, Jr, Howell JF, Flynn WF, Moorhead DT. Operative risk in patients with previous coronary artery bypass. Ann Thorac Surg 1978;26:215–221.

67. Reul GJ, Jr., Cooley DA, Duncan JM, et al. The effect of coronary bypass on the outcome of peripheral vascular operations in 1093 patients. J Vasc Surg 1986;3:788–798.

68. Charlson ME, MacKenzie CR, Gold JP, Ales KL, Topkins M, Shires GT. Preoperative characteristics predicting intraoperative hypotension and hypertension among hypertensives and diabetics undergoing noncardiac surgery. Ann Surg 1990;212:66–81.

69. Stone JG, Foex P, Sear JW, Johnson LL, Khambatta HJ, Triner L. Risk of myocardial ischaemia during anaesthesia in treated and untreated hypertensive patients. Br J Anaesthes 1988;61:675–679.

70. Magnusson J, Thulin T, Werner O, Jarhult J, Thomson D. Haemodynamic effects of pretreatment with metoprolol in hypertensive patients undergoing surgery. Br J Anaesthes 1986;58:251–260.

71. Bonow RO, Carabello B, de Leon AC, et al. ACC/AHA guidelines for the management of patients with valvular heart disease. A report of the American College of Cardiology/American Heart Association. Task Force on Practice Guidelines (Committee on Management of Patients with Valvular Heart Disease). J Am Coll Cardiol 1998;32:1486–1588.

72. Rahimtoola SH. Catheter balloon valvuloplasty of aortic and mitral stenosis in adult. Circulation 1987; 75:895–901.

73. O'Kelly B, Browner WS, Massie B, Tubau J, Ngo L, Mangano DT. Ventricular arrhythmias in patients undergoing noncardiac surgery: the Study of Perioperative Ischemia Research Group. JAMA 1992;268:217–221.

74. Kennedy HL, Whitlock JA, Sprague MK, Kennedy LJ, Buckingham TA. Long-term follow-up of asymptomatic healthy subjects with frequent and complex ventricular ectopy. N Engl J Med 1985;312: 193–197.

75. Pastore JO, Yurchak PM, Janis KM, Murphy JD, Zir LM. The risk of advanced heart block in surgical patients with right bundle branch block and left axis deviation. Circulation 1978;57:677–680.

76. Gregoratos G, Cheitlin MD, Conill A, et al. ACC/AHA guidelines for implantation of cardiac pacemakers and antiarrhythmia devices: a report of the American College of Cardiology/American Heart Association Task Force on Practice Guidelines (Committee on Pacemaker Implantation). J Am Coll Cardiol 1998;31:1175–1209.

77. Christopherson R, Beattie C, Frank SM, Norris EJ, Meinert CL. Perioperative morbidity in patients randomized to epidural or general anesthesia for lower extremity vascular surgery. Perioperative Ischemia Randomized Anesthesia Trial Study Group. Anesthesiology 1993;79:422–434.

78. Slogoff S, Keats AS. Randomized trial of primary anesthetic agents on outcome of coronary artery bypass operations. Anesthesiology 1989;70:179–188.

79. Rahimtoola SH, Loeb HS, Ehsani A, Sinno MZ, Chuquimia R, Lal R. Relationship of pulmonary artery to left ventricular diastolic pressures in acute myocardial infarction. Circulation 1972;46: 283–290.

80. Isaacson IJ, Lowdon JD, Berry AJ, et al. The value of pulmonary artery and central venous monitoring in patients undergoing abdominal aortic reconstructive surgery: a comparative study of two selected, randomized groups. J Vasc Surg 1990;12:754–760.

81. Joyce WP, Provan JL, Ameli FM, McEwan MM, Jelenich S, Jones DP. The role of central haemodynamic monitoring in abdominal aortic surgery. A prospective randomised study. Eur J Vasc Surg 1990;4:633–636.

82. Polanczyk CA, Rohde LE, Goldman L, et al. Right heart catheterization and cardiac complications in patients undergoing noncardiac surgery: an observational study. JAMA 2001;286:309–314.

83. Barone JE, Tucker JB, Rassias D, Corvo PR. Routine perioperative pulmonary artery catheterization has no effect on rate of complications in vascular surgery: a meta-analysis. Am Surg 2001;67:674–679.

84. London MJ, Tubau JF, Wong MG, Layug E, Hollenberg M, Krupski WC. The "natural history" of segmental wall motion abnormalities in patients undergoing noncardiac surgery. S.P.I. Research Group. Anesthesiology 1990;73:644–655.

85. Eisenberg MJ, London MJ, Leung JM, et al. Monitoring for myocardial ischemia during noncardiac surgery: a technology assessment of transesophageal echocardiography and 12-lead electrocardiography: the Study of Perioperative Ischemia Research Group. JAMA 1992;268:210–216.
86. Mathew JP, Fleisher LA, Rinehouse JA, et al. ST segment depression during labor and delivery. Anesthesiology 1992;77:635–641.
87. Yeager RA, Moneta GL, Edwards JM, Taylor LM, McConnell DB, Porter JM. Late survival after perioperative myocardial infarction complicating vascular surgery. J Vasc Surg 1994;20:598–604.

15 Special Consideration for the Diabetic Foot

Gary W. Gibbons, MD and
Geoffrey Habershaw, DPM

CONTENTS

INTRODUCTION

The incidence of diabetes mellitus worldwide is increasing at an alarming rate. In the United States approx 16 million people (6% of the population) have diabetes mellitus, half of whom do not know they have the disease. The prevalence of this disease has increased across all racial groups over the last decade, although those at highest risk are African-Americans, Hispanics, and American Indians. Diabetes is the seventh leading cause of death in the United States, primarily due to cardiovascular complications.

Lower extremity ulcers leading to amputation are an associated complication and increasing problem among individuals with diabetes. It is estimated that 15% of diabetics will develop a foot ulcer during their lifetime, which precedes nontraumatic amputation 85% of the time *(1,2)*. Not surprisingly, more than half of all lower limb amputations in the United States occur in people with diabetes—86,000 last year. Furthermore, it is estimated that half of these amputations are preventable. Not only is amputation the diabetic patient's greatest fear, but there is decreased physical, emotional, and social function following an amputation. Amputation rates are greater with increasing age, in men compared to women, and among members of racial and ethnic minorities. Access to care, and the quality and comprehensiveness of the care delivered, are major variables affecting the outcome of diabetic foot care and amputation prevention. Despite our best efforts, the incidence of lower extremity amputation in people with

From: *Contemporary Cardiology: Peripheral Arterial Disease: Diagnosis and Treatment*
Edited by: J. D. Coffman and R. T. Eberhardt © Humana Press Inc., Totowa, NJ

diabetes continues to rise. The economic impact on patients, families, and society is staggering, with hospital costs alone estimated at 860 million dollars annually *(3)*.

WOUND HEALING

It is well established that wound healing is impaired in people with diabetes mellitus. The faulty healing of wounds in people with diabetes has been attributed to three key predisposing factors *(4,5)*:

- Peripheral neuropathy
- Abnormal cellular/inflammatory pathways
- Vascular disease/tissue hypoxia

Peripheral Neuropathy

Symmetric distal polyneuropathy of diabetes mellitus has three major effects on the lower extremity: sensory, motor, and autonomic. After about 10 yr of diabetes mellitus, there is loss of the protective sensations including pressure, pain, and temperature. This blunts or abolishes the warning signals of potential dangerous conditions or events and may result in injury without detection. This may lead to more extensive injury because of failure to protect the limb *(6)*.

Motor polyneuropathy results in weakness and atrophy of the intrinsic muscles of the foot, leading to changes in foot structure, frank deformity, and altered biomechanics. Atrophy of the intrinsic muscles of the foot allows a hammering disfiguration of the digits and enhancement of pressure points on the toes and metatarsal heads. The altered shape of the foot into a relative "cavus" attitude increases the pressure at the heel. These changes place the foot at high risk, which needs to be identified early so the foot can be protected from skin breakdown, infection, and ulceration. Proximal muscle weakness may also contribute to foot-drop deformity. This will usually occur slowly and may be noted by the patient because of increased stumbling and tripping. The inability to maintain proper balance may also be noticed, especially while standing still. Bracing may become necessary to allow for safe and effective ambulation.

Autonomic neuropathy impairs the normal maintenance of skin integrity and vascular tone, leading to arteriovenous shunting, which lessens oxygen and nutrients available to the tissues. It leads to dryness and cracking of the skin as a result of sweat and sebaceous gland dysfunction. Thickening and drying of the skin and nails may be difficult to care for without professional help. Decreased vascular tone in the lower limbs may contribute to the development of edema.

Neuropathy also impairs the neuroinflammatory response, the hyperemic response, and a proper thermoregulatory response, all of which can interfere with normal wound healing.

Abnormal Cellular/Inflammatory Pathways

Acute wounds normally respond in an orderly and predictable sequence during the healing phases *(7)*. The diabetic wound, however, appears to be stuck in the inflammatory/proliferative phase, allowing for repeated injury, infection, and further inflammation. Abnormalities in cellular function, particularly among fibroblasts and neutrophils, have been found in people with diabetes. The humoral responses to wound healing, such as extracellular matrix production and cytokine production, are adversely affected by advanced glycosylation end products preventing the normal sequence of wound healing phases.

Vascular Disease/Tissue Hypoxia

Peripheral arterial disease (PAD) is among the many etiologies contributing to ischemic pain, nonhealing ulceration, and amputation in individuals with and without diabetes. The incidence of PAD in diabetic patients is at least four times that of nondiabetic individuals and increases with age and duration of diabetes. Severe impairment in limb perfusion can lead to tissue hypoxia with subsequent tissue damage and loss. The severity of PAD is worse among those with diabetes. Critical ischemia is associated with 62% of nonhealing ulcers and a causal factor for 46% of amputations. It is imperative therefore that a basic understanding of diabetic PAD, its diagnosis, and treatment be a prerequisite for successful management of diabetic lower extremity problems.

DIABETIC PAD

PAD decreases arterial perfusion to the lower extremity and foot. PAD may lead to limb pain, ulceration, and impaired wound healing, and decreases the ability to fight infection by delaying or preventing delivery of oxygen, nutrients, the components of a proper immune response, and antibiotics to the infected area. This problem is more dramatic in the patient with diabetes, as will be discussed.

Risk Factors and Prevention

Diabetic PAD is more common, occurs at a younger age, and advances more rapidly with a roughly equal male-to-female ratio compared with nondiabetic PAD. While diabetes is an important risk factor for PAD, other well-established risk factors such as hypertension, smoking, and hyperlipidemia act synergistically, contributing additional risk for the diabetic patient. Preventing or delaying the onset of PAD is best achieved by the elimination of risk factors including the cessation of cigarette smoking, good control of diabetes, control of hypertension and hyperlipidemia, maintaining ideal weight, and regular exercise. Periodic clinical vascular examination, including noninvasive testing when appropriate, identifies diabetic patients at especially high risk so that they can be observed more carefully or referred to a vascular specialist.

Pathologic Arterial Changes

Although the pathology of atherosclerosis is similar in diabetic and nondiabetic patients, there are several distinguishing features characterizing diabetic PAD. Although atherosclerotic occlusive disease can involve any artery in the diabetic patient, especially in those who smoke, there is a predilection for the disease to primarily involve the tibial and peroneal arteries between the knee and the foot (8). The foot vessels, especially the dorsalis pedis artery and the distal posterior tibial and plantar arteries, are usually spared. There continues to be a misconception, even published in the literature, that there is an occlusive microvascular disease affecting the diabetic foot that precludes revascularization and wound healing. This, unfortunately, leads to inappropriate or no vascular evaluation and care in many diabetic patients who could benefit from an aggressive treatment including revascularization. Because there is sparing of the foot arteries, tissue perfusion in the ischemic diabetic foot can usually be restored with appropriate vascular reconstructions.

It is true that the diabetic patient is particularly prone to develop a nonocclusive microcirculatory impairment that involves the capillaries and arterioles, especially those of the kidneys, retinae, and peripheral nerves *(9)*. This microvascular dysfunction begins early in the diabetic individual's life. There is increased microvascular pressure and flow leading to endothelial injury with sclerosis (basement membrane thickening) and a resultant limited capillary capacity with loss of autoregulatory function including the abolition of a vasoconstrictor response. Basement membrane thickening may impede leukocyte migration and impair diffusion, resulting in a metabolic blockage of oxygen utilization. Increased arteriovenous shunting, an impaired hyperemic response to heat and inflammation, the loss of a postural vasoconstrictor response, an increased capillary permeability leading to edema formation, as well as the diminished or loss of neurogenic regulatory responses, alters the diabetic patient's ability to respond to injury with a proper and orderly sequence of healing.

Peculiar to the diabetic is the development of calcification involving the intimal plaque and media (medial calcinosis/Mönckeberg's sclerosis) that frequently involves diabetic arteries at all levels. Medial calcinosis is the most common reason noninvasive testing results are only complementary to clinical judgment in assessing diabetic PAD. Medial calcinosis leads to falsely high segmental pressures and erroneously elevated ankle–brachial index (ABI). Medial calcinosis can also complicate surgical bypass techniques and adversely affects laser, atherectomy, and balloon angioplasty treatment.

Diabetic patients also have a diminished ability to establish collateral circulation, especially around the infrageniculate arterial branches at the knee level. This is one reason why it is better to directly bypass to an artery that has continuity all the way down to the foot when one is trying to heal extensive tissue loss in the diabetic patient.

Clinical Presentation and Evaluation

Similar to that of nondiabetic individuals, the clinical presentation of diabetic patients with major artery occlusions or hemodynamically significant stenoses varies depending on their activity level and the adequacy of collateral pathways *(1,10)*. Intermittent claudication (IC), the inability to walk a given distance (usually described in blocks) because of an ache or pain in the muscles of the leg, is the earliest symptomatic manifestations of PAD (*see* Chapter 3). The stenosis or blockage can usually be determined by the group of muscles involved and is generally one level higher. Patients with calf claudication usually have superficial femoral artery disease. Patients with buttock, hip, or thigh claudication have disease involving the aorta and iliac arteries. Remembering that the diabetic patient has a predilection for tibial/peroneal disease, significant foot pain while walking may be the first presentation and not calf claudication. Diagnosing IC in the diabetic patient is made more difficult by the presence of peripheral and autonomic neuropathy. Diabetic patients may state that they just have to stop walking and are really not able to describe classic IC. As PAD worsens, rest pain occurs and is often described as a deep aching pain of muscles in the foot that is present at rest or at night—so-called rest pain, indicative of critical limb ischemia (see Chapter 6). Relief is obtained by hanging the feet in a dependent position or walking, especially at night. As the disease progresses further, tissue ulceration and/or gangrene can develop. Because of sensory neuropathy, diabetic patients often present with tissue loss or gangrene as the first sign of severe PAD.

Clinical evaluation, judgment, and experience remain the most important means for determining the degree of vascular compromise in the diabetic lower extremity. Noninvasive testing, by whatever means, is only complementary to the clinical evaluation. Doppler-derived arterial pressures are measured at the ankle to determine the systolic pressure and ABI (*see* Chapter 4). Results of the systolic ankle pressure and ABI correlate well with the degree of ischemia in nondiabetic patients—a systolic arterial ankle pressure of < 50 mmHg and ABI < 0.4 suggest severe perfusion abnormality and support critical limb ischemia. However, the systolic ankle pressure and the ABI are often falsely elevated in diabetic patients secondary to medial calcification. Because medial calcinosis frequently spares the foot and toe arteries, measurement of the toe systolic pressure is often useful. A systolic toe–brachial pressure index < 0.7 is considered abnormal while an absolute toe pressure of < 30 mmHg is considered inadequate for wound healing.

Transcutaneous oxygen tension ($TcPO_2$) may also be used to assess the degree of ischemia and likelihood of healing an ulcer, particularly in the diabetic individual *(11)*. Normal $TcPO_2$ is defined as 55 mmHg or greater. In general, if the $TcPO_2$ is 30 mmHg or greater, then the arterial blood supply should be adequate for wound healing, while those below 15 mmHg are inadequate for healing. Measuring $TcPO_2$, however, is dependent on many variables and, like other noninvasive tests, is only complementary to clinical judgment, especially when one is trying to heal extensive tissue loss and/or gangrene. A good rule of thumb is that an experienced vascular consultation and contrast arteriography or magnetic resonance angiography (MRA) are indicated when there is uncertainty as to whether ischemia is contributing to the diabetic foot problem.

Arteriography is still considered the gold standard for defining the anatomic location and extent of atherosclerotic occlusive disease affecting the arteries of the lower leg and foot (*see* Chapter 5). More than 90% of diabetic patients presenting with ischemic foot ulcerations/gangrene have demonstrated surgically correctable occlusive disease with current arteriographic techniques, especially digital subtraction arteriography. It is important to visualize the arterial tree all the way down and include the foot vessels, remembering that diabetic PAD more typically affects the tibial/peroneal arteries. While there is an increased risk of contrast-induced renal insufficiency in the diabetic patient, proper hydration remains the best means for preventing or minimizing this complication. Further advances in MRA may make it the procedure of choice in the future, especially in patients with renal compromise. Proper individualized treatment alternatives require communication with the radiologist to ensure complete visualization all the way to the foot vessels.

Treatment Initiatives

The treatment of diabetic PAD depends on its severity as determined by the patient's presenting symptoms and physical examination, including a detailed vascular evaluation. The patient's general medical conditions and associated risk factors must be taken into consideration, as well as the patient's own interpretation of his or her functional status and well being. Motivation and compliance need to be addressed. Mild to moderate claudication is best treated by controlling risk factors such as the cessation of smoking, weight reduction, control of lipid levels and hypertension, good diabetes control, and an exercise program (*see* Chapters 8 and 9). Protective footwear and regular foot inspections are important during and after exercise. Diabetic patients should inspect their feet daily and have their feet examined at every doctor's visit. Those who cannot see well, as is common among diabetic patients because of retinopathy, should have a family member inspect their feet regularly. Diabetic individuals can often live with significant PAD without a problem until some type of traumatic event initiates a blister or ulcer. This most commonly happens with improperly fitting shoes. A running shoe, cross-trainer, or some other type of athletic sneaker should be worn during exercise. Diabetic patients with significant neuropathy, and especially those with ischemia, should not wear old, worn out shoes for exercise or even daily wear *(12,13)*.

Antiplatelet agents (clopidogrel, aspirin, dipyridamole) should be used to prevent ischemic cardiovascular events, even in the diabetic (*see* Chapter 9). However, the efficacy of antiplatelet agents for alleviating claudication has not been confirmed in clinical trials. The use of the hemorheologic agent pentoxifylline to reduce blood viscosity has not been generally successful for dramatically improving walking distance (*see* Chapter 10). Cilostazol is both a vasodilator and antiplatelet agent that has been found to be effective in improving the walking distance of patients with intermittent claudication.

Indications for arteriography and vascular reconstruction in diabetic patients are similar to those for the nondiabetic individuals and include disabling claudication, ischemic rest pain/night pain, tissue ulceration, gangrene, or an inability of a surgical procedure to heal because of associated ischemia. It should be reiterated that if a health care professional believes that ischemia may be complicating management of a diabetic wound, then the patient should be referred to a vascular specialist knowledgeable about diabetic vascular disease and its treatment. If one is providing the appropriate wound care and the wound is still not healing, then reassessment for the adequacy of the circulation to allow proper wound healing should be undertaken.

Revascularization Techniques

ENDOVASCULAR PROCEDURES

Endovascular procedures include percutaneous transluminal angioplasty (PTA) with and without stent placement, atherectomy, and laser-assisted angioplasty (*see* Chapter 12). It was hoped that endovascular procedures would be less costly, require shorter hospitalizations, and be associated with less morbidity than traditional vascular reconstruction surgeries. Unfortunately, the long-term results of laser-assisted angioplasty and atherectomy have been disappointing, especially in the treatment of diabetic infrainguinal (outflow) disease.

PTA with and without stent placement remains the most common endovascular revascularization procedure. The success of PTA depends on the location of the diseased artery being treated, the length of the diseased artery being treated, whether the disease is localized or diffuse, and the amount of calcium associated with the plaque. Balloon angioplasty (PTA) results are best with short, isolated stenotic areas in high-flow arteries such as the iliac. Diminishing success is associated with more extensive or distal occlusive disease, especially if it is diffuse and heavily involved with calcium. This finding has important implications for diabetic arterial occlusive disease because it tends to be complicated by all of these conditions. Our most frequent use of PTA is in management of short, isolated stenotic segments in the aortoiliac segment, especially prior to a distal revascularization. The routine use of stents following balloon angioplasty may improve patency but further clinical studies are needed before it is recommended in the treatment of diabetic infrainguinal (outflow) disease.

SURGICAL VASCULAR RECONSTRUCTION

Diabetic patients tolerate surgical revascularization procedures extremely well with excellent outcomes, and morbidity and mortality rates equal to those of nondiabetic individuals. Both inflow (aortoiliac and aortofemoral) procedures and outflow (infrainguinal, including femoral, popliteal, tibial/peroneal, and pedal) procedures can be tailored to individual patient's needs depending on the location and extent of disease, associated risk factors, and the patient's overall well being. Patients who have severe dementia or mental deterioration and who do not ambulate are certainly not candidates for revascularization. Patients with extensive tissue destruction with questionable limb salvage, even if the circulation was restored, must be carefully evaluated as to whether they would be better served by performing a primary amputation. Advanced age is not a contraindication to revascularization. It is important to assess the patient's functional status, motivation, compliance, and general medical condition including risk factors and comorbid conditions that might affect graft patency and overall success. The preoperative assessment and preparation helps determine the particular procedure that a patient may successfully tolerate (*see* Chapter 14).

Coronary artery disease and left ventricular dysfunction are the leading causes of morbidity and mortality in all major revascularization procedures. Because of diabetic sensory and autonomic neuropathy, underlying cardiac disease may be asymptomatic. An abnormal electrocardiogram or a history of significant coronary artery disease or left ventricular dysfunction (congestive heart failure) requires further preoperative cardiac evaluation including possible risk stratification testing.

If arteriography has affected renal function, it should return to baseline, if at all possible, prior to any revascularization procedure. Compromised pulmonary function must be evaluated and treated because it may influence not only the type of revascularization procedure recommended but also the administration of anesthesia. Medications are reviewed and adjusted, especially those affecting the clotting cascade. Control of blood sugar is a prerequisite prior to any revascularization procedure unless it is an emergency.

All active infection must be controlled prior to surgical revascularization. Infected wounds must be carefully probed and all necrotic tissue and pus debrided and dependently drained *(14)*. It should be remembered that infection travels along the course of lymphatics that lie adjacent to the vein most commonly harvested for the bypass. Appropriate adjunctive intravenous antibiotics should be administered throughout the perioperative period. Dressings should be appropriate for the wound being treated. Once infection is controlled, immediate arteriography (or MRA) and revascularization is undertaken to minimize any further ischemic necrosis.

Invasive intraoperative and perioperative monitoring may reduce the intraoperative and immediate postoperative complications (mainly cardiac) (*see* Chapter 14). Nutritional replenishment, control of edema, and proper blood sugar control are extremely important throughout the perioperative period. It is generally best to keep the blood sugar < 200 during the perioperative period.

While early ambulation is now the norm, it must be delayed in patients with open dependent ulcers or after reconstructive foot surgery or a local forefoot amputation. Active and passive physical therapy including range of motion exercises are encouraged. For the diabetic it is preferred to increase weight bearing slowly in the prolonged non-weight bearing patient to prevent the development of an acute Charcot foot, disruption of a local reconstructive foot procedure, or aggravation of a locally debrided ulcer or minor amputation.

Inflow Procedures. The management of aortoiliac occlusive disease is basically the same for diabetic and nondiabetic patients and most often requires the use of synthetic bypass grafts *(15)* (*see* Chapter 13).

Infrainguinal (Outflow) Procedures. Unrecognized and/or untreated lower extremity ischemia increases the risk for major amputation. The indications for infrainguinal revascularization in diabetics include disabling claudication, rest pain, tissue loss, gangrene, and failure of ulcers to heal *(16)*.

Autogenous vein (usually saphenous or arm vein) is the conduit of choice. Synthetic grafts are used only as a last resort. The surgery can usually be tailored depending on the amount, size, and quality of vein available, the patient's indications, associated risk factors, and the actual anatomic setup as determined by complete arteriography or MRA visualizing the foot vessels. It is important to discuss the purpose of the bypass with everyone involved in the patient's care including the patient and his or her family. Is there a need to cure claudication or to restore foot perfusion to heal extensive tissue loss or a previously performed foot procedure?

The simplest and most effective vascular bypass would be one that bypasses a blockage in the superficial femoral artery with restoration of flow to the popliteal, tibial/peroneal vessels down and into the dorsalis pedis and plantar arteries. Unfortunately, this bypass is not usually an option for diabetic patients who need to heal extensive tissue loss. Restoration of pulsatile blood flow to the foot has been found to be most important to achieve the most rapid and durable healing of extensive tissue loss, gangrene, or incisions from local forefoot procedures. For claudication and/or rest pain, a more proximal infrainguinal bypass usually suffices.

A flexible approach to distal surgical revascularization (especially when there is limited vein) allows for the use of an inflow source that is most distal, such as the popliteal artery, when it is available. The decision to place the vein in the reverse, non-reversed, or *in situ* position depends on the anatomy, the size, and the quality of the vein, and the amount of vein that is needed. In general, the larger part of the vein should be placed in the more proximal larger artery and the smaller end used for the distal anastomosis. The *in situ* technique (in which the vein is left in its anatomical position) or nonreversed vein technique, requires vein valve lysis for the creation of a suitable conduit.

Once the circulation is restored, more localized debridement and/or reconstructive foot surgery and/or minor amputation can be performed, or a previously performed debridement may be left open to heal. By restoring foot perfusion, direct foot-sparing surgery such as local excision of ulcerations and infected bony prominences, osteotomies, and/or arthroplasties, have eliminated the need for even minor amputations in the diabetic foot. There is rapid and durable healing with return of function and well being for most patients *(16)*.

MANAGEMENT OF THE DIABETIC FOOT

Advances in the management of the diabetic foot have accelerated since World War II. Prior to that time, the first diabetic foot operation was a below-knee or above-knee amputation. In many areas of the world this is still the case. The first "diabetic foot operation" in the United States was the transmetatarsal amputation (17). When extensive infection and tissue loss affected the forefoot, transmetatarsal amputation and early antibiotics, such as penicillin and sulfa, were potential solutions to salvage a walking foot in the patient who would have previously lost it. As a result, thousands of patients have been able to avoid a major amputation because of this procedure alone (10).

The treatment of PAD with bypass surgery was first addressed and applied to the patient with diabetic foot problems in the 1950s. The femoral–popliteal bypass graft, when performed on the limb having a transmetatarsal amputation, was more likely to heal owing to the enhanced blood supply. Further advances in arteriography, use of antibiotics, cardiac and renal care, microscopic distal bypass surgery, diabetes management, reconstructive foot surgery, wound care, orthotics and bracing, and shoes have made it more likely than not that a limb can be saved from amputation.

A "team approach" is the mainstay for the modern approach to limb salvage. This and other essential concepts for the management of the diabetic foot were explored in depth by the American Diabetes Association in 1999 when it convened a panel of experts in many fields from around the world (14,18). This panel determined that the evaluation and treatment of this problem was multiple and varied. There was a paucity of scientific data to support most treatments, many of which were supported only by anecdotal experience. They determined that the treatments that were most effective were:

1. Effective management of diabetes mellitus, cardiac and renal disease (e.g. good glycemic control).
2. Aggressive surgical debridement of necrotic tissue, including reconstructive foot surgery as needed.
3. Bypass grafting to treat vascular disease.
4. Effective use of antibiotics.
5. Shoes and orthotics.

It is estimated that 60–70% of diabetic foot ulceration occurs because of neuropathy and 30–40% because of ischemia in combination with neuropathy.

Pathophysiology of Ulcer Formation

Three factors lead to skin break down and ulceration: (1) high stress, (2) low continuous stress, and (3) repetitive moderate stress.

High stress, 700–1000 lb/in.^{2}, will interrupt the skin integrity due the skin's inability to withstand this acute event. An example of this would be stepping on a nail or a broken piece of glass when barefoot. Although this can cause severe injury, it is not the most common cause of ulceration in patients with diabetes and neuropathy.

Low continuous stress, 2–3 lb/in.^{2}, causes ulceration usually over a bony prominence in a nonambulatory patient. This is the decubitus ulceration seen most commonly in the heels, buttocks and scapulas of the bedridden patient. Patients with diabetes mellitus and neuropathy who are walking do not develop decubitus ulcers of their lower extremities.

Repetitive moderate stress, 40–60 lb/in.², is the force most responsible for the breakdown of the skin in a neuropathic foot. This force causes enough irritation of the skin to allow for a response and repair before ulceration occurs and calluses are the result. Eventually, these calluses become painful in the patient without neuropathy. Thinning the callus and adjustment of shoe and gait result in improvement in the level of comfort. The patient with neuropathy, however, does not feel this discomfort, thus fails to limp, and places recurrent pressure at these focal points. This results in the formation of a sub-callus blister, which eventually breaks and becomes infected with skin flora bacteria. This infection leads to further tissue destruction and ulcer formation *(4,10)*.

Healing Ulcerations

The essential elements for healing of foot ulcers are restoration of blood flow, control of infection, general medical care, and relief of pressure *(19)*. Pulsatile arterial flow to the foot is best. Bypass grafts taken to the dorsalis pedis artery or the posterior tibial artery should be considered if the foot pulses are absent in the face of a nonhealing ulcer. Infection must be adequately controlled. Ulcers that probe to subcutaneous structures or bone must be rapidly and aggressively opened and debrided *(20)*. Patients with diabetes mellitus may not mount an appropriate response to sepsis owing to immunosuppression. Regular mechanical debridement of wounds of all necrotic tissue is a mainstay of treatment.

Adequate medical management of the patient is imperative. Control of blood sugar maintains an adequate cellular response to sepsis. Maintenance of optimal perfusion of the tissues is important, as is treatment of underlying coronary artery disease and congestive heart failure. Chronic renal insufficiency will delay healing from the consistently high concentrations of metabolic byproducts and fluid balance disturbances. Adequate nutrition is imperative for wound healing. Pressure must be relieved from the ulcerated site. Repetitive mechanical irritation of the ulcerated site will cause additional tissue destruction.

Management of Ulcers and Neuropathic Feet

Patients with foot ulcers will be managed either as inpatients or outpatients; the decision is based on whether the ulceration is mild or severe (Figs. 1 and 2). Individuals with mild ulcerations can be managed as outpatients and those with severe ulcers must be admitted for more aggressive treatment *(10,12)*.

Pressure relief of the ulcerated foot becomes the challenge once arterial flow has been deemed adequate or restored, infection controlled by antibiotics/surgery and metabolic control is adequate. There is no substitute for non-weight-bearing ambulation. Crutches, walkers, or wheelchairs are the most effective means for relieving weight. Neuropathic patients will bear weight on their ulcerated foot when they are not hospitalized. This being the case, some other technique must be used to relieve pressure. The felted foam dressing, total contact cast, healing sandals, and braces are a few of these techniques.

- Healing sandals and braces may be removed easily by patients; thus they are not reliable as or effective as other pressure relieving techniques.
- The total contact cast is an effective pressure-relieving technique. It works very well for those with experience in its application, maintenance, and removal. However, the process is labor intensive, time consuming, and potentially risky. Con-

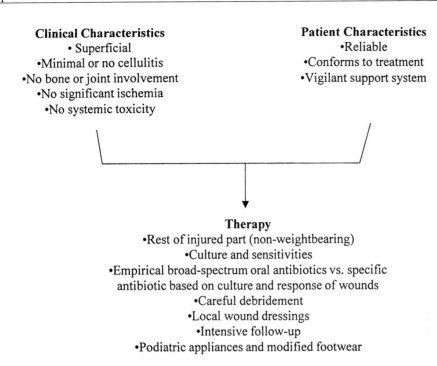

Clinical Characteristics
• Superficial
•Minimal or no cellulitis
•No bone or joint involvement
•No significant ischemia
•No systemic toxicity

Patient Characteristics
•Reliable
•Conforms to treatment
•Vigilant support system

Therapy
•Rest of injured part (non-weightbearing)
•Culture and sensitivities
•Empirical broad-spectrum oral antibiotics vs. specific
antibiotic based on culture and response of wounds
•Careful debridement
•Local wound dressings
•Intensive follow-up
•Podiatric appliances and modified footwear

Fig. 1. Management of non-limb-threatening diabetic foot ulcers. Clinical and patient characteristics used to guide potential therapies.

founding issues such as a disturbance in fluid balance or a recent distal bypass graft, as well as a propensity to irritate other bony prominences, makes it a less desirable technique.
•   Felted foam dressing have been used at the Joslin Diabetes Center for > 20 yr and are often a mainstay of efficient, reliable, and safe pressure relief from the ulcerated site. Pedal barographic measurements have shown a 60–80% vertical force pressure relief at the site of plantar ulceration with felted foam dressing in place (10).

Patients should be instructed to remain off the foot and bear weight only when absolutely necessary. A postoperative shoe should be used with a molded orthotic. The pad may be left in place for up to 1 wk, until the patient returns for debridement of the wound and replacement of the pad. A sock is worn over the pad at all times except when the dressing is changed. The rubber cement used comes off the skin when the pad is removed and will not tear the skin if carefully removed. The ulcer should be measured and probed at each change. If healing is progressing, the process is continued. If not, reassessment of vascular status, infection, diabetic control, and compliance are necessary. No ulcer should take more than 12 wk to heal. Aggressive frequent debridement of the ulcer has proven valuable to overall healing *(10,12)*.

SHOES FOR THE NEUROPATHIC FOOT

There is no perfect shoe for the neuropathic foot *(21,22)*. Any shoe worn has the potential to cause an abrasion that can lead to infection. The shoes that are worn should

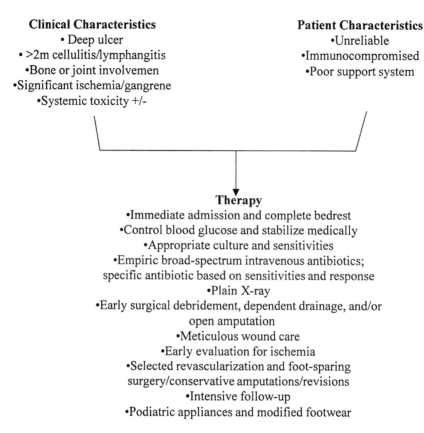

Clinical Characteristics
- Deep ulcer
- >2m cellulitis/lymphangitis
- Bone or joint involvemen
- Significant ischemia/gangrene
- Systemic toxicity +/-

Patient Characteristics
- Unreliable
- Immunocompromised
- Poor support system

Therapy
- Immediate admission and complete bedrest
- Control blood glucose and stabilize medically
- Appropriate culture and sensitivities
- Empiric broad-spectrum intravenous antibiotics; specific antibiotic based on sensitivities and response
- Plain X-ray
- Early surgical debridement, dependent drainage, and/or open amputation
- Meticulous wound care
- Early evaluation for ischemia
- Selected revascularization and foot-sparing surgery/conservative amputations/revisions
- Intensive follow-up
- Podiatric appliances and modified footwear

Fig. 2. Management of limb-threatening diabetic foot ulcers. Clinical and patient characteristics used to guide potential therapies.

have characteristics that make them least likely to cause abrasions. The toe box should be round and pliable, the midsole cushioned, and the sole made of nonslip material. Lacing or Velcro fasteners should close the toes to allow for swelling. There should be a cushioned insole that may be replaced with an orthotic, if necessary. The modern day athletic shoe fits this design reasonable well.

The extra-depth shoe has all these features but the room in the toe box is maximized. The best way to avoid shoe-related foot problems is to instruct neuropathic patients to rotate their shoes and socks every 3–4 hr. There are three reasons for this: (1) it gives the insensate patient the brief moment to inspect the foot for undetected injury; (2) pressure points are altered by rotating to another pair of shoes; and (3) all shoes begin to lose cushioning and support after 3–4 hr of use, thus increasing friction *(10,12)*.

Rotating shoes is a simple task that will minimize the development of skin breakdown. Custom-molded shoes should be used when the foot deformity is severe enough that it precludes the use of over-the-counter shoes. A Charcot foot that has healed with deformity may benefit from the use of a molded shoe. These shoes can be built around the deformed foot and leave room for extra support and cushioning from orthotics. The orthotics should be at least 1/2 in. thick. They can be low cut or chukka height to give the ankle support.

ORTHOTICS

Orthotics serve to alter musculoskeletal dynamics and cushion vertical forces. The use of soft rather than rigid orthotics is preferred with the neuropathic foot. Heat molded Plastizode, in various densities, is easily adapted to athletic, extra-depth and molded shoes. The orthotics may also be covered with soft materials to minimize shearing and twisting forces.

THE CHARCOT FOOT

Charcot neuropathic arthropathy occurs in about 1 in 700 patients with diabetes mellitus (23). It will not develop without the presence of peripheral neuropathy and is not exclusive to the patient with diabetes mellitus. It can occur in any disease that damages the peripheral nerves or posterior column of the central nervous system. In the United States diabetes is certainly the most common cause, with alcoholic-induced neuropathy second and hereditary insensitivity to pain third. Other causes of Charcot foot include syringomyelia and tabes dorsalis.

The development of Charcot joint disease is thought to be a result of a combination of vascular dysfunction and somatosensory nerve dysfunction. Some investigators have also implicated excessive nonenzymatic glycosylation of collagen.

Patients remember an injury in about 40% of cases, but usually just note unilateral unexplained swelling of one foot that may or may not be painful. Early in the course of the disorder, the swelling may be minimal in the morning but recur and progress during the day. Later in the course of Charcot foot, the swelling is always present and, indeed, may begin to become painful.

The foot is warm and swollen but will usually not show deformity in the early stages. When there is deformity, crepitus may be felt at the level of the midfoot most commonly. This is pathognomonic for an active fracture. When deformity occurs it is usually in the midfoot at the tarsometatarsal junction, which occurs at this level in 60% of cases. The remaining 40% will occur at the metatarsophalangeal joints, talonavicular joint level, talocalcaneal joints and the ankle joint. The more proximal the fracture, that is, closer to the ankle joint, the more severe the fracture is in terms of treatment and rehabiltation.

A high index of suspicion is essential for the effective diagnosis of a Charcot fracture. A unilateral swollen foot in a neuropathic patient without foot ulceration should be considered to be Charcot fracture until proven otherwise. Infection and deep venous thrombosis also need to be ruled out. Plain radiographs will many times be negative early because Charcot fracture begins as a ligamentous injury with no overt evidence of bone disruption on X-ray film. However, bone scans will be useful at this time owing to its high sensitivity and the presence of accelerated bone metabolism. It is not necessary to obtain a bone scan if fracture is seen on plain films. Although unilateral Charcot foot is the most common presentation, it occurs in the contralateral foot in about 30–40% of patients within a year.

The mainstay of treatment continues to be non-weight-bearing. There is no better substitute for crutches, walker, or a wheelchair. Casting may be done but it should be a non-weight-bearing cast. A removal bivalve cast will permit daily inspection of the skin and may work as well as closed casting provided that weight bearing is restricted. Patients who cannot be non-weight-bearing may be placed in off-the-shelf walking casts, which will give some protection and allow healing at a slower rate. The duration of non-weight-

Table 1
Advice for Patients

Patients should not:
1. Go barefoot at any time, even inside the house.
2. Wear tight or worn out shoes.
3. Use any sharp instruments on the foot to trim calluses and nails.
4. Wear medicated corn pads.
5. Use any form of external heat including heating pads and hot water bottles.
6. Soak feet in hot water.
7. Smoke or be near people who are smoking.

Patients should:
1. Wash their feet and dry them well and use a mild soap.
2. Uses padded socks to help absorb friction.
3. Wear shoes that fit and ones that do not have to be broken in.
4. Change their shoes and socks twice a day.
5. Check their feet for any breaks in the skin and report it to their physician.
6. Keep the blood sugar level in good control.
7. Make sure to remind their primary doctor to check their feet at each visit.
8. Have the primary doctor refer them to a podiatrist if self-care.

bearing is typically 3 mo, but this time may be adjusted up or down depending on the clinical situation.

Signs of healing will be temperature reduction, resolution of swelling, and absence of crepitus on clinical examination. Serial X-ray films taken each month should show fracture healing with evidence of sclerotic bone changes. An active fracture will give way to coalescence as non-weight-bearing is continued. Crepitus must be gone before weight-bearing begins. Swelling and temperature increase may persist owing to the inevitable degenerative arthritis that will now develop. It may take a full year for all of the swelling to diminish. Resumption of weight-bearing should be gradual and partial. Osteopenia of adjacent bony structures will be inevitable as a side effect. Partial, gradual weight-bearing over 4–6 wk is necessary to help to avoid further injury *(10,12)*.

SUMMARY

Foot-related problems, especially ulceration, are a serious concern among patients with diabetes mellitus. Although a "small" percentage of the population, diabetic individuals account for nearly half of all lower extremity amputations. Given these concerns, in 1999 the American Diabetes Association published a consensus position to provide guidance to health care professionals who manage foot wounds in people with diabetes *(14,18)*. There are six approaches that are supported by clinical trials or well-established principles of wound healing: offloading, debridement, dressings, antibiotics, vascular reconstruction, and amputation when necessary. Adjunctive medical therapies included normalization of blood sugar, treatment of comorbid conditions, control of edema, nutritional repletion and support, and physical and emotional therapy. While the assessment and management of ischemia is important for the diabetic patient, it must be a part of the total treatment algorithm to ensure wound healing and prevent amputation. Our own algorithms for treatment of non-limb-threatening and limb-threatening infections are outlined in Figs. 1 and 2.

REFERENCES

1. Pecoraro RE, Reiber GE, Burgess EM. Pathways to diabetic limb amputation: basis for prevention. Diabetes Care 1990;13:513–521.
2. Ramsey SD, Newton K, Blough D, et al. Incidence, outcomes, and cost of foot ulcer in patients with diabetes. Diabetes Care 1999;22:382–387.
3. Reiber GE, Lipsky BA, Gibbons GW. The burben of diabetic foot ulcers. Am J Surg 1998;176(Suppl 2A):5S–10S.
4. Laing P. The development and complications of diabetic foot ulcerations. Am J Surg 1998; 176(Suppl 2A):11S–19S.
5. Stadelmann WK, Digenis AG, Tobin GR. Impediments to wound healing. Am J Surg 1998; 176(Suppl 2A):39S–47S.
6. Caputo GM, Cavanaugh PR, Ulbrecht JS, Gibbons GW, Karchmer AW. Assessment and management of foot disease in patients with diabetes. N Engl J Med 1994;33: 854–860.
7. Stadelmann WK, Digenis AG, Tobin GR. Physiology and healing dynamics of chronic cutaneous wounds. Am J Surg 1998; 176(Suppl 2A):26S–36S.
8. Rosenblum BI, Pomposelli FB, Giurini JM, et al. Maximizing foot salvage by a combined approach of foot ischemia and neuropathic ulceration in patients with diabetes mellitus: a five year experience. Diabetes Care 1994;17:983–987.
9. Tooke JE. Microcirculation and diabetes. Br Med Bull 1989;45:206–233.
10. Gibbons GW. The diabetic foot. In: Becker KL, Kahn RC, eds. Principles and Practice of Endocrinology and Metabolism, 2nd edit. Philadelphia: JB Lippincott, 1995, pp.1313–1316.
11. Wyss CR, Matsen FA, Simmons CW, Burgess EM. Transcutaneous oxygen tension measurements on limbs of diabetic and nondiabetic patients with peripheral vascular disease. Surgery 1984;95:339–346.
12. Gibbons GW, Habershaw GM, Marccacio EJ. Management of the diabetic foot. In: Callow AD, Ernst C, eds. Vascular Surgery: Theory and Practice. Norwich, CT: Appleton and Lange, 1995, pp.167–179.
13. Mayfield JA, Reiber GE, Sanders LJ, Farrise D, Pogach, LM. Technical review: preventive foot care in people with diabetes. Diabetes Care 1998;21:2161–2177.
14. Cavanaugh PR, Buse JB, Frykberg RG, et al. Consensus development conference on diabetic foot wound care. Diabetes Care 1999;22:1354–1360.
15. Faries PL, LoGerfo FW, Hook SC, et al. The impact of diabetes on arterial reconstructions for multi-level arterial occlusive disease. Am J Surg 2001;181:251–255.
16. Gibbons GW, Burgess AM RN, Guadagnoli E, et al. Return to wellbeing and function after infrainguinal revascularization. J Vasc Surg 1995;21:35–45.
17. Habershaw GM, Gibbons GW, Rosenblum BI. A historical look at the transmetatarsal amputation and its changing interactions. J Am Podiatr Med Assoc 1993;83:79–81.
18. American Diabetes Association: Position Statement. Preventive foot care in people with diabetes. Diabetes Care 1998;21:2178–2179.
19. Steed DL. Foundations of good ulcer care. Am J Surg 1998; 76(Suppl 2A):20S–25S.
20. Grayson ML, Gibbons GW, Balogh K, Levin E, Karchmer AW. Probing to bone in infected ulcers: a clinical sign of underlying osteomyelitis in diabetic patients. JAMA 1995;273:721–723.
21. Sarnow MR, Veves A, Giurini JM, Rosenblum BI, Chrzan JS, Habershaw GM. In-shoe foot pressure measurements in diabetic patients with at-risk feet and in healthy subjects. Diabetic Care 1994;17:1002–1006.
22. Habershaw GM. Outcomes of preventive care in a diabetic foot specialty clinic. J Foot Ankle Surg 1999;38:81.
23. Giurini JM, Chrzan Js, Gibbons GW, Habershaw GM. Charcot joint disease in diabetic patients: correct diagnosis can prevent progressive deformity. Postgrad Med 1991;89:163–169.

16 Arterial Vascular Disease in Women

Marie Gerhard-Herman, MD

CONTENTS

INTRODUCTION

Vascular disease is a significant, often unrecognized, source of morbidity in women. Furthermore, the presence or absence of peripheral arterial disease (PAD) provides important prognostic information concerning a patient's risk of heart attack and death. Instituting proven therapies for atherosclerosis, thrombosis, and vasculitis may significantly improve the life expectancy and quality of life of patients. This chapter discusses the vascular diseases that are commonly seen in women, and creates a framework for diagnosis and treatment.

Acquired arterial stenoses and occlusions may be chronic or acute. The most common cause of PAD is atherosclerosis. Other etiologies must be considered in women without risk factors for atherosclerosis, or in those with an unusual distribution of arterial occlusive disease (Table 1).

These entities affect the vessels from the aorta to distal extremity, and can be categorized by the size of vessels affected. The majority of the patients with large vessel arteritis, including Takayasu's arteritis, are women. In contrast, only 30% of the individuals with thromboangiitis obliterans are female. Arterial occlusion also occurs as a consequence of embolism or thrombosis *in situ*. Emboli originating in the heart may travel to the aorta and distal sites in the extremities. Thrombosis can develop acutely in diseased arteries or occur in normal arteries in patients with hypercoagulable states or trauma.

From: *Contemporary Cardiology: Peripheral Arterial Disease: Diagnosis and Treatment*
Edited by: J. D. Coffman and R. T. Eberhardt © Humana Press Inc., Totowa, NJ

Table 1
Etiologies of Occlusive Arterial Disease

Atherosclerotic vascular disease
Arterial emboli
Hypersensitivity arteritis (includes collagen vascular disease)
Polyarteritis nodosa arteritis
Giant cell arteritis[a]
Fibromuscular dysplasia[a]
Takayasu's arteritis[a]
Thromboangiitis obliterans (Buerger's disease)
Radiation-induced arterial damage
Arterial (mycotic) infections
Popliteal entrapment syndrome
Hyperviscosity syndrome
Homocysteinemia

---

[a]Denotes female predominance.

LOWER EXTREMITY ATHEROSCLEROSIS

Current data document an increasing number of women with PAD *(1)*. It is projected that by the year 2020 women > 65 yr old will constitute up to 15% of the population. The number of women with PAD will continue to increase as these demographic changes occur. The trend of the aging female population combined with that of increased cigarette smoking in women suggests that women will represent the majority of patients with peripheral atherosclerosis in the next century.

In general medical practice, PAD affects 23% of women 55 and older, and may be difficult to diagnose with traditional history and physical examination. Only one third of women with an abnormal ankle–brachial index (ABI) report symptoms of intermittent claudication (IC) *(2)*. The biennial incidence rate of IC was 3.5 per 1000 for women and 7.1 per 1000 for men in the Framingham Study over a 20-yr period as ascertained by questionnaire. The prevalence of IC ranges from 1.2% to 14.1% in women as compared to 2.2–14.4% in men *(3,4)*.

The prevalence of PAD can also be measured using objective measures such as ABI, rather than by questionnaires. The Edinburgh Artery Study found that 25% of the population 55–74 yr of age had PAD as determined by an ABI < 0.9 *(5)*. Men and women of this population were affected almost equally. In a recent observational study, 35% of all women over age 65 were found to have an ABI < 0.9 *(6)*.

More than 60% of women with objective evidence of PAD do not have symptoms of arterial insufficiency. Yet, the diagnosis of even asymptomatic PAD identifies an individual with a fivefold increase in the risk of cardiovascular death *(7)*. Atherosclerotic changes occur in all blood vessels, and it is the cardiac manifestations of this disease that are largely responsible for patient mortality. Symptoms of PAD can range from IC, described as discomfort in the muscles of the legs with activity that disappears with rest, to critical limb ischemia (CLI), rest pain, and gangrene. Recent literature suggests that asymptomatic cases are more prevalent in women than in men, and that women with CLI may be more likely to progress to limb loss *(8)*.

Risk Factors for PAD in Women

As with men, diabetes mellitus and cigarette smoking are the strongest risk factors for the development of atherosclerosis in women *(3)*. Glucose intolerance is associated with a fourfold increase in risk in women for the development of atherosclerotic disease compared with a 2.4-fold increase in risk in men. Even more disturbing is the observation that frank glycosuria increases the risk of IC eightfold in women and fourfold in men. These findings suggest that diabetes may have a greater impact on the symptomatic progression of peripheral atherosclerosis in women than in men. In addition, hyperlipidemia and hypertension are clear risk factors for PAD.

The impact of cigarette smoking on the incidence and progression of PAD in women cannot be overstated. As with diabetes, cigarette smoking increases the duration, progression, and extent of symptomatic arterial stenoses *(9)*. Women who quit smoking have an improved prognosis as measured by stroke-free survival, decreased incidence of myocardial infarction, and limb salvage when compared to the prognosis of those women who continue to smoke *(7)*. It is quite ominous that the fastest growing population of cigarette smokers is teen-age girls. Women who smoke become symptomatic from PAD an average of 10 yr earlier than nonsmoking women *(3)*, and appear to have more aortoiliac occlusive disease. The hypoplastic aortoiliac syndrome has been described as "an entity peculiar to women" and is perhaps the most dramatic example of early onset arterial occlusive disease *(10)*. This syndrome is characterized by disabling IC occurring in female smokers in their 30s and 40s, and marked narrowing of the distal aorta and iliac bifurcation on angiography.

The role of menopause, loss of ovarian function, in the development and progression of peripheral atherosclerosis is not entirely understood. In animal models of atherosclerosis, ovariectomy is associated with accelerated atherosclerosis whereas sham ovariectomy is not *(11)*. In women, early menopause has been associated with an increased incidence of aortoiliac disease, an association first noted over 30 yr ago. The incidence of claudication increases in women in their postmenopausal years, and is identical to that of men by the ninth decade. These findings suggest that there is decreased atherogenesis with intact ovarian function, perhaps via the hormones associated with intact ovarian function. In animal models of atherosclerosis, the increased atherosclerosis associated with ovariectomy is attenuated by replacing estrogen. In the first randomized controlled trial of hormone replacement in postmenopausal women, the Heart and Estrogen/Progestin Replacement Study, there was no difference in cardiovascular events at 5 yr between the active and placebo treatments, and a trend toward less peripheral arterial procedures in the women in the active treatment arm *(12,13)*. Females in the Rotterdam Study were questioned about hormone use and underwent objective evaluation for PAD at baseline *(14)*. Follow-up evaluation demonstrated 52% decreased risk of PAD among long-term users even after adjusting for age, smoking, lipid profile, health care maintenance, and socioeconomic status. These findings suggest that hormone replacement use of at least 1-yr duration after menopause protected women from developing PAD in later life. This disparity between the animal observations, human observations, and the first randomized clinical trial may be due in part to differences in replacement regimens used. Ongoing primary and secondary prevention trials of hormone replacement therapy in postmenopausal women, including those with soy and selective estrogen receptor modulators, may further clarify the role of estrogens in peripheral atherosclerosis.

Treatment of PAD (Table 2)

Risk Factor Treatment and Pharmacotherapy

Treatment of modifiable risk factors for atherosclerosis is an important goal in women as in men. Smoking cessation is associated with a significant decrease in the risk of cardiovascular events, but only a modest change in the symptoms of claudication and walking distance in women *(9)*. Smoking cessation does appear to halt the progression of PAD. Aggressive blood sugar control in the treatment of diabetes has also had similar results. In the United Kingdom Prospective Diabetes Study, men and women receiving intensive therapy had a trend for fewer myocardial infarctions than those on diet therapy *(15)*. Nonetheless, there was no change in limb loss or risk of PAD with intensive therapy. Clearly, the relationship of intensive blood glucose control to symptoms of PAD is poorly understood.

Patients with hypertension are treated to reduce systolic blood pressure to < 130 mmHg and diastolic blood pressure to < 85 mmHg in order to decrease cardiovascular risk *(16)*. It has been hypothesized that large decreases in systemic blood pressure may decrease limb pressure and shorten pain free walking distance but supervised exercise training may reduce blood pressure and improve pain free walking distance. However, few women have been included in these trials of supervised exercise.

Antiplatelet agents do not decrease claudication symptoms, but they have a profound beneficial effect on cardiovascular events in men with IC. The trials of secondary prevention of vascular disease by antiplatelet treatment were reviewed by the Antiplatelet Trialists' Collaboration *(17)*. Unfortunately, the impact of these agents on cardiovascular events and the secondary prevention of PAD in women is still unknown, as women were not included in most of these trials. One exception is the randomized trial of clopidogrel vs aspirin in patients at risk of ischemic events (CAPRIE) *(18)*. Greater than 30% of the population in this trial were women. In this study the long-term administration of clopidogrel to patients with atherosclerotic vascular disease was slightly more effective than aspirin in reducing the combined cardiovascular endpoint. This suggests that both antiplatelet agents will decrease cardiovascular mortality in women with PAD.

Pharmacological therapy for symptomatic relief of PAD is discussed thoroughly in Chapter 10. Cilostazol therapy results in improvement in both pain-free and absolute walking distance, and ABI *(20)*. Importantly, the randomized trials of this medication have included women (up to 30%). The inclusion of women in significant numbers allows clinicians to make recommendations for women without extrapolating from exclusively male trials. Propionyl-l-carnitine improves muscle metabolism and has been observed to improve pain-free walking distance in men *(21)*. It is approved for this indication in Europe and under investigation in the United States. Prostaglandins are also being evaluated in patients with critical limb ischemia and in those with claudication. The intravenous preparations hold promise, but treatment is complicated by flushing, myalgias, headache, and gastrointestinal cramping.

Revascularization for PAD

Women afflicted with PAD account for one third of all distal revascularization procedures and amputations. Women and men undergoing these procedures have similar risk factors, but the women are consistently 3–5 yr older than their male counterparts *(22)*. In a meta-analysis of population-based studies on limb ischemia, men were more likely to

Table 2
Treatment of Peripheral Atherosclerosis

Evaluate and treat systemic atherosclerosis:
  Smoking cessation
  Lipid lowering (19)
  Blood pressure (16)
  Diabetes

Antithrombotic/antiplatelet therapies are mandatory:
  Aspirin or clopidogrel

Supervised exercise program

Pharmacologic therapy
  Cilostazol

Revascularization

develop disease progression than women *(7)*. Despite the wealth of literature on the outcome of lower extremity revascularization and risk factor analysis for graft failure, few have clearly addressed the issue of gender. Two studies have identified female gender as an independent predictor of graft failure *(23,24)*. Arterial size appears to have a significant impact on the success of these reconstructions. In a randomized multicenter controlled trial comparing prosthetic above knee femoropopliteal bypass grafting, the choice of smaller graft diameter was associated with a dramatic decrease in 5-yr patency.

TAKAYASU'S ARTERITIS

Takayasu's arteritis is a chronic inflammatory disease affecting the aorta and its proximal branches (*see* Chapter 19) *(25)*. This arteritis occurs predominantly in women < 40 yr of age; 85% of all cases occur in women. It is a periarteritis that begins with inflammation throughout the vessel wall and occasional giant cells at sites where the elastic lamina is destroyed. Fibrosis of the vessel occurs in the chronic phase. This results in the typical angiographic appearance of stenoses as long, smooth, narrowed segments. The pattern of arteries that are affected varies according to the patient's geographic location. In North American and Japanese patients, the aortic arch and its branches are often involved, while in Indian and Mexican patients, the abdominal aorta and its branches are more often involved.

Clinical Presentation and Diagnosis

The disease often begins with fevers, malaise, myalgias, and occasionally pain over the affected vessels (e.g., carotodynia). Over time symptoms of arterial occlusive disease with arterial insufficiency develop. These include IC, cerebrovascular ischemia, and visceral pain. Aortic aneurysm or aortic dissection can also occur. Takayasu's arteritis should be suspected in individuals with unequal pulses or blood pressures in their extremities, and in young women with carotid and subclavian bruits.

Diagnostic Tests

There is no laboratory test to diagnose Takayasu's arteritis. The American College of Rheumatology has reporting criteria for studies of Takayasu's arteritis (Table 3). Having

Table 3
Clinical Evidence of Takayasu's Arteritis

Female < 40 yr old
Diminished brachial pulse
10 mmHg difference in brachial blood pressure
Subclavian artery bruit
Extremity claudication
Narrowing of the aorta or proximal branches on angiography

three of the six criteria indicates high specificity and sensitivity for the diagnosis. In addition, angiography using computed tomography and magnetic resonance can demonstrate artery wall inflammation. The erythrocyte sedimentation rate is a marker for disease activity. It is used in combination with systemic complaints or new symptoms of arterial insufficiency.

Management

Medical treatment with corticosteroids is effective in 60% of the patients. Methotrexate and cyclophosphamide can be added if prednisone is ineffective or poorly tolerated. These drugs may decrease clinical and angiographic evidence of Takayasu's arteritis. Percutaneous transluminal angioplasty with stenting has been used successfully in few patients with short, concentric stenoses *(26)*. Surgical arterial bypass is often employed for patients with symptomatic ischemia. When surgery is performed during periods of active disease, however, there are dramatically higher complication and restenosis rates *(27,28)*.

GIANT CELL ARTERITIS

Giant cell arteritis, or temporal arteritis, occurs typically in individuals older than 50 yr (*see* Chapter 19). The mean age at onset is 70 yr, with the highest prevalence in Caucasian females of Northern European ancestry. It is found in the arteries throughout the body *(29)*. This arteritis begins with lymphocyte infiltration throughout the arterial wall and intimal thickening. The classic pathologic findings are granuloma with multinucleated giant cells and focal necrosis in the region of the disrupted elastic lamina. The pattern is described as one of "skip" lesions. Therefore many arterial sections must be examined before excluding this diagnosis. Temporal, carotid, vertebral, subclavian, brachial, and coronary arteries and the aorta are often involved.

Clinical Presentation and Diagnosis

Symptoms of giant cell arteritis include visual changes, headache, scalp tenderness, fever, weight loss, and malaise. Claudication of the jaw, tongue, arms, and legs may occur. The presentation can be dramatic, as with aortic dissection. Half of these patients will have clinical findings of polymyalgia rheumatica *(30)*. Elevated erythrocyte sedimentation rate is common, but not required to make the diagnosis. The diagnosis is based on clinical presentation (Table 4), with confirmation by pathologic or angiographic examination.

Table 4
Giant Cell Arteritis

Elderly white female
3:1 Female/male ratio
Propensity for carotid artery and branches but may involve any artery.
Symptoms include visual disturbances and blindness.
Diagnosis requires artery biopsy.

Management

Steroids are the main treatment, and their use has dramatically decreased the incidence of blindness with temporal arteritis. Treatment begins with prednisone 40–60 mg/d. The prednisone dose can typically be tapered in 2–4 wk. Remission can occur, and may not happen until after 1–2 yr of therapy. Surgical intervention is indicated for limb salvage and may be needed to decrease mortality from aortic aneurysm or dissection. Death is rare and results from stroke, myocardial infarction, ruptured aortic aneurysms, and aortic dissection.

FIBROMUSCULAR DYSPLASIA

Fibromuscular dyplasia occurs predominantly in women in the third and fourth decades. The female-to-male ratio is 9:1. It results from fibroplasia of the medial layer in most cases. The angiographic appearance has been described as a "string of beads." The "beads" are larger than the normal caliber of the vessel. Four distinct pathologic types have been identified: intimal fibroplasia, medial fibroplasia, medial hyperplasia, and perimedial fibroplasia.

Fibromuscular dyplasia affects predominantly the distal renal and carotid arteries *(31,32)*. The clinical presentations include renovascular hypertension and transient ischemic attacks. The diagnosis is made by angiography and exclusion of collagen vascular disease. Revascularization is the only treatment option for symptomatic disease (*see* Chapter 3).

THROMBOANGIITIS OBLITERANS

Thromboangiitis obliterans, also known as Buerger's disease, results in intimal inflammation and thrombosis in the small and medium arteries in the extremities (*see* Chapter 18). Migratory superficial thrombophlebitis also occurs. The disease historically affected young male cigarette smokers, but is now reported with increasing frequency in young female cigarette smokers *(33)*.

Clinical Presentation

Patients present with a variety of symptoms including Raynaud's phenomenon, foot claudication, and digital gangrene. Severe ischemia may result in peripheral neuropathy. There are segmental occlusions of small and medium arteries on angiography. These are usually at the distal part of the upper and lower extremities, and accompanied by corkscrew collaterals.

Management

There is no effective treatment without abstinence from tobacco. New lesions develop less often if the patient stops smoking. Digital ulcers may require debridement. Pharmacologic therapy is designed to decrease the vasospasm that accompanies the arterial narrowings. It includes calcium channel blockers, α-adrenergic blockers, and vasodilator prostaglandin infusion to decrease vasospasm. The use of aspirin has also been advocated in these patients.

RAYNAUD'S PHENOMENON

Raynaud's phenomenon refers to episodes of vasospasm resulting in digital ischemia. Episodes of well-demarcated digital cyanosis or pallor follow cold exposure and emotional distress. The diagnosis is based on the patient's history *(34)*. Simple office maneuvers such as cold water immersion do not reliably induce episodes of digital ischemia. Primary Raynaud's phenomenon (no underlying etiology apparent) occurs in up to 20% of all women. The prevalence is highest in those populations living in colder climates. Unique features of digital arterial innervation contribute to the occurrence of Raynaud's phenomenon. The cutaneous vessels of the fingers and toes have only sympathetic adrenergic vasoconstrictor fibers. The increased sympathetic efferent activity that normally causes vasoconstriction can cause profound vasospasm in individuals with Raynaud's phenomenon. Decreased perfusion, digital arterial narrowing, and increased blood viscosity also alter digital blood flow and can contribute to Raynaud's phenomenon.

Classification

Raynaud's phenomenon is classified as primary, that is, not associated with another disease, or secondary, that is, occurring as a consequence of another disease or treatment *(34)*. Criteria of primary Raynaud's phenomenon (Table 5) include history of bilateral episodes of digital pallor or cyanosis; symptoms for longer than 2 yr, strong, symmetric pulses on physical examination, and no digital pitting, ulcerations, or gangrene. The tests for antinuclear antibody, the erythrocyte sedimentation rate, and nail fold capillaroscopy are normal in primary Raynaud's phenomenon. Primary Raynaud's phenomenon is associated with a favorable prognosis. A secondary cause of Raynaud's phenomenon is suggested by the presence of prolonged digital ischemia with findings such as digital ulcers (Table 6).

There are other causes of secondary Raynaud's phenomenon including thermal or vibration injury, arterial occlusive disease, neurologic disorders, and toxins. Most secondary causes of Raynaud's phenomenon are obvious before the episodes of digital ischemia begin. One exception to this rule is scleroderma. In patients with scleroderma the Raynaud's phenomenon can precede evidence of scleroderma by years.

In secondary Raynaud's phenomenon, the arterial supply to the digits can be evaluated to determine the degree of fixed arterial occlusion. Such testing includes digital systolic pressure measurements, digital plethysmography, or Doppler flow studies of the digits. When abnormal arterial flow is seen, the test can be repeated following warming of the patient. If the arterial flow appears normal after warming, vasospasm rather than

Table 5
Primary Raynaud's Phenomenon

Bilateral episodes of digital cyanosis or pallor
Absence of digital ulceration, pitting, or gangrene
Symmetric and strong peripheral pulses
Symptoms for > 2 yr
No evidence of disease or drugs associated with secondary Raynaud's
Normal ESR (erythrocyte sedimentation rate)
Normal ANA (antinuclear antibody test)
Normal nail fold capillaroscopy

Table 6
Some Secondary Causes of Raynaud's Phenomenon

Collagen diseases
   Scleroderma
   Systemic lupus erythematosus
   Dermatomyositis
   Polyarteritis

Drugs
   β-Receptor blocking drugs
   Bromocriptine
   Ergot derivative
   Dopamine
   Vinyl chloride
   Bleomycin and vincristine
Frostbite, immersion foot
Carpal tunnel syndrome
Thoracic outlet syndrome
Blood dyscrasias (cryoglobulinemia and cold agglutinins)
Occupational trauma
Thromboangiitis obliterans

fixed arterial occlusion is present. Arteriography is indicated only if an obstructive lesion requiring revascularization is suspected.

Management

The mainstay of treatment is teaching the patient to avoid stimuli that precipitate digital ischemic attacks. This includes instructions to dress warmly, and means wearing not only gloves, but also sweaters, coats, and hats. Reflex sympathetic vasoconstriction occurs in the digits in response to cold exposure in other parts of the body (e.g., head). Calcium channel blockers (except verapamil) and α-adrenergic blockers are used to decrease symptoms. Intravenous iloprost improves digital ulcer healing in patients with scleroderma but is not approved for this use in the United States. Selective digital sympathectomy and microarteriolysis may also result in ulcer healing and symptom improvement in severe cases. Cervical and lumbar sympathectomy have been performed, but with very limited long-term success.

ACROCYANOSIS

Acrocyanosis is an unusual disorder in the general population, but is seen in 20% of the women with anorexia nervosa *(35)*. Acrocyanosis presents as episodes of coldness and cyanosis in the hands and feet. Unlike Raynaud's phenomenon, the cyanosis extends beyond the digits to the palms and occasionally above the wrist.

The clinical presentation is attributed to arteriolar spasm. The cyanosis increases with cold exposure and is relieved by warming. There may be mild edema and excess sweating of the hands and feet on physical examination. There are no trophic changes or ulceration of the digits. If the patient is examined during an episode, pallor is seen when the extremity is raised above the heart level, indicating that the findings are not attributable to venous obstruction. Patients with acrocyanosis have no physical evidence of central cyanosis, and routine laboratory evaluation is normal. The disorder is self-limited, and does not indicate worsened prognosis from the underlying starvation. The acrocyanosis generally resolves as weight gain occurs in patients with anorexia nervosa.

SUMMARY

PAD continues to be a challenging diagnostic dilemma in women. There are an increasing number of women with atherosclerotic vascular disease, and it is often asymptomatic. Although asymptomatic, it is a powerful predictor of myocardial infarction, stroke, and mortality. Risk factors in women are similar to men but diabetes may have a greater impact on the disease in women. The role of estrogens in atherosclerotic vascular disease in women needs to be clarified owing to contrasting study results. Treatment has not been as well studied in women as in men but antiplatelet agents and cilostazol are beneficial for prevention of ischemic events and IC, respectively. With revascularization procedures, female gender is an independent predictor of graft failure.

Although the predominant cause of PAD in women is atherosclerosis, other etiologies must be considered. Scleroderma, giant cell arteritis, fibromuscular dysplasia, and Takayasu's arteritis occur more frequently in women than in men. Careful history and physical examination, combined with selective testing, can elucidate the cause of arterial insufficiency.

REFERENCES

1. Vogt MT, Wolfson SK, Kuller LH. Lower extremity arterial disease and the aging process: a review. J Clin Epidemiol 1992;45:529–542.
2. Stoffers HE, Rinkens PE, Kester AD, Kaiser V, Knottnerus JA. The prevalence of asymptomatic and unrecognized peripheral arterial occlusive disease. Int J Epidemiol 1996;25:282–290.
3. Kannel WB, McGee DL. Update on some epidemiologic features of intermittent claudication: the Framingham Study. J Am Geriatr Soc 1985;33:13–18.
4. Agner E. Natural history of angina pectoris, possible previous myocardial infarction and intermittent claudication during the eighth decade: a longitudinal epidemiologic study. Acta Med Scand 1981;210: 271–276.
5. Fowkes FG, Housley E, Cawood EH, Macintyre CC, Ruckley CV, Prescott RJ. Edinburgh Artery Study: prevalence of asymptomatic and symptomatic peripheral arterial disease in the general population. Int J Epidemiol 1991;20:384–392.
6. McDermott MM, Fried L, Simonsick E, Ling S, Guralnik JM. Asymptomatic peripheral arterial disease is independently associated with impaired lower extremity functioning: the women's health and aging study. Circulation 2000;101:1007–1012.

7. Hooi JD, Stoffers HE, Knottnerus JA, van Ree JW. The prognosis of non-critical limb ischaemia: a systematic review of population-based evidence. Br J Gen Pract 1999;49:49–55.

8. Tunis SR, Bass EB, Klag MJ, Steinberg EP. Variation in utilization of procedures for treatment of peripheral arterial disease: a look at patient characteristics. Arch Intern Med 1993;153: 991–998.

9. Jonason T, Ringqvist I. Changes in peripheral blood pressures after five years of follow-up in non-operated patients with intermittent claudication. Acta Med Scand 1986;220:127–132.

10. Jernigan WR, Fallat ME, Hatfield DR. Hypoplastic aortoiliac syndrome: an entity peculiar to women. Surgery 1983;94:752–757.

11. Guetta V, Cannon RO 111. Cardiovascular effects of estrogen and lipid lowering therapies in post-menopausal women. Circulation 1996;93:1928–1937.

12. Hulley S, Grady D, Bush T, et al. Randomized trial of estrogen plus progestin for secondary prevention of coronary heart disease in postmenopausal women. Heart and Estrogen/progestin Replacement Study (HERS) Research Group. JAMA 1998;280:605–613.

13. Hsia J, Simon JA, Lin F, et al. Peripheral arterial disease in randomized trial of estrogen with progestin in women with coronary heart disease: the Heart and Estrogen/Progestin Replacement Study. Circulation 2000;102:2228–2232.

14. Westendorp IC, in't Veld BA, Grobbee DE, et al. Hormone replacement therapy and peripheral arterial disease: the Rotterdam study. Arch Intern Med 2000;160:2498–2502.

15. Nathan DM. Some answers, more controversy, from UKPDS. United Kingdom Prospective Diabetes Study. Lancet 1998;352:832–833.

16. The sixth report of the Joint National Committee on prevention, detection, evaluation, and treatment of high blood pressure. Arch Intern Med 1997;157:2413–2446.

17. Secondary prevention of vascular disease by prolonged antiplatelet treatment. Antiplatelet Trialists' Collaboration. Br Med J (Clin Res Ed) 1988;296:320–331.

18. A randomised, blinded, trial of clopidogrel versus aspirin in patients at risk of ischaemic events (CAPRIE). CAPRIE Steering Committee. Lancet 1996;348:1329–1339.

19. Gould AL, Rossouw JE, Santanello NC, Heyse JF, Furberg CD. Cholesterol reduction yields clinical benefit: impact of statin trials. Circulation 1998;97:946–952.

20. Dawson DL, Cutler BS, Meissner MH, Strandness DE, Jr. Cilostazol has beneficial effects in treatment of intermittent claudication: results from a multicenter, randomized, prospective, double-blind trial. Circulation 1998;98:678–686.

21. Brevetti G, Perna S, Sabba C, Martone VD, Condorelli M. Propionyl-l-carnitine in intermittent claudication: double-blind, placebo-controlled, dose titration, multicenter study. J Am Coll Cardiol 1995; 26:1411–1416.

22. Norman PE, Semmens JB, Lawrence-Brown M, Holman CD. The influence of gender on outcome following peripheral vascular surgery: a review. Cardiovasc Surg 2000;8:111–115.

23. Enzler MA, Ruoss M, Seifert B, Berger M. The influence of gender on the outcome of arterial procedures in the lower extremity. Eur J Vasc Endovasc Surg 1996;11:446–452.

24. Magnant JG, Cronenwett JL, Walsh DB, Schneider JR, Besso SR, Zwolak RM. Surgical treatment of infrainguinal arterial occlusive disease in women. J Vasc Surg 1993;17:67–76.

25. Kerr GS, Hallahan CW, Giordano J, et al. Takayasu arteritis. Ann Intern Med 1994;120:919–929.

26. Bali HK, Jani S, Jain A, Sharma BK. Stent supported angioplasty in Takayasu arteritis. Int J Cardiol 1998;66:S213–217.

27. Robbs JV, Abdool-Carrim AT, Kadwa AM. Arterial reconstruction for nonspecific arteritis (Takayasu's Disease): medium to long term results. Eur J Vasc Surg 1994;8:401–407.

28. Kerr G. Takayasu's arteritis. Rheum Dis Clin North Am 1995;21:1041–1058.

29. Mohan N, Kerr G. Spectrum of giant cell vasculitis. Curr Rheumatol Rep 2000;2:390–395.

30. Epperly TD, Moore KE, Harrover JD. Polymyalgia rheumatica and temporal arthritis. Am Fam Physician 2000;62:789–796.

31. Begelman SM, Olin JW. Fibromuscular dysplasia. Curr Opin Rheumatol 2000;12:41–47.

32. Begelman SM, Olin JW. Nonatherosclerotic arterial disease of the extracranial cerebrovasculature. Semin Vasc Surg 2000;13:153–164.

33. Olin JW, Young JR, Graor RA, Ruschhaupt WF, Bartholomew JR. The changing clinical spectrum of thromboangiitis obliterans (Buerger's disease). Circulation 1990;82(Suppl 5):IV3–8.

34. Wigley FM. Raynaud's phenomenon. Curr Opin Rheumatol 1993;5: 773–784.

35. Bhanji S, Mattingly D. Acrocyanosis in anorexia nervosa. Postgrad Med J 1991;67:33–35.

17

Atheromatous Embolism

Jay D. Coffman, MD

CONTENTS

INTRODUCTION

Atheromatous embolization is due to the travel of atheromatous debris from large arteries to wedge into the microcirculation of body parts or organs. It may present as a blue toe syndrome or as malignant embolization to body organs such as the kidneys and brain. The most common cause is manipulation of a severely athermatous aorta or artery by catheterization or surgery. Treatment modalities of atheroemblism are inadequate, and many patients continue to suffer excess morbidity and even mortality.

ETIOLOGY

The origin of atheromatous emboli is usually large blood vessels that are extensively involved with atherosclerosis. The aorta often has a shaggy and irregularly ulcerated inner lining although only plaques may be seen, especially in the proximal aorta *(1)*. Erosions of the vessel intima allow soft atheromas to perforate into the vessel lumen. Cholesterol crystals and amorphous atherosclerotic material then embolize to distal sites. An aortic aneurysm may also be the source of the emboli. Depending on the involved blood vessel, emboli may travel to the brain, upper and lower extremities, but-

From: *Contemporary Cardiology: Peripheral Arterial Disease: Diagnosis and Treatment*
Edited by: J. D. Coffman and R. T. Eberhardt © Humana Press Inc., Totowa, NJ

tocks, any organ in the abdomen, spinal cord, and the prostate. Emboli to the pancreas, gastrointestinal tract, adrenals, thyroid, bone marrow, and testes may occur.

A clinical picture consistent with emboli composed of fibrin and platelets has been described *(2,3)*. These patients had few embolic episodes and unilateral extremity involvement. They did not have severe atherosclerosis of the aorta. Peculiarly, livedo reticularis was not seen. The fibrinoplatelet emboli were thought to originate from a high-grade focal stenosis of an artery supplying the lower extremity, as demonstrated by arteriography. It is difficult to prove these are cases of fibrinoplatelet emboli, as they cannot be seen in pathological specimens, as the emboli disappear with the fixation process. However, these patients were treated successfully with antiplatelet agents or anticoagulation and with transluminal angioplasty, which is different from the unsuccessful treatment of cholesterol emboli. Two of these patients had embolic complications following the administration of thrombolytic therapy *(3)*.

EPIDEMIOLOGY

There is male predominance of atheromatous embolism in the cases reported in the literature and most patients are > 50 yr of age. In the Dutch population, the average frequency of the disease is 6.2 cases per million population per year *(4)*. In one autopsy study of 100 men in this age group, 4% revealed atheromatous emboli *(5)*. Another postmortem study of more than 2000 patients found a prevalence of only 0.79%, but the diagnosis was apparently dependent on the number, size, and site of tissue blocks examined *(6)*. The most recent autopsy study reported a prevalence of 0.31% (4). In this study, the most frequently involved sites were the kidney, skin, and gastrointestinal tract, in that order.

INSTIGATING CAUSES

An underlying cause of spontaneous embolization often cannot be established. It has been hypothesized that increasing intrathoracic pressure by coughing and straining cause the atherosclerotic debris to break loose *(7)*. In the last three decades, catheterization of atherosclerotic blood vessels has become the most common cause *(8)*; one study reported an incidence of 12% in 60 patients *(9)*. Evidently the catheter disrupts the diseased intima of the blood vessels. If patients' extremities are carefully examined following cardiac catheterization, many will show evidence of showers of emboli (petechiae) which are usually asymptomatic. Although symptomatic emboli may occur 3–6 wk following catheterization in some cases *(10)*, symptoms and signs typically appear within the first few days after the procedure. Surprisingly atherosclerotic emboli are not more common using a femoral artery approach as opposed to a brachial artery approach for catheters. In the large CASS study, microembolization occurred in 0.17% with the catheterization approach via the brachial artery approach compared to 0.08% via the femoral artery *(11)*. Manipulation of the thoracic aorta during cardiac surgery is another common cause of atheromatous emboli, particularly if that segment of the aorta is involved with extensive atherosclerotic disease. Cardiac surgeons attempt to avoid manipulation of these aortas. Atheroembolism of the kidneys has been reported following aortic angiography or renal artery angioplasty *(12)*. It may occur in 1.4–3% patients following angioplasty or aortorenal bypass surgery. Thrombolytic therapy has been blamed for emboli but many of these patients had undergone catheterization previously *(13,14)*. In 60 patients with cholesterol embolism following an acute myocardial infarction (MI), 29 had received tissue plasminogen activator; cholesterol embolization proven by muscle and skin biopsies was not more frequent than in the 31 patients treated conservatively for an acute MI *(9)*.

Patients have also developed atheroembolism within several weeks of starting coumarin derivatives, and cessation of embolization has occurred when the drug was stopped. The original description was of six patients with purple toes; because skin biopsies were negative, coumarin was blamed *(15)*. Muscle biopsies were not performed. The role of coumarin in causing atheromatous embolism remains speculative for this reason. Once lesions from microemboli are present, anticoagulation could cause hemorrhage into the affected sites and delay healing.

PATHOLOGY

Histological examination of involved tissue reveals needle-shaped cholesterol clefts in small arteries or arterioles (200–900 μm). The cholesterol crystals are dissolved by the fixative process. Inflammatory infiltrates, intimal thickening, and perivascular fibrosis may be present *(9,16)*. Lymphocytes, neutrophils, and even eosinophils may be seen with the red blood cells in the vessel lumen. Giant cells may also invade the vessel wall, confusing the diagnosis with polyarteritis nodosa if cholesterol clefts cannot be seen. Lipid-laden or vacuolated macrophages are not uncommon.

CLINICAL PRESENTATION AND PHYSICAL EXAMINATION (TABLE 1)

Unilateral or bilateral painful, discolored toes are the most common presentation. A rash may occur on the legs and feet. Calf pain with tender muscles is not unusual. Skin involvement of the buttocks may also occur.

Patients may present with transient ischemic attacks, strokes, peripheral palsies, coronary insufficiency or acute MI, renal failure, hemorrhagic pancreatitis, splenic infarction, hemorrhagic cystitis, necrotizing cholecystitis, prostatitis, ischemia or ulceration of the gastrointestinal tract, and ischemic lesions or ulceration of the upper extremities. Patients have been described with disseminated intravascular coagulation *(17)*, restless leg syndrome *(18)*, or acute polymyositis *(19)*. When many organs are involved, it has been called a "malignant embolic syndrome" because most patients die within 1 yr *(7)*.

Physical examination reveals bluish-red, sometimes hemorrhagic, mottled discoloration of the toes. One or more digits may be involved. The soles and lateral aspects of the feet are often affected. The lesions are very painful and tender and may evolve into infarcted areas. Extensive infarcts of the skin of the buttocks and thighs may occur. Pedal pulses are usually present. The cyanotic areas blanch with pressure and are surrounded by normally perfused skin. Petechiae and livedo reticularis may be seen on the legs and feet (Fig. 1). Elevated plaques occur occasionally in the skin. One study reported that 35% of patients had cutaneous manifestations *(20)*. Livedo reticularis occurred in 49%, gangrene in 35%, cyanosis in 28%, ulceration in 17%, nodules in 10%, and purpura in 7% of those with cutaneous signs. Livedo reticularis is a mottled discoloration of the extremities or trunk of the body in a reticular, fishnet or lacelike pattern. The webs of the fishnet are reddish-violet or blue with the skin color appearing

Table 1
Clinical Manifestations of Atheromatous Emboli

Mottled reddish-blue, painful toes
Petechiae
Livedo reticularis
Usually normal pulses
Elevated skin plaques
Tender calf muscle

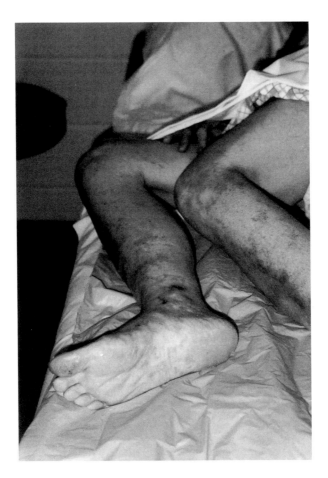

Fig. 1. Atheromatous emboli to the limbs in a patient with extensive atheromatous disease of the aorta. Livedo reticularis is present on the leg. Areas of skin necrosis and ulceration have occurred at the medial ankle.

normal or pale between the webs. The calf muscles may be tender. With renal involvement, transient hypertension may occur, which may be difficult to control. It is probably due to renal ischemia causing the release of renin. In a few patients, cholesterol emboli may be seen in the retinal arterioles (Hollenhorst plaques); these may originate in the aorta or internal carotid arteries.

DIFFERENTIAL DIAGNOSIS

The differential diagnosis includes several other diseases that can cause ischemic toes or renal failure (Table 2). History and physical examination help to exclude connective tissue diseases with Raynaud's phenomenon, polyarteritis nodosa, or vasculitis. In some patients skin or muscle biopsies with the demonstration of cholesterol clefts are necessary to exclude these diseases. Polycythemia or thrombocytosis may present with one or more blue toes and can be ruled out by complete blood and platelet counts. A normal partial thromboplastin time rules against a circulating anticoagulant causing microcirculatory thrombi. Arterial thromboses due to tumors usually occur in patients with advanced manifestations of the oncological disease *(21)*. To determine cardiac sources of emboli, history and physical examination may not be sufficient; echocardiograms, cardiac monitoring, or blood cultures may be needed. Renal failure from atheroembolism must be distinguished from contrast-induced nephropathy from the procedures performed on the patients. Nephropathy from radiographic dye usually occurs immediately following the catheterization with a few days of oliguria. The serum creatinine level peaks within 2 wk. In microembolization, the creatinine level may not rise for 2 wk to 3 mo and the renal dysfunction is often progressive. An oliguria phase is not common.

LABORATORY STUDIES

The sedimentation rate is often elevated but is a nonspecific test. The white blood cell count is usually normal or increased especially if the toe lesions are infected. Eosinophilia of 6–18% may be present *(8)*. It is an important finding occurring in up to 80% of patients with renal involvement *(22)*. Eosinophiluria also may occur *(23)* and hypocomplementemia and thrombocytopenia have been reported *(24)*. A slowly rising serum creatinine also implicates renal atheroembolism. Many other laboratory tests may suggest involvement of other organs when symptoms are present such as liver function tests and serum amylase.

DIAGNOSIS

The clinical picture shown in Table 1 is classical but a definitive diagnosis is made by skin, muscle, or kidney biopsy. Skin biopsies are better tolerated by patients and often reveal the diagnosis *(10)*. However, deep skin biopsies should be performed *(8)*. Areas on the toes should be avoided because nonhealing ulcers may be induced. If skin biopsies do not demonstrate the characteristic findings, biopsy of the gastrocnemius or quadriceps muscles is necessary *(5,16)*. Muscle biopsy has been reported to have a 95–100% sensitivity, whereas skin biopsy has only a 41% sensitivity for the diagnosis *(5,16)*. The skin or muscle biopsies show elongated needle-shaped clefts in small arterial vessels, often accompanied by inflammatory infiltrates, intima thickening, and perivascular fibrosis *(9,16)*. The presence of giant cells may confuse the diagnosis with polyarteritis nodosa.

With the characteristic clinical picture and other causes of the lesions ruled out, diffuse atherosclerosis of the proximal vessels demonstrated by angiography and cholesterol clefts on skin or muscle biopsy, the diagnosis is usually determined. Transesophageal echocardiography (TEE) may be necessary to detect thoracic aortic plaques or debris when this could be the embolic source. In 20 patients with severe cholesterol emboli, Ferrari and colleagues found aortic plaques or debris, seen by TEE, were

Table 2
Differential Diagnosis of the Blue (Purple) Toe Syndrome

Atheromatous emboli
Vasculitis or polyarteritis
Connective tissue diseases with Raynaud's phenomenon
Endocarditis, intracardiac thrombi, arrhythmias
Polycythemia
Thrombocytosis
Circulating anticoagulants
Malignancy with or without cryoglobulins or macroglobulins

significantly more common in the patients than in a control group *(25)*. They were found predominantly in the descending aorta.

PROGNOSIS

In most patients with atheromatous emboli to the lower limbs, the showers of emboli spontaneously cease within a 3-mo period *(26)*. The toe lesions are very slow to heal over a period of 6 wk to 6 mo. Loss of tissue or toes may occur if infections cannot be controlled. Amputation of limbs has been necessary in rare patients. If there is kidney involvement, renal failure is a distinct possibility and patients have required dialysis either for a limited time or permanently. Patients with the malignant syndrome have involvement of multiple organs and usually do not live more than a year, succumbing to the brain or renal lesions. A 60% mortality has been reported in patients whose emboli originate from blood vessels above the diaphragm compared to 11% with emboli from vessels below the diaphragm *(27)*.

TREATMENT

Surgical Treatment

Removal or exclusion of the source of emboli by surgery would seem most logical. In patients with aortic atherosclerosis, aortoiliac or axillofemoral bypass of the abdominal aorta is performed. However, there are reports that surgery does not always prevent recurrences; extraanatomic bypasses with ligation of the external iliac arteries has been recommended *(1)*. More distal bypasses or endarterectomy may stop the embolic showers if the source is femoral or popliteal disease. With renal involvement, proximal abdominal aortic bypasses with renal artery arms are used. The high mortality in patients with emboli from diffuse involvement of the entire aorta (the malignant syndrome) requires replacement of the whole aorta when the patient is a suitable candidate.

Medical Treatment

Therapeutic successes have been reported with antiplatelet agents, aspirin, and dipyridamole, but control studies have not been performed *(2,3,28,29)*. Heparin may also be beneficial *(30)*, although one study of two patients claimed that emboli occurred during low-molecular-weight heparin treatment *(31)*. It has been postulated that heparin or warfarin would prevent a thrombin or fibrin coating of ulcerated atherosclerotic plaques, and therefore cholesterol embolization would occur or recur *(1)*. Corticorteroids have also been advocated for the treatment of cholesterol emboli on the basis that the pathological picture around the cholesterol crystals resembles vasculitis *(25,32,33)*. Renal involvement has also been reported to improve *(34–36)*. Cholesterol lowering agents (HMG-CoA inhibitors), simvastatin *(37–39)*, and lovastatin *(40)*, but also low-density lipoprotein apheresis *(41)* have been reported as efficacious for the treatment of cholesterol embolism. Control studies are lacking and small numbers of patients have been treated. Pentoxifylline was evidently effective in one patient *(42)*.

Warfarin has been avoided because its use appeared to be associated with the onset of the disease. However, anticoagulants would benefit patients with fibrinoplatelet emboli *(3)* and have been reported to stop emboli in patients with thoracic aortic plaques *(43,44)*. Embolization from thoracic aortic plaques or debris seems to behave like a separate entity from more distal sources of cholesterol emboli because large and small emboli may occur and it responds to pharmacological intervention. These patients usually have complex thoracic aortic plaques > 4 mm thick and may also show mobile components. Thoracic atheroma have been reported to be successfully treated with warfarin *(44)* but not antiplatelet agents *(43)*, although there are no controlled studies.

SUMMARY

Atheromatous emboli usually originate from atherosclerotic large blood vessels or aortic aneurysms. Cholesterol crystals and amorphous atherosclerotic materials may embolize to any distal organ. Affected patients are usually males > 50 yr of age. Most frequently the kidney, skin, and gastrointestinal tract are involved. The most common cause is the catheterization of atherosclerotic blood vessels but idiopathic cases occur. Patients often present with painful, discolored toes or feet, tender calf muscles, petechiae, and livedo reticularis. However, any organ in the body except perhaps the lungs can be affected. Renal failure is common. Laboratory studies are nonspecific. However, eosinophilia should strongly suggest renal involvement. A definitive diagnosis is made by finding elongated needle-shaped clefts in small arterial vessels of a skin or muscle biopsy. The prognosis depends on the organs involved; renal failure is a threat in patients who continue to embolize, and patients with multiple organ involvement usually do not live more than a year. Treatment of atheromatous emboli has not been consistently successful with any pharmacological agent but surgical removal or exclusion of the source of emboli offers the best possibility for stopping the embolization.

REFERENCES

1. Hollier LH, Kazmier FJ, Ochsner J, Bowen JC, Procter CD. "Shaggy" aorta syndrome with atheromatous embolization to visceral vessels. Ann Vasc Surg 1991,5:439–444.
2. Kumpe DA Zwerdlinger S, Griffin DJ. Blue toe syndrome: treatment with percutaneous transluminal angioplasty. Radiology 1988;166:37–44.
3. Brewer ML, Kinnison ML, Perler BA, White RI Jr. Blue toe syndrome: treatment with anticoagulants and delayed percutaneous transluminal angioplasty. Radiology 1988;166:31–36.
4. Moolenaar W, Lamers CBHW. Cholesterol crystal embolization in the Netherlands. Arch Int Med 1996;156:653–657.
5. Maurizi CP, Barker AE, Trueheart RE. Atheromatous emboli. Arch Pathol 1968;86:528–534.
6. Kealy WF. Atheroembolism. J Clin Pathol 1978;31:984–989.
7. Eliot RS, Kanjuh VI, Edwards JE. Atheromatous embolism. Circulation 1964;30:611–618.
8. Colt HG, Begg RJ, Saporito JJ, Cooper WM, Shapiro AP. Cholesterol emboli after cardiac catheterization. Medicine 1988;67:389–400.

9. Blankenship JC, Butler M, Garbes A. Prospective assessment of cholesterol embolization in patients with acute myocardial infarction treated with thrombolytic vs. conservative therapy. Chest 1995;107: 662–668.

10. Hyman BT, Landas SK, Ashman RF, Schelper RL, Robinson RA. Warfarin-related purple toes syndrome and cholesterol microembolization. Am J Med 1987;82:1233–1237.

11. Davis K, Kennedy JW, Kemp HG Jr., Judkins M, Gosselin AJ, Killip T. Complications of coronary arteriography from the collaborative study of coronary artery surgery (CASS). Circulation 1979;59: 1105–1112.

12. Gafter U, Chagnac A, Levi J. Cholesterol emboli in atherosclerotic patients: reports of four cases occurring spontaneously or complicating angioplasty and aortorenal bypass. J Am Geriat Soc 1987;35:357–359.

13. Schwartz MW, McDonald GB. Cholesterol embolization syndrome. JAMA 1987;258:1934–1935

14. Ben-Chitrit S, Korzets R, Hershovitz R, Bernheim J, Schneider M. Cholesterol embolization following thrombolytic therapy with streptokinase and tissue plasminogen activator. Nephrol Dial Transplant 1994;9:428–430.

15. Feder W, Auerbach R. "Purple toes": an uncommon sequela of oral coumarin drug therapy. Ann Intern Med 1961;55:911–917.

16. Anderson WR, Richards AM. Evaluation of lower extremity muscle biopsies in the diagnosis or atheroembolism. Arch Pathol 1968;86:535–541.

17. Leroy D, Michel M, Mandard J, Elie H, Deschamps P. Association of disseminated intravascular coagulation and cutaneous crystal emboli. Ann Dermatol Venereal 1981;108:665–673.

18. Harvey JC. Cholesterol microembolization: a cause of restless leg syndrome. South Med J 1976;69:269–272.

19. Haywood TA, Fessel WJ, Strange DA. Atheromatous microembolism simulating polymyositis. JAMA 1968;203:135–137.

20. Falanga V, Fine MJ, Kapoor WN. The cutaneous manifestations of cholesterol crystal embolization. Arch Dermatol 1986;122:1194–1198.

21. Comerford JA, Broe PJ, Wilson IA, Bourchier-Hayes DJ. Digital ischaemia and palpable pedal pulses. Br J Surg 1987;74:93–95.

22. Kasinath BS, Corwin HL, Bidani AK, Korbet SM, Swartz MM, Lewis EJ. Eosinophilia in the diagnosis of atheroembolic renal disease. Am J Nephrol 1987;7:173–177.

23. Wilson DM, Salazer TL, Farkouh ME.Eosinophiluria in atheroembolic renal disease. Am J Med 1991;91:186–189.

24. Cosio FG, Zager RA, Sharma HM. Atheroembolic renal disease causes hypocomplementemia. Lancet 1985;2:118–121.

25. Ferrari E, Taillan B, Drai E, Morand P Baudouy M. Investigation of the transthoracic aorta in cholesterol embolization by transesophageal echocardiography. Heart1998;79:133–136

26. Deschamps P, LeRoy D, Mandard JC, Heron JF, Lawret P. Livedo reticularis and nodules due to cholesterol embolism in the lower extremities. Br J Dermatol 1977;97:93–97.

27. Kvilekval K, Yunis JP, Mason RA, Giron F. After the blue toe: prognosis of non-cardiac arterial embolization in the lower extremities. J Vasc Surg 1993;17:328–335.

28. Morris-Jones W, Preston FE, Greeney M, Chatterjee DK. Gangrene of the toes with palpable pulses: response to platelet suppressive therapy. Ann Surg 1981;193:462–466.

29. Benvegna S, Cassina I, Giuntini G, Rusignuolo F, Talarico F, Florena M. Atherothrombotic microembolism of the lower extremities (the blue toe syndrome) from atherosclerotic nonaneurysmal aortic plaques. J Cardiovasc Surg 1990;31:87–91.

30. Coffman JD. Clinical forum: atheroembolism after cardiac surgery. J Vasc Med Biol 1989;1:37–41.

31. Belenfant X, D'Auzac C, Bariéty J, Jacquot C. Embolies de cristaux de cholesterol au cours de traitements par héparine de bas poids moléculaire. Presse Med 1997;26:1236–1237.

32. Vacher-Coponat H, Pache X, Dussol B, Bertrand Y. Pulmonary-renal syndrome responding to corticosteroids: Consider cholesterol embolization. Nephrol Dial Transplant 1997;12:1977–1979.

33. Belenfant X, Meyrier A, Jacquot C. Supportive treatment improves survival in multivisceral cholesterol crystal embolism. Am J Kidney Dis 1999;33:840–845

34. Fabbian F, Catalano C, Lambertini D, Bordin V, DiLandro D. A possible role of corticosteroids in cholesterol crystal embolization. Nephron 1999;83:189–190.

35. Stabellini N, Rizzioli E, Trapassi MR, Fabbian F, Catalano C, Gillis P. Renal cholesterol microembolization: is steroid therapy effective? Nephron 2000:86:239–240.

36. Graziani G, Stanostasi S, Angelini C, Badalamenti S. Corticosteroids in cholesterol emboli syndrome. Nephron 2001;87:371–373.
37. Woolfson RG, Lachmann H. Improvement in renal cholesterol emboli syndrome after simvastatin. Lancet 1998;351:1331–1332.
38. Finch TM, Ryatt KS. Livedo reticularis caused by cholesterol embolization may improve with simvastatin. Br J Dermat 2000;143:1319–1320.
39. Rumpf KW, Schult S, Mueller GA. Simvastatin treatment in cholesterol emboli syndrome. Lancet 1998;352:321–322.
40. Cabali S, Hochman I. Goor Y. Reversal of gangrenous lesions in the blue toe syndrome with lovastatin: a case report. Angiology 1993;44: 821–825.
41. Tsunoda S, Daimon S, Miyazaki R, Fujii H, Imazu A, Mabarchi. LDL apheresis as intensive lipid-lowering therapy for cholesterol embolization. Nephrol Dial Transplant 1999;14: 1041–1042.
42. Carr ME Jr, Sanders K, Todd WM. Pain relief and clinical improvement temporally related to the use of pentoxifylline in a patient with documented cholesterol emboli—a case report. Angiology 1994;45:65–69.
43. Ferrari E, Vidal R, Chevalier T, Baudony M. Atherosclerosis of the thoracic aorta and aortic debris as a marker of poor prognosis: benefit of oral anticoagulants. J Am Coll Cardio 1999;33:1317–1322.
44. Dressler FA, Craig WR, Castello R, Labovitz AJ. Mobile aortic atheroma and systemic emboli: efficacy of anticoagulation and influence of plaque morphology on recurrent stroke. J Am Coll Cardiol 1998;31:134–138.

18

Thromboangiitis Obliterans (Buerger's Disease)

Jeffrey W. Olin, DO

CONTENTS

INTRODUCTION
EPIDEMIOLOGY
ETIOLOGY AND PATHOGENESIS
PATHOLOGY
BUERGER'S DISEASE IN BLOOD VESSELS IN UNUSUAL LOCATIONS
CLINICAL FEATURES
LABORATORY TESTS AND ARTERIOGRAPHIC FINDINGS
DIFFERENTIAL DIAGNOSIS
TREATMENT
CONCLUSION
REFERENCES

INTRODUCTION

Felix von Winiwater described the first case of thromboangiitis obliterans in 1879 *(1)*. A 57-yr-old man had a 12-yr history of foot pain resulting in gangrene leading to amputation. On examination of the amputated specimen, there were endarteritis and endophlebitis that were distinct from atherosclerosis *(1)*. Twenty-nine years later, Leo Buerger described the pathology in 11 amputated limbs and called this disease "thromboangiitis obliterans," which later became more commonly know as Buerger's disease *(2)*. The pathological description in 1908 was so accurate and detailed that little has been added over the last century.

Thromboangiitis obliterans (TAO) is a segmental inflammatory disease that most commonly affects the small and medium-sized arteries and veins in both the upper and lower extremities. In many of the earlier published reports and those originating from Japan, TAO was almost exclusively encountered in young men *(3)*. However, in the more recent Western literature, the prevalence of TAO has increased in women. Virtually all patients are heavy users of tobacco, usually cigarette smoking.

TAO is a vasculitis but differs from other forms of vasculitis in three important ways: histopathologically, there is a highly cellular and inflammatory thrombus with relative sparing of the blood vessel wall; acute phase reactants such as the Westergren sedimen-

From: *Contemporary Cardiology: Peripheral Arterial Disease: Diagnosis and Treatment*
Edited by: J. D. Coffman and R. T. Eberhardt © Humana Press Inc., Totowa, NJ

tation rate and C-reactive protein (CRP) are usually normal as are many serologic immunologic markers (circulating immune complexes, complement levels, cryoglobulins); and commonly measured autoantibodies (antinuclear antibody, rheumatoid factor) are normal or negative *(4,5)*. Yet an immune reaction has been demonstrated in the endothelium and arterial intima and a sensitivity to type III collagen has been described *(6–9)*.

EPIDEMIOLOGY

While Buerger's disease has a worldwide distribution, it is more prevalent in the Middle, Near, and Far East regions than in North America and Western Europe *(10,11)*. This difference may be due in part to a genetic predisposition to the disease and in part to different diagnostic criteria used in different parts of the world. At the Mayo Clinic the prevalence rate of patients with the diagnosis of Buerger's disease has steadily declined from 104 per 100,000 patient registrations in 1947 to 12.6 per 100,000 patient registrations in 1986 *(11,12)*. Prevalence rates have varied from as low as 0.5–5.6% of all peripheral arterial disease patients in Western European countries to as high as 45–63% in India, 16–66% in Korea and Japan, and 80% in Israel among Jews of Ashkenazim ancestry *(13–15)*.

The reported prevalence of Buerger's disease in women was 1–2% in most published series of cases before 1970. Several recently published series showed a much higher prevalence of women with the disease *(4,12,16,17)*. We have demonstrated that 42 (26%) of 160 patients with Buerger's disease from 1970 to 1996 at the Cleveland Clinic Foundation were women *(4,16)*. The reason for the apparent increased number of women with Buerger's disease is unknown, but could possibly be attributed to the increased number of women smokers. The prevalence of Buerger's disease in Japanese women remains relatively low compared to the increased number of female smokers *(3,18)*, and in a recent study from Hong Kong all 89 of the patients were men *(19)*. The reported prevalence will vary depending on the criteria used to diagnose TAO.

ETIOLOGY AND PATHOGENESIS

The etiology of Buerger's disease is unknown. While TAO is a vasculitis *(20)*, there are two features that distinguish it from other forms of vasculitis. Pathologically, the thrombus in TAO is highly cellular and there is much less intense cellular activity in the wall of the blood vessel. In addition, TAO differs from many other types of vasculitis in that the usual markers of inflammation and immunologic activation (elevation of acute phase reactants such as Westergren sedimentation rate and CRP), the presence of circulating immune complexes, and the presence of commonly measured autoantibodies (antinuclear antibody, rheumatoid factor, complement levels, etc.) are usually normal or negative.

Smoking

It is not known if cigarette smoking causes or contributes to the development of Buerger's disease. However, tobacco use is a major factor in the activity of the disease. The progression and continued symptoms associated with TAO are closely linked with continued use of tobacco *(4,21)*. Matsuhita and colleagues have shown that there was a very close relationship between active smoking and an active course of Buerger's disease using the level of cotinine (a metabolite of nicotine) as a measurement of active smoking *(22)*. It has been demonstrated that passive smoking can cause endothelial dysfunction in healthy young adults *(23)*. While passive smoking (secondary smoke) has not been shown to be associated with the onset of TAO, it may be an important factor in the continuation of symptoms in patients during the acute phase of Buerger's disease. Although there have been several cases of TAO in users of smokeless tobacco or snuff *(24–26)*, the disease is more commonly associated with heavy tobacco use *(4,27)*. Kjeldsen and Mozes *(28)* have demonstrated that patients with TAO had higher tobacco consumption and carboxyhemoglobin levels than patients with atherosclerosis or a control group of patients. The incidence of TAO is higher in countries where the consumption of tobacco is large. There is a higher incidence of TAO in India among individuals of a low socioeconomic class who smoke bidis (homemade cigarettes containing raw tobacco) *(29–31)*.

Although there are investigators who believe that Buerger's disease can occur in non-smokers *(32)* most believe that current or past smoking is a requirement for the diagnosis *(3,4,17,18)*. Lie described one case of pathologically proven Buerger's disease affecting the upper extremities of a 62-yr-old man who had "allegedly" discontinued smoking 15 yr earlier *(33)*. However, this report did not contain urinary nicotine measurements, cotinine measurements, or carboxyhemoglobin levels. Therefore, it is possible that this person was still smoking.

Central to disease initiation and progression is tobacco use or exposure. However, only a small number of smokers worldwide eventually develop TAO; therefore, other etiologic factors may play a role as a triggering mechanism for the development of TAO in susceptible individuals.

Immunologic Mechanisms

Several studies have examined the immunologic mechanisms in patients with TAO. Adar and colleagues studied 39 patients with Buerger's disease and measured the cell-mediated sensitivity for type I and III collagen by an antigen-sensitive thymidine-incorporation assay *(7)*. There was an increased cellular sensitivity to type I and III collagen (normal constituents of human arteries) in patients with TAO compared to patients with arteriosclerosis obliterans or healthy male controls. There was a low, but significant, level of anticollagen antibody in 7 of 39 serum samples from patients with TAO, whereas this antibody was not detected in the control group of patients. Circulating immune complexes have been found in the peripheral arteries of some patients with TAO *(34–36)*.

Hypercoagulability and Endothelial Function

There have been conflicting data on the presence of hypercoagulability in Buerger's disease *(16,37–42)*. A recent report showed that patients with TAO had an increased likelihood of having the prothrombin gene mutation 20210A (odds ratio 7.98) *(37)*. The endothelium plays a very important role in patients with TAO. Eichhorn and colleagues demonstrated that one might predict disease activity by measuring antiendothelial cell antibody (AECA) titers *(8)*. Seven of 28 patients with active TAO had AECA titers of 1857 ± 450 arbitrary units (AU) compared with 126 ± 15 AU in 30 normal control subjects ($p < 0.001$) and 461 ± 41 AU in the 21 patients in remission ($p < 0.01$). Antibodies from the sera of patients with active disease reacted not only with surface epitopes but also with sites within the cytoplasm of human endothelial cells. If this study can be confirmed, it may be possible to objectively follow the disease activity in patients with Buerger's disease.

There is impaired endothelium-dependent vasorelaxation in the peripheral vasculature of patients with Buerger's disease *(43)*. Forearm blood flow (FBF) was measured plethysmographically in the nondiseased limb during the infusion of acetylcholine (an endothelium-dependent vasodilator), sodium nitroprusside (an endothelium-independent vasodilator), and occlusion-induced reactive hyperemia. The increase in FBF to intraarterial acetylcholine was lower in patients with TAO than in healthy controls (14.1 $\pm$ 2.8 mL/min per dL of tissue volume vs 22.9 $\pm$ 2.9 mL/min per dL, $p < 0.01$). There was no significant increase in FBF response to sodium nitroprusside (13.1 $\pm$ 4 mL/min per dL vs 16.3 $\pm$ 2.5 mL/min per dL). There was no significant difference between the two groups during reactive hyperemia. These data indicate that endothelium-dependent vasodilatation is impaired even in the nondiseased limb of patients with TAO.

Genetics

Although no gene has been identified to date, there may be an as of yet unidentified genetic predisposition to developing TAO. There is no consistent pattern in HLA haplotypes among patients with Buerger's disease.

In summary, there is no single etiologic mechanism present in patients with TAO. Tobacco seems to play a central role both in the initiation and continuance of the disease. Other etiologic factors such as genetic predisposition, immunologic mechanisms, endothelial dysfunction, and abnormalities in coagulation may play a role in some patients.

PATHOLOGY

Buerger's disease is an inflammatory thrombosis that affects both arteries and veins, and the histopathology of the involved blood vessels varies according to the chronologic age of the disease. The histopathology is most likely to be diagnostic at the acute phase of the disease. It evolves to changes being consistent with or suggestive of the disease in the appropriate clinical setting at the immediate stage or subacute phase, and becomes indistinguishable from other vascular diseases at end-stage or chronic phase when all that remains is organized thrombus and fibrosis of the blood vessels *(2,10,44,45)*. The histologic distinction between Buerger's disease and atherosclerosis is clear cut and the differentiation can be made with a high degree of accuracy *(44)*. It should also be emphasized that the small blood vessels in the hand and foot are not usually affected by atherosclerosis.

Acute Phase Lesions

The early, or acute, phase lesion is characterized by acute inflammation involving all layers of the vessel wall, especially of the veins, in association with occlusive cellular thrombus. Around the periphery of the thrombus, there are frequently what appear to be collections of polymorphonuclear leukocytes with karyorrhexis, the so-called "microabscesses," in which one or more multinucleated giant cells may be present (Fig. 1). The prominent inflammatory thrombotic lesion occurs more often in veins than in arteries. If the acute superficial phlebitic lesion of the skin is biopsied at an early stage, it is most common to find the acute pathological abnormalities of TAO *(46)*. However, there may be different lesions in segments of the same vein such as acute phlebitis without throm-

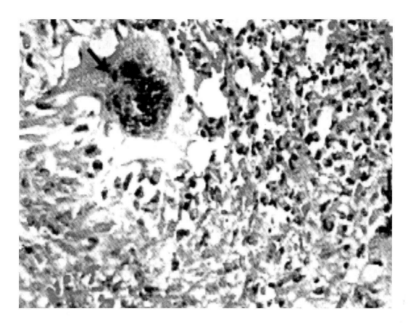

Fig. 1. Typical acute histologic lesion of Buerger's disease in a vein with intense thromboangiitis showing a microabscess in the thrombus and a multinucleated giant cells (*arrow*) (X400 H & E). (Reproduced with permission of the publisher from Lie JT. Thromboangiitis obliterans [Buerger's disease] revisited. Pathol Annual 1988;23(Part 2):257–291).

bosis, acute phlebitis with thrombosis, and acute phlebitis with thrombus containing microabscess and giant cells (48).

Intermediate Phase and End-Stage Lesions

In the intermediate (or subacute) phase there is progressive organization of the occlusive thrombus and continued presence of the prominent inflammatory cell infiltrate within the thrombus but less so in the vessel wall. The chronic phase or end stage is characterized by further organization of the occlusive thrombus with extensive recanalization, prominent vascularization of the media, and adventitial and perivascular fibrosis. "In all three stages, the normal architecture of the vessel wall subjacent to the occlusive thrombus and including the internal elastic lamina remains essentially intact. These findings distinguish thromboangiitis obliterans from arteriosclerosis and from other systemic vasculitides in which there is usually more striking disruption of the internal elastic lamina and the media, disproportional to those attributable to aging change" *(47)*.

It should be noted that both Buerger's disease and arteriosclerosis may coexist and thus create further diagnostic uncertainty and controversy. Buerger's disease does not protect against atherosclerosis.

BUERGER'S DISEASE OF BLOOD VESSELS IN UNUSUAL LOCATIONS

While Buerger's disease is almost exclusively a disease of the small and medium-sized blood vessels in the lower and upper limbs, there have been only occasional reports, usually without adequate histologic proof, of involvement of larger arteries such as the aorta, the pulmonary artery, and iliac arteries. Although Buerger (2) had noted that typical histologic findings could be present in blood vessels other than those of the limbs, the involvement of the cerebral arteries, coronary arteries, renal arteries, and mesenteric arteries has been documented in only a few patients, almost all as single case reports (2,48–51). The most extreme case of Buerger's disease with peripheral and visceral involvement was that of an 18-yr-old male cigarette smoker who, in a span of 15 yr, underwent bilateral sympathectomies, two bowel resections, and 13 amputations, including bilateral above-elbow and above-knee amputations, before he succumbed at age 33 to another episode of bowel infarction from recurrent Buerger's disease of the mesenteric arteries and veins (52). Buerger's disease has also been demonstrated pathologically in other unusual sites (53) such as saphenous vein bypass grafts (54), temporal arteries (55) and testicular and spermatic arteries and veins (56).

CLINICAL FEATURES

Buerger's disease typically occurs in young male smokers with symptom onset before age 45. However recent reports have demonstrated an increased prevalence of TAO in women (4,6,12,17). This does not appear to be the case, however, in the Japanese literature (3,18,19). Buerger's disease usually begins with distal limb ischemia. As the disease progresses, it may involve more proximal arteries such as the superficial femoral or brachial artery. Large artery involvement has been reported in TAO but this is unusual and rarely occurs in the absence of small vessel involvement (53).

TAO is often not diagnosed in the early stages because patients may present with foot or arch claudication and this symptom is often mistaken for an orthopedic problem. As the disease progresses, patients may develop ischemic ulcerations on the distal portion of the toes and/or fingers (Fig. 2).

At the Cleveland Clinic Foundation, 112 patients with Buerger's disease were evaluated between 1970 and 1987 (4). The presenting clinical signs and symptoms are shown in Table 1. Intermittent claudication occurred in 70 patients (63%) and 76% of patients had ischemic ulcerations at the time of presentation. The age and gender distribution and the presenting signs and symptoms were virtually identical in a follow-up series of an additional 40 patients evaluated from 1988 to 1996 (16).

A helpful clue in differentiating TAO from other diseases is that two or more limbs are almost always involved. In Shionoya's series, two limbs were affected in 16% of patients, three limbs in 41%, and all four limbs in 43% of patients (3). Therefore, when angiography is performed, it has been our practice to evaluate both upper extremities and/or lower extremities in patients who clinically present with involvement of only one limb. Angiographic abnormalities consistent with Buerger's disease are frequent in limbs that are not yet clinically involved.

In patients with lower extremity ulceration in whom Buerger's disease is a consideration, an Allen's test should be performed to assess the circulation in the hands and fingers (57,58). An abnormal Allen's test in a young smoker with lower extremity ulcerations is highly suggestive of TAO, as it demonstrates small vessel involvement in both the upper and lower extremities. In one large series, 63% of all patients demonstrated an abnormal Allen's test (4). Except in patients with end-stage renal disease and

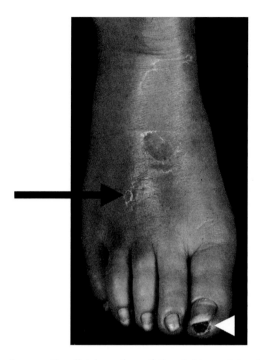

Fig. 2. Ischemic ulcer on the distal portion of the right great toe (*arrow*) in a patient with acute Buerger's disease. Note the superficial thrombophlebitis on the dorsum of the foot (*arrowhead*). (Reproduced from Olin JW, Lie JT. Thromboangiitis Obliterans. In: Cooke JP, Frohlich ED, eds. Current Management of Hypertension and Vascular Disease.BC Decker, 1992, pp. 265–271.)

diabetes, atherosclerosis does not occur in the hand and rarely occurs distal to the subclavian artery. This feature helps to differentiate TAO from atherosclerosis.

Superficial thrombophlebitis occurred in approximately 40% of patients with TAO (Fig. 2) *(4)*. The thrombophlebitis may be migratory and may parallel disease activity *(27)*. Biopsy of an acute superficial thrombophlebitis will often demonstrate the typical histopathological lesions of acute Buerger's disease (Fig. 1).

Cold sensitivity is common and may be one of the earliest manifestations of TAO. In addition, Raynaud's phenomenon has been reported in approx 40% of patients. The extremities of patients with Buerger's disease often have an erythematous or cyanotic appearance *(59)*.

LABORATORY TESTS AND ARTERIOGRAPHIC FINDINGS

There are no specific laboratory tests to aid in the diagnosis of TAO. Excluding other diseases that can present in a similar fashion to Buerger's disease often is helpful in making the diagnosis. A complete serologic profile should be obtained and include the following: complete blood count with differential, liver function, renal function, fasting blood sugar, urinalysis, acute phase reactants (Westergren sedimentation rate and CRP), antinuclear antibody, rheumatoid factor, complement measurements, serologic markers for CREST syndrome and scleroderma (anticentromere antibody and SCL70), and a complete hypercoagulability screen to include antiphospholipid antibodies. A proximal

Table 1
Thromboangiitis Obliterans: Demographic Characteristics, Presenting Symptoms and Signs

Variable	Series from 1970 to 1987[a]
Patients (n)	112
Mean age (yr)	42
Men	86 (77%)
Women	26 (23%)
Intermittent claudication	70 (63%)
Rest pain	91 (81%)
Ischemic ulcers	85 (76%)
Upper extremity	24 (28%)
Lower extremity	39 (46%)
Both	22 (26%)
Thrombophlebitis	43 (38%)
Raynaud's phenomenon	49 (44%)
Sensory findings	77 (69%)
Abnormal Allen test	71 (63%)

[a]From Olin JW et al. Circulation 1990; (Suppl): IV-3-IV-8.

source of emboli may be excluded by performing echocardiography (two-dimensional and/or transesophageal) and arteriography.

An arteriogram is often required to be certain that there is no proximal disease and that no other possible disease is mimicking TAO. While the findings on arteriography may be suggestive of TAO, there are no pathognomonic angiographic findings in TAO (60–62). Proximal arteries should be normal demonstrating no evidence of atherosclerosis, aneurysm, or other source of proximal emboli. To diagnose Buerger's disease with proximal artery involvement, a pathological specimen is necessary. The disease is confined most often to the distal circulation and is almost always infrapopliteal in the lower extremities and distal to the brachial artery in the upper extremities. There is small and medium-sized vessel involvement such as the digital arteries in the fingers and toes; the palmar and plantar arteries in the hand and foot; as well as the tibial, peroneal, radial, and ulnar arteries (27,47). Isolated disease below the popliteal artery almost never occurs in atherosclerosis except in the patient with diabetes mellitus. However, because diabetes is exclusionary for the diagnosis of TAO (in the absence of a pathological specimen), there should be no confusion between these two diseases.

TAO is a segmental disorder, demonstrating areas of diseased vessels interspersed with normal blood vessel segments. There is often evidence of multiple vascular occlusions with collateralization around the obstructions (corkscrew collaterals) (Fig. 3). Corkscrew collaterals are not pathognomonic of Buerger's disease as they may be present in other small vessel occlusive diseases such as CREST syndrome or scleroderma. In fact, the arteriographic appearance of Buerger's disease may be identical to that seen in patients with scleroderma, CREST syndrome, systemic lupus erythematosus, rheumatoid vasculitis, mixed connective tissue disease, and antiphospholipid antibody syndrome. However, the clinical and serological manifestations of these other immunologic diseases should help to differentiate them from TAO. Irregularity or calcification of the blood vessel wall should be exclusionary for the diagnosis of Buerger's disease.

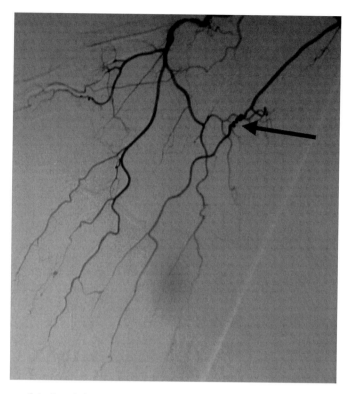

Fig. 3. Angiogram of the hand demonstrating multiple digital artery occlusions with collateralization ("corkscrew collaterals") (*arrows*) around the areas of occlusion.

DIFFERENTIAL DIAGNOSIS

The diagnosis of TAO should not be difficult if diseases that mimic TAO are excluded. The most important diseases to exclude are atherosclerosis, emboli, and autoimmune diseases as discussed above. Under most circumstances, with the use of echocardiography and arteriography, atherosclerosis and emboli can be excluded with a high degree of clinical certainty.

It should not be difficult to differentiate patients with TAO from those with Takayasu's arteritis or giant cell arteritis (*see* Chapter 19). Whereas patients with TAO manifest distal extremity ischemia, patients with Takayasu's arteritis or giant cell arteritis present with proximal vascular involvement. The arteriographic features of Takayasu's disease or giant cell arteritis are quite distinctive.

In the presence of lower extremity involvement, the possibility of popliteal artery entrapment syndrome or cystic adventitial disease should be considered, both of which are readily apparent on arteriography, computed tomography (CT) scan, or magnetic resonance imaging (MRI). An aneurysm of the popliteal artery should be easily diagnosed by physical examination.

A careful history should be taken for the possibility of ergotamine use (abuse) as this may cause severe ischemia in multiple limbs. Ergotamine ingestion and TAO may cause both lower and upper extremity ischemia. Even if the patient denies a history of migraine headaches or previous ergotamine use, ergotamine blood levels should be obtained in some patients to exclude this condition. Other drugs such as cocaine *(63)* and marijuana *(64)* have been implicated in causing a syndrome very similar to Buerger's disease. If there is isolated involvement of the upper extremity, occupational hazards such as vibratory tool use and hypothenar hammer syndrome should be considered.

Several different diagnostic criteria have been proposed for the diagnosis of TAO *(25,65)*. The criteria of Shionoya *(66,67)* and Olin *(4)* are shown in Table 2. The algorithm shown in Fig. 4 may be helpful in the diagnosis of TAO *(47)*.

TREATMENT

Discontinue Tobacco Use or Exposure

The only definitive method to halt disease progression and prevent amputations is the complete discontinuation of cigarette smoking or the use of tobacco in any form *(4,68–70)*. Even small amounts of cigarette smoking, or the use of smokeless tobacco (chewing tobacco, snuff), have been reported to not only cause Buerger's disease but also to keep it active once it has already occurred *(24,26)*. One hundred and twenty-nine patients have been followed long term at the Cleveland Clinic Foundation, and 55 (43%) were able to discontinue cigarette smoking (Fig. 5). If irreversible tissue loss was not present at the time the patient stopped smoking, amputation did not occur. Ninety-four percent of patients avoided amputation in the ex-smoking group. In the 74 patients who continued to smoke, 41% required one or more amputations. There is an extremely strong correlation between smoking cessation and disease activity (ischemic ulcer healing and avoidance of amputation). Therefore, if the patient has stated that he or she has stopped using tobacco products and the disease remains active, a urine nicotine and cotinine level should be measured to determine if the patient is still smoking or is being exposed to high amounts of environmental (secondary) tobacco smoke *(22)*. Frequent education and counseling are extremely important on the physician's part to encourage the patient to discontinue using tobacco products. The patient should be reassured that if he or she is able to discontinue tobacco use, the disease will become quiescent and amputation will not occur as long as irreversible tissue loss has not already occurred. However, patients may continue to experience intermittent claudication or Raynaud's phenomenon because the occluded arterial segments will remain occluded.

Drug Therapy

Other than discontinuation of cigarette smoking, all other forms of therapy are palliative. In a prospective, randomized, double-blind trial comparing a 6-h daily infusion of iloprost (a prostaglandin analog) to aspirin, iloprost was superior in causing total relief of rest pain and complete healing of ischemic ulcerations. At 6 mo, 88% of the patients receiving iloprost responded to therapy as compared to only 21% of the aspirin-treated group *(71)*. The European TAO Study Group has also studied an oral extended release preparation of iloprost. Although there was some benefit, oral iloprost is not nearly as effective as the intravenous form *(72)*. A recent report suggested that there might be a role for immunosuppressive therapy with cyclophosphamide in the acute phase of Buerger's disease *(73)*. This will need to be studied in much greater detail before it can be recommended as standard therapy.

Table 2
Criteria for the Diagnosis of TAO

Shionoya's criteria	*Olin's criteria*
Onset before age 50	Onset before age 45
Smoking history	Current (or recent past) tobacco use
Infrapopliteal arterial occlusions	Distal extremity ischemia (claudication, rest pain, ischemic ulcers, gangrene) documented with noninvasive testing
Upper limb involvement or phlebitis migrans	Laboratory tests to exclude autoimmune diseases, hypercoagulable states, and diabetes mellitus
Absence of atherosclerotic risk factors other than smoking	Exclude a proximal source of emboli with echocardiography and arteriography. Demonstrate consistent arteriographic findings in the involved and clinically noninvolved limbs.

A biopsy is rarely needed to make the diagnosis unless the patient presents with unusual characteristics such as large artery involvement or age > 45.

[a]From Olin JW. Current treatment of thromboangiitis obliterans (Buerger's disease). Harrison's, On Line 2001, in press.

Thrombolytic Therapy

Several studies have reported on the use of intraarterial thrombolytic therapy as an adjunct for the treatment of Buerger's disease *(74,75)*. Eleven patients with long-standing Buerger's disease who had gangrene or pregangrenous lesions of the toes or feet were treated with selective low-dose intraarterial streptokinase (10,000 U bolus followed by 5000 U/h) *(74)*. The authors reported an overall success rate (defined as amputation being avoided or altered) of 58.3%. Other reports on the use of thrombolytic therapy have not been as favorable. Further study will be required to determine the role of thrombolytic therapy in patients with Buerger's disease.

Surgical Procedures

Surgical revascularization for Buerger's disease is often not a feasible alternative owing to the diffuse segmental involvement and distal nature of the disease. There is often not a distal target vessel available for bypass surgery. However, if a distal target is available and the patient is facing limb loss, bypass surgery should be considered with the use of autogenous vein *(76–79)*. Sasajima and colleagues reported a 5-yr primary patency of 66.8% in those who discontinued smoking and 34.7% in patients who continued to smoke *(78)*. Another surgical approach that has been reported to be successful in Buerger's disease is that of omental transfer *(80,81)*. Surgical therapy for TAO is not commonly performed in the United States, primarily because a reasonable target vessel for bypass is often not available and most patients will do very well if they are able to discontinue smoking.

The role of sympathectomy in preventing amputations or in treating pain is unclear *(4)*. Sympathectomy may be helpful in the healing of superficial ischemic ulcerations. We have recently treated one patient with a spinal cord stimulator resulting in complete healing of all upper extremity ulcerations when all other conservative measures had failed *(82)*.

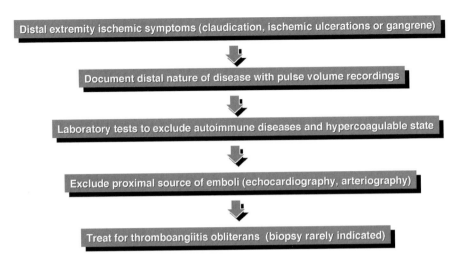

Fig. 4. Diagnostic algorithm for the diagnosis of thromboangiitis obliterans. (From Olin JW, Lie JT. Thromboangiitis obliterans [Buerger's disease]. In: Loscalzo J, Creager MA, Dzau VJ, eds. Vascular Medicine. Boston: Little, Brown, 1996, pp. 1033–1049.)

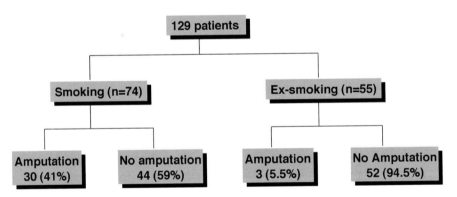

Fig. 5. Smoking status related to amputation. (From Olin JW. Thromboangiitis obliterans [Buerger's disease]. In: Rutherford RB, ed. Vascular Surgery, 4th edit. Philadelphia: WB Saunders, 2000, pp. 350–364.

Therapeutic Angiogenesis

Isner and colleagues *(83)* reported on seven limbs in six patients with TAO using intramuscular injection of plasmid DNA (ph VEGF 165). Of the ulcers that were non-healing for more than 1 mo, the ulcers healed completely in three of five limbs after intramuscular VEGF$_{165}$ gene therapy. In the remaining two patients, nocturnal rest pain was relieved. It is too early to tell what role gene therapy will play in patients with TAO but it appears to be a promising therapeutic modality.

General Measures

Good general vascular care is essential in the treatment of patients with ischemia secondary to TAO. A reverse Trendelenburg (vascular) position should be used in patients who have severe ischemic rest pain. Adequate narcotics should be made available during the time period of severe ischemia. Anticoagulation is generally not efficacious in the treatment of Buerger's disease unless the patient has recurrent episodes of superficial thrombophlebitis. Good foot and hand care should be undertaken. A calcium channel-blocking agent such as nifedipine or amlodipine should be used in patients with vasospasm. Pentoxifylline has not been adequately studied in patients with TAO. A preliminary report indicates that cilostazol may be helpful in digital ischemia *(84)*. The mechanism for such an effect is not clearly understood. Heel protectors should be used in patients with severe ischemia to prevent pressure ulcers from developing.

CONCLUSION

TAO (Buerger's disease) is an inflammatory, nonatherosclerotic disease affecting the small and medium-sized arteries and veins in both the upper and lower extremities. Tobacco use plays a central role in both the initiation and the continuance of the disease, and discontinuation of tobacco use in any form is the mainstay of treatment. Amputation almost never occurs in patients who are able to discontinue using tobacco.

REFERENCES

1. von Winiwater F. Ueber eine eigenthumliche Form von Endarteritis und Endophlebitis mit Gangran des Fusses. Arch Klin Chir 1879;23:202–226.
2. Buerger L. Thromboangiitis obliterans: a study of the vascular lesions leading to presenile spontaneous gangrene. Am J Med Sci 1908;136;567–580.
3. Shionoya S. Buerger's disease (thromboangiitis obliterans). In: Rutherford RB, ed. Vascular Surgery. Philadelphia: WB Saunders, 1989, pp. 207–217.
4. Olin JW, Young JR, Graor RA, Ruschaupt WF, Bartholomew JR. The changing clinical spectrum of thromboangiitis obliterans (Buerger's disease). Circulation 1990;82(Suppl IV):3–8.
5. Olin JW. Thromboangiitis obliterans (Buerger's disease). Curr Opin Rheumat 1994;6:44–49.
6. Olin JW. Thromboangiitis obliterans (Buerger's disease). N Engl J Med 2000;343:864–869.
7. Adar R, Papa MC, Halperin Z, et al. Cellular sensitivity to collagen and thromboangiitis obliterans. N Engl J Med 1983;308:1113–1116.
8. Eichhorn J, Sima D, Lindschau C, et al. Antiendothelial cell antibodies in thromboangiitis obliterans. N Engl J Med 1983;308:1113-6.
9. Kobayashi M, Ito M, Nakagawa A, Nishikimi N, Nimura Y. Immunohistochemical analysis of arterial wall cellular infiltration in Buerger's disease (endarteritis obliterans). J Vasc Surg 1999;29:451–458.
10. Lie JT. Thromboangiitis obliterans (Buerger's disease) revisited. Pathol Annual 1988;23:(Part 2): 257–291.
11. Lie JT. The rise and fall and resurgence of thromboangiitis obliterans (Buerger's disease). Acta Pathol Jpn 1989;39:153–158.
12. Lie JT. Thromboangiitis obliterans (Buerger's disease) in women. Medicine 1987;64:65–72.
13. Cachovan M. Epidemiologie und geographisches Verteilungsmuster der Thromboangiitis obliterans. In: Heidrich H, ed. Thromboangiitis Obliterans Morbus Winiwarter-Buerger. Stuttgart, New York: Georg Thieme, 1988, pp. 31–36.
14. Ishikawa K, ed. Annual report of the Buerger's Disease Research Committee of Ministry of Health and Welfare of Japan, Tokyo, 1976, pp. 3–15, 86–97.
15. Matsushita, M, Nishikimi N, Sakurai T, Nimura Y. Decrease in prevalence of Buerger's disease in Japan. Surgery 1998;124:498–502.
16. Olin JW, Childs MB, Bartholomew JR, Calabrese LH, Young JR. Anticardiolipin antibodies and homocysteine levels in patients with thromboangiitis obliterans. Arthritis Rheum 1996;39:S-47.
17. Mills JL, Taylor LM, Porter JK. Buerger's disease in the modern era. Am J Surg 1987;154:123–154.
18. Shionoya S. Buerger's disease. Pathology, diagnosis and treatment. Nagoya: The University of Nagoya Press, 1990, pp. 261.
19. Lau H, Cheng SWK. Buerger's disease in Hong Kong: a review of 89 cases. Aust N Z J Surg 1997;67: 264–269.

20. Lie JT. Diagnostic histopathology of major systemic and pulmonary vasculitic syndromes. Rheum Clin N Am 1990;16:269–292.
21. Olin JW. Thromboangiitis obliterans (Buerger's disease). In: Rutherford RB, ed. Vascular Surgery, 4th edit. Rutherford RB, Philadelphia, WB Saunders, 2000, pp. 350–364.
22. Matsushita M, Shionoya S, Matsumoto T. Urinary cotinine measurements in patients with Buerger's disease: effects of active and passive smoking on the disease process. J Vasc Surg 1991;14:53–58.
23. Otuska R, Watanabe H, Hirata K, et al. Acute effects of passive smoking on the coronary circulation in healthy young adults. JAMA 2001;286:436–441.
24. Lie JT. Thromboangiitis obliterans (Buerger's disease) and smokeless tobacco. Arthritis Rheum 1988; 31:812–813.
25. Mills JL, Porter JM. Buerger's disease: a review and update. Semin Vasc Surg 1993;6:14–23.
26. Joyce JW. Buerger's disease (thromboangiitis obliterans). Rheum Dis Clin N Am 1990;116:463–470.
27. Papa MZ, Adar R. A critical look at thromboangiitis obliterans (Buerger's disease). Vasc Surg 1992;5: 1–21.
28. Kjeldsen K, Mozes M. Buerger's disease in Israel: investigations on carboxyhemoglobin and serum cholesterol levels after smoking. Acta Chir Scand 1969;135:495–498.
29. Rahman M, Chowdhury AS, Fukui T, Hira K, Shimbo T. Association of thromboangiitis obliterans with cigarette and bidi smoking in Bangladesh: a case-control study. Int J Epidemiol 2000;29:266–270.
30. Grove WJ, Stansby GP. Buerger's disease and cigarette smoking in Bangladesh. Ann Roy Coll Surg Eng 1992;74:115–118.
31. Jindal RM, Patel SM. Buerger's disease in cigarette smoking in Bangladesh. Ann Roy Coll Surg Eng 1992;74:436–437.
32. Sasaki S, Sakuma M, Kunihara T, Yasuda K. Current trends in thromboangiitis obliterans (Buerger's disease) in women. Am J Surg 1999;177:316–320.
33. Lie JT. Thromboangiitis obliterans (Buerger's disease) in an elderly man after cessation of cigarette smoking: case report. Angiology 1987;38:864–867.
34. De Albuquerque RR, Delgado L, Correia P, Torrinha JF, Serrao D, Braga A. Circulating immune complexes in Buerger's Disease-endarteritis obliterans in young men. J Cardiovasc Surg 1989;30:821-825.
35. Gulati SM, Madhra K, Thusoo TK, Nair SK, Saha K. Autoantibodies in thromboangiitis obliterans. Angiology 1982;33:642–650.
36. Gulati SM, Saha K, Kant L Thusoo TK, Prakash A. Significance of circulating immune complexes in thromboangiitis obliterans (Buerger's disease). Angiology 1984;35:276–281.
37. Avcu F, Akar E, Demirkilic U, Yilmac E, Akar N, Yaloin A. The role of prothrombotic mutations in patients with Buerger's disease. Thromb Res 2000;100:143–147.
38. Casellas M, Perez A, Cabero L. Buerger's disease and antiphospholipid antibodies in pregnancy. Ann Rheum Dis 1993;52:247–248.
39. Craven JL, Cotton RC. Haematological differences between thromboangiitis obliterans and atherosclerosis. Br J Surg 1967;54:862–867.
40. Chaudhury NA, Pietraszek MH, Hachiya T, et al. Plasminogen activators and plasminogen activator inhibitor 1 before and after venous occlusion of the upper limb in thromboangiitis obliterans (Buerger's disease). Thromb Res 1992;66:321–329.
41. Siguret V, Alhenc-Gelas M, Aiach M, Friessinger JN, Gaussen P. Response to DDAVP stimulation in thirteen patients with Buerger's disease. Thromb Res 1997;86:85–87.
42. Pietraszek MH, Chaudhury NA, Koyano K, et al. Enhanced platelet response to serotonin in Buerger's disease. Thromb Res 1990;60:241–246.
43. Makita S, Nakamura M, Murakami H, Komoda K, Kawazoe K, Hiramori K. Impaired endothelium dependent vasorelaxation in peripheral vasculature of patients with thromboangiitis obliterans (Buerger's disease). Circulation 1996;94(Suppl II):II-211–II-215.
44. Dible JH. The Pathology of the Limb Ischaemia. Edinburgh: Oliver & Boyd, 1966, pp. 79–96.
45. Leu HJ. Early inflammatory changes in thromboangiitis obliterans. Pathol Microbiol 1975;43: 151–156.
46. Leu HJ, Bollinger A. Phlebitis saltans sive migrans, Vasa 1978;7:440-442.
47. Olin JW, Lie JT. Thromboangiitis Obliterans (Buerger's disease). In: Loscalzo J, Creager MA, Dzau VJ, eds. Vascular Medicine Boston: Little, Brown, 1996, pp. 1033–1049.
48. Deitch EA, Sikkema WW. Intestinal manifestation of Buerger's disease. Am Surg 1981;47:326–28.
49. Siddiqui MZ, Reis ED, Soundararajan K, Kerstein MD. Buerger's disease affecting mesenteric arteries: a rare cause of intestinal ischemia: a case report. Vasc Surg 2001;35:235–238.

50. Donatelli F, Triggiani M, Nascimbene S, et al. Thromboangiitis obliterans of coronary and internal thoracic arteries in a young woman. J Thor Cardiovasc Surg 1997;113:800–802.
51. Rosen N, Sommer I, Knobel B. Intestinal Buerger's disease. Arch Pathol Lab Med 1985;109:962–963.
52. Cebezas-Moya R, Dragstedt LR III. An extreme example of Buerger's disease. Arch Surg 1970;101: 632–634.
53. Shionoya S, Ban I, Nakata Y, Matsubara J, Hirai M, Kawai S. Involvement of the iliac artery in Buerger's disease (pathogenesis and arterial reconstruction). J Cardiovasc Surg 1978;19:69–76.
54. Lie JT. Thromboangiitis obliterans (Buerger's disease) in a saphenous vein arterial graft. Hum Pathol 1987;18:402–404.
55. Lie JT, Michet CJ Jr. Thromboangiitis obliterans with eosinophilia (Buerger's disease) of the temporal arteries. Hum Pathol 1988;19:598–602.
56. Buerger L. The Circulatory Disturbance of the Extremities: Including Gangrene, Vasomotor and Trophic Disorders. Philadelphia: WB Saunders, 1924.
57. Olin JW, Lie JT. Thromboangiitis obliterans (Buerger's disease). In: Cooke JP, Frohlich ED, eds. Current Management of Hypertension and Vascular Disease. St Louis: Mosby Yearbook, 1992, pp. 265–271.
58. Allen EV. Thromboangiitis obliterans: methods of diagnosis of chronic occlusive arterial lesions distal to the wrist with illustrative cases. Am J Med Sci 1929;178:237–244.
59. Kimura T, Yoshizaki S, Tsushima N et al. Buerger's colour. Br J Surg 1990;77:1299–1301.
60. Lambeth JT, Yong NK. Arteriographic findings in thromboangiitis obliterans with emphasis on femoropopliteal involvement. Am J Radiol 1970;109:553–562.
61. McKusick VA, Harris WS, Ottsen OE, et al. Buerger's disease: a distinct clinical and pathologic entity. JAMA 1962;181:93–100.
62. McKusick VA, Harris WS, Ottsen OE, Goodman RM. The Buerger syndrome in the United States. Arteriographic observations with special reference to involvement of the upper extremities and the differentiation from atherosclerosis and embolism. Bull Johns Hopkins Hosp 1962;110:145–176.
63. Marder VJ, Mellinghoff IK. Cocaine and Buerger disease. Arch Intern Med 2000;160:2057–2060.
64. Disdier P, Granel B, Serratrice J, et al. Cannabis arteritis revisited: ten new case reports. Angiology 2001;52:1–5.
65. Papa MZ, Rabi I, Adar R. A point scoring system for the clinical diagnosis of Buerger's disease. Eur J Vasc Endovasc Surg 1996;11:335–339.
66. Shionoya S. Diagnostic criteria of Buerger's disease. Int J Cardiol 1998;66 (Suppl 1): S243–S245.
67. Shionoya S. What is Buerger's disease? World J Surg 1983;7:544–551.
68. Corelli F. Buerger's disease: cigarette smoker disease may always be cured by medical therapy alone: uselessness of operative treatment. J Cardiovasc Surg 1973;14:28–36.
69. Gifford RW, Hines EA. Complete clinical remission in thromboangiitis obliterans during abstinence from tobacco: report of a case. Proc Staff Meet Mayo Clin 1951;26:241–245.
70. Hooten WM, Bruns HK, Hays JT. Inpatient treatment of severe nicotine dependence in a patient with thromboangiitis obliterans (Buerger's disease). Mayo Clin Proc 1998;73:529–532.
71. Fiessinger JN, Schafer M for the TAO Study. Trial of iloprost vs. aspirin: treatment for critical limb ischemia of thromboangiitis obliterans. Lancet 1990;335:555–557.
72. The European TAO Study Group. Oral iloprost in the treatment of thromboangiitis obliterans (Buerger's disease): a double-blind, randomized, placebo-controlled trial. Eur J Vasc Endovasc Surg 1998;15:300–307.
73. Saha K, Chabra N, Gulati SM. Treatment of patients with thromboangiitis obliterans with cylophosphamide. Angiology 2001;52:399–407.
74. Hussein EA, Dorri AE. Intra-arterial streptokinase as adjuvant therapy for complicated Buerger's disease: early trials. Int Surg 1993;78:54–58.
75. Kubota Y, Kichikawa K, Uchida H, Nishimine K, Hirohashi R, Ohishi H. Superselective urokinase infusion therapy for dorsalis pedis artery occlusion in Buerger's disease. Cardiovasc Intervent Radiol 1997;20:380–382.
76. Inada K, Iwashima Y, Okada A, Matsumoto K. Non-atherosclerotic segmental arterial occlusion of the extremities. Arch Surg 1974;108:663–667.
77. Sayin A, Bozkurt AK, Tuzun H, Vural FS, Erdog G, Ozer M. Surgical treatment of Buerger's disease: experience with 216 patients. Cardiovasc Surg 1993;1:377–380.
78. Sasajima T, Kubo Y, Inaba M, Goh K, Azuma N. Role of infrainguinal bypass in Buerger's disease: an eighteen year experience. J Vasc Endovasc Surg 1997;13:186–192.

79. Shindo S, Saka A, Kubota K et al. Staged vascular reconstruction along with repeatedly performed angiography to prevent ischemic limb loss with Buerger's disease: report of a case. Surg Today 2001; 31:754–758.

80. Singh I, Ramteke VK. The role of omental transfer in Buerger's disease: New Delhi's experience. Aust NZ J Surg 1996;66:372–376.

81. Talwar S, Jain S, Porwal R, Laddha BL, Prasad P. Free versus pedicled omental grafts for limb salvage in Buerger's disease. Aust N Z J Surg 1998;68:38–40.

82. Swigris JJ, Olin JW, Mekhail NA. Implantable spinal cord stimulator to treat the ischemic manifestations of thromboangiitis obliterans (Buerger's disease). J Vasc Surg 1999;29:928-935.

83. Isner JM, Baumgartner I, Rauh G, et al. Treatment of thromboangiitis obliterans (Buerger's disease) by intramuscular gene transfer of vascular endothelial growth factor: preliminary clinical results. J Vasc Surg 1998;28:964–973.

84. Dean SM, Satiani B. Three cases of digital ischemia treated with cilostazol. Vasc Med 2001;6: 245–248.

19 Large-Vessel Vasculitis

Eugene Y. Kissin, MD and
Peter A. Merkel, MD, MPH

INTRODUCTION

Autoimmune inflammation of large-caliber arteries is an unusual cause of vascular insufficiency. Owing to its rarity, the diagnosis of large-vessel vasculitis (LVV) is often initially missed, leading to excess morbidity and mortality. Clues to the diagnosis of LVV include systemic signs of illness such as malaise, weight loss, or fever, with an unusual distribution of ischemic symptoms. Other cases are diagnosed serendipitously at the time of revascularization when inflammation is seen, leading to a search for the underlying cause and altering treatment for these patients.

LVV occurs as a defining manifestation of Takayasu's arteritis, a rare disease, and as an uncommon manifestation of giant cell arteritis, a much more frequent ailment. LVV also arises as an unusual manifestation in conditions such as ankylosing spondylitis, Behçet's disease, relapsing polychondritis, retroperitoneal fibrosis, and Cogan's syndrome.

Diagnosis of diseases causing LVV can be aided by radiographic examination of the vascular system with ultrasound, magnetic resonance imaging, and angiography. Furthermore, radiography can help monitor disease activity and evaluate the effects of therapy.

LVV is thought to develop as a result of autoimmune dysregulation. Thus, therapeutic options for LVV include various antiinflammatory and immunosuppressive medications such as high-dose glucocorticoids, methotrexate, azathioprine, and cyclophosphamide. Revascularization is employed for advanced, limb-threatening cases. However, insufficient control of the underlying inflammatory process may lead to revascularization failure.

From: *Contemporary Cardiology: Peripheral Arterial Disease: Diagnosis and Treatment*
Edited by: J. D. Coffman and R. T. Eberhardt © Humana Press Inc., Totowa, NJ

This chapter describes the clinical presentations of various LVV with an emphasis on giant cell arteritis and Takayasu's arteritis. New information on the utility of vascular imaging systems is also discussed.

GIANT CELL ARTERITIS
History of Giant Cell Arteritis

Dr. Jonathan Hutchinson is credited with the initial scientific description of giant cell arteritis (GCA) in 1890 when he described a man over 80 yr old who was seen due to "red 'streaks on his head' which were painful and prevented his wearing his hat." These streaks were over inflamed and swollen temporal arteries that, over time, lost pulsation *(1)*. In 1935, Barnard described the first case of temporal arteritis leading to vision loss *(2)*. Numerous synonyms exist for GCA, including temporal arteritis, cranial arteritis, and Horton's disease, although Horton was not the first to describe GCA. In 1948, Harrison had already noted that "the disease is far too widespread in its distribution for either 'temporal' or 'cranial' to be accurate" names for the disease *(2)*. Furthermore, biopsies frequently fail to reveal giant cells and other vasculitidies also show giant cell perivascular infiltrate *(3)*. Part of the difficulty in naming this disease stems from its varied presentations, including involvement of extracranial arteries such as the aorta *(4)*, internal carotids, or iliacs *(5)*; the occasional absence of systemic symptoms *(6)*; and sporadic absence of confirmatory histological findings on temporal artery biopsy *(7,8)*. Although glucocorticoids had not yet been discovered, Harrison noted that temporal artery biopsy could give symptomatic relief of headache without changing the course of disease *(2)*.

Epidemiology of GCA

GCA is one of the most common causes of vaculitis, with population-based studies suggesting an incidence of 2–76 per 100,000. GCA may be even more common than these studies indicate. A necropsy series from Sweden found 1.2% of 1326 temporal artery biopsies showed evidence of prior GCA. Of the 16 cases found, only 2 had been diagnosed prior to death, while 9 of the16 had documented symptoms of GCA but did not receive the diagnosis *(9)*.

One of the most characteristic features of GCA is its predilection for the elderly *(10)*. Indeed, one of the criteria for diagnosis is age over 50 *(11)*, and those aged 70–80 are 10 times as likely to develop GCA as those in their 50s *(10)*. Furthermore, women are 1.6–7.0 times as likely as men to develop this disease, possibly because of the increased proportion of women in the elderly population.

Interesting geographic patterns of disease incidence have been noted for GCA, with it being more common among populations in northern climates. The yearly incidence in populations over age 50 ranges from 76 per 100,000 in Denmark to only 1.6 per 100,000 in Tennessee *(12–17)*. Unfortunately, there are no epidemiological studies from countries on the equator or in the Southern hemisphere. Speculation on possible causes for the predilection of GCA for populations in higher longitudes includes migration patterns of a genetically predisposed group or ultraviolet radiation exposure *(18)*.

Histology of GCA

The diagnosis of GCA usually depends on biopsy of a temporal artery *(19)*. Common histological features include intimal hyperplasia as well as inflammation of the arteries and capillaries in the adventitia, media, and intima *(20)*. However, to interpret a biopsy as positive for GCA, fragmentation of the internal elastic lamina in association with an inflammatory infiltrate must be seen. Changes associated with aging can produce progressive intimal thickening, medial atrophy, and disruption of the internal elastic lamina, thus mimicking GCA *(21)*. The presence of multinucleated giant cells is helpful diagnostically but is absent in 40–45% of cases *(22)*. Small-vessel vasculitis surrounding a normal temporal artery is also suggestive of GCA *(23)* (Fig. 1).

Reliance on temporal biopsy for confirmation of the diagnosis of GCA can sometimes lead to confusion when a normal biopsy result is obtained. "Skip lesions" as close as 330 μm apart are a well-recognized feature of GCA *(20)*. Consequently, normal biopsies can be obtained in up to 15% of cases *(7,8,20)*. A 2- to 4-cm unilateral temporal artery biopsy in a patient with GCA will be diagnostic in 85% of cases. Biopsy of the contralateral artery increases the yield by about 5%. The recommendation of serial, multilevel sectioning of temporal artery specimens to increase sensitivity has been somewhat overstated. When examined in a rigorous manner, multilevel sectioning leads to additional diagnoses of GCA in only 2% of cases *(3)*. In addition to skip lesions, the absence of suggestive histological changes on biopsy may be due to milder disease. Patients with negative temporal artery biopsies are substantially less likely to have symptoms of jaw claudication, visual changes, or temporal artery abnormalities on examination *(24,25)*.

Concern is often raised about the effect of glucocorticoid therapy on the subsequent diagnostic yield in temporal artery biopsy. A study by Achkar and colleagues reviewed 535 temporal artery biopsies in a blinded fashion and collected information on length of glucocorticoid use. This study suggests that the diagnostic yield of temporal artery biopsy is not decreased by up to 2 wk of glucocorticoid therapy *(26)*.

Pathogenesis of GCA

While the etiology of GCA is not yet known, there is evidence that GCA develops as a maladaptive response to arterial injury *(27)*. Antigen-selected CD4 T cells are recruited to inflamed blood vessels and produce interferon-γ (INF-γ) along with other inflammatory cytokines. INF-γ, in particular, has been linked to ischemic complications in this disease. INF-γ may induce ischemia by stimulating multinucleated giant cells to produce platelet-derived growth factor (PDGF) and vascular endothelial growth factor (VEGF). This response may be an attempt to repair injury but instead leads to intimal hyperplasia and luminal obstruction. Macrophage response to IFN-γ may also depend on the local environment, with adventitial macrophages producing interleukin-6 (IL-6), medial macrophages producing metalloprotinases, and intimal macrophages producing nitric oxide (NO) and PDGF *(28,29)*. These responses may cause the characteristic histological findings of inflammation, disruption of the elastic lamina, medial atrophy, and intimal injury/hyperplasia.

Clinical Findings of GCA

Manifestations of GCA can be subcategorized into those due to systemic inflammation and those due to vascular compromise (Table 1). The most common systemic symptoms include those of polymyalgia rheumatica (PMR), which are fever, weight loss, malaise, morning joint stiffness, and proximal limb girdle pain *(30)*. While 40% of patients with GCA develop classical PMR symptoms during the course of this disease,

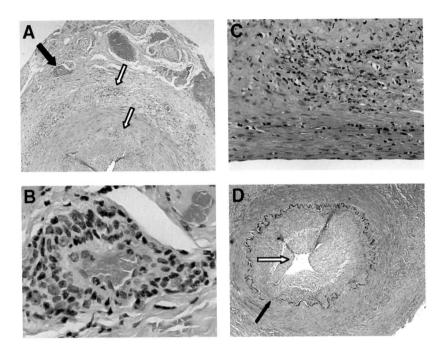

Fig. 1. Biopsy specimen from the temporal artery of a patient with GCA. **(A)** Low-power view showing small-vessel vasculitis around the vasa vasorum in the adventitia (*solid arrow*) and mononuclear inflammatory cells in the adventitia, media, and intima (*open arrows*). **(B)** High-power view of small-vessel vasculitis. **(C)** High-power view of the intima–media junction showing infiltration by inflammatory cells. **(D)** Elastin stain demonstrating fragmentation of the internal elastic lamina (*solid arrow*) and hypertrophy of the intima causing luminal stenosis (*open arrow*)

Table 1
Clinical Manifestations of GCA

Clinical finding	Percent of GCA patients
New headache	87–93
Temporal artery abnormality	47–73
Jaw claudication	42–50
Polymyalgia rheumatica	29–57
Fever	27–37
Ophthalmologic features	26–60
Blurred vision	43
Amaurosis fugax	6–33
Permanent visual loss	15
Diplopia	4–10
Eye pain	5–8
Neurologic symptoms	17
Synovitis	6
Stroke	2

Data from refs. *8,24,25,36,37,42.*

23% will also develop peripheral joint or soft tissue abnormalities *(31)*. Although arthralgias (joint pain without effusion) are most common, true synovitis occurs in 13% of patients. Thus, PMR with arthritis can be difficult to differentiate from elderly-onset rheumatoid arthritis.

Vascular symptoms of GCA are limited to external cranial arteries in 90% of patients *(32,33)*. The resulting symptoms of headache, temporal artery tenderness, and jaw claudication commonly occur and are predictive of future vascular compromise if left untreated *(34–37)*. Other manifestations of cranial artery involvement include toothache (3%), tongue pain and claudication (5%), facial pain (16%), and vertigo or hearing loss (7%) *(38)*. Cranial arteritis can be so extensive as to cause scalp or tongue necrosis. Blindness is the most feared and common permanent end-organ complication of GCA, and occurs mainly due to occlusion of the ophthalmic (81%), cilioretinal (22%), or central retinal artery (14%) *(39)*.

Prior to the availability of glucocorticoid treatment, vision loss occurred in 50–60% of patients with GCA *(35,40)*. With glucocorticoid use this complication has decreased to 8–22%. While only 50% of GCA patients report visual symptoms, an autopsy study found evidence of posterior ciliary arteritis in 75% of GCA cases *(41)*. Importantly, up to 65% of permanent vision loss is preceded by more subtle visual abnormalities such as blurred vision, amaurosis fugax, diplopia, eye pain, or visual hallucinations (Charles Bonnet syndrome) (Table 1) *(42)*. From 37% to 64% of transient visual abnormalities are followed by permanent vision loss *(35,38)*.

Predisposing factors for vision loss include transient visual symptoms, other cranial vascular compromise such as jaw claudication, HLA type (DRB1*04), and temporal artery biopsy positivity *(8,34,35)*. Interestingly, fever, weight loss, elevated liver enzymes, and a negative temporal artery biopsy are negative predictors of eye involvement *(34,35,37)*. Permanent vision loss developed a mean of 15 d after the first visual symptom *(36)*. However, these are not strong predictors and patients may present with monocular blindness and no other symptoms of GCA *(6)*.

Stroke is another serious complication of GCA. Patients with visual manifestations are at a much higher lifetime risk of stroke *(35)*. Fifty percent of GCA-associated strokes involve the vertebral–basilar territory, while only 15–20% of atherosclerotic strokes arise from these arteries. Strokes tend to occur 1–3 wk after visual symptoms and treatment with high-dose glucocorticoids may fail to prevent these dreaded events.

GCA can involve large noncranial arteries in 10% of cases *(32,33)*. The aorta is the most commonly involved noncranial artery in GCA (Fig. 2), followed by upper extremity arteries *(4,33)*, with only occasional reports of lower extremity involvement *(43)*. Similarly to patients with other causes of LVV, these manifestations are associated with claudicatory symptoms, auscultatory bruits over the arteries, and pulse deficits. One study found 23 of 248 (9%) GCA patients to have definite large-vessel involvement *(33)*. A population-based retrospective study found the incidence of thoracic aneurysms in patients with GCA to be increased 17 times and abdominal aneurysms 2.4 times that of an age-matched population *(4)*. In this series, the diagnosis of aortic aneurysm was made 2–10 yr after the initial diagnosis of GCA.

Patients with GCA and LVV present somewhat differently than classic GCA and share common clinical characteristics as well as HLA haplotype associations with patients afflicted with Takayasu's arteritis *(5)*. Only 10% of patients with GCA and LVV present with headache and only 1% develop symptoms of visual changes or jaw claudi-

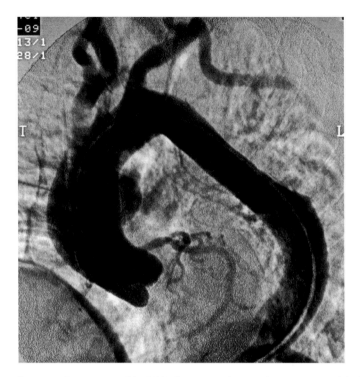

Fig. 2. Aortic angiogram of a woman with GCA demonstrating aortic aneurysm with dissection.

cation. Other patients have an abdominal aortic aneurysm and no symptoms of classic GCA but have periaortic inflammation that is noted during surgery and GCA found in surgical specimens of the aortic wall *(44)*. How to classify patients with aortic vasculitis and no other signs or symptoms of disease is debatable, as is the necessity of immunosuppressive therapy. Perhaps the most rational approach would be to regularly screen these patients for other areas of vascular involvement with history, physical examination, and radiographic studies and make treatment decisions based on the results.

Laboratory Findings in GCA

An elevated erythrocyte sedimentation rate (ESR) remains the laboratory test most closely associated with PMR and GCA. However, 5–15% of patients with GCA will have a normal or minimally elevated ESR *(45)*. These patients are also less likely to exhibit systemic signs or symptoms of disease and most have a blunted inflammatory response to other stimuli. In patients with a high ESR, the ESR may fail to completely normalize even with successful treatment *(46)*. Furthermore, there is some evidence that the ESR and other markers of systemic inflammation are raised to a lesser degree in patients with GCA and ischemic complications than in those patients without such complications *(37)*.

Other markers of inflammation such as the C-reactive protein (CRP) have been used to complement the ESR, with the combination of studies providing the highest specificity for GCA of 97% *(46,47)*. CRP has also been found to respond more promptly to therapy, but is a less-sensitive marker of relapse compared to ESR (44% vs 52%) *(46)*.

Neither test is able to consistently predict clinical relapse of disease, as elevation of ESR and CRP occurs prior to relapse in only 20% and 26% of patients, respectively.

Other markers for inflammation seen in GCA include a normocytic anemia, thrombocytosis, hyperfibrinogenemia, and elevated alkaline phosphatase *(30,37)*. Thrombocytosis of $> 400 \times 10^9$ /L is associated with twice the risk of vision loss in GCA with the increased risk correlating with the degree of thrombocytosis *(34)*. The increased risk of vision loss may be a direct effect of increased platelets and may warrant anticoagulant therapy. Alternatively, thrombocytosis may be a surrogate marker of increased PDGF levels produced by macrophages and multinucleated giant cells, correlating with the degree of intimal hyperplasia *(29)*.

Other cytokines have also been investigated in GCA. One study found IL-2 levels to be inversely related to the risk for cranial ischemic complications *(48,49)*. In addition, levels of IL-6 have been found to correlate with disease activity and may be responsible for inducing an acute-phase response *(50)*.

Diagnosis of GCA

The diagnosis of GCA is established by combining clinical history, physical examination findings, laboratory abnormalities, and temporal artery biopsy. The American College of Rheumatology criteria for classification of GCA serve as a useful guide for clinicians faced with the possibility of GCA in a patient *(11)*. The five criteria for diagnosis of GCA include age over 50, new onset of localized headache, temporal artery tenderness or decrease in pulse, ESR over 50, and temporal artery biopsy with necrotizing arteritis comprised of mononuclear or granulomatous infiltrate. Meeting three of five criteria gives a sensitivity of 93% and a specificity of 91% in differentiating GCA from other forms of vasculitis. Temporal artery biopsy may be virtually diagnostic for GCA but is not absolutely required. Although diagnostic imaging techniques such as ultrasound are intriguing, they are not yet accepted as replacements for arterial biopsy.

Treatment of Giant Cell Arteritis

Glucocorticoids are the mainstay of therapy for all aspects of GCA and are effective for both symptomatic relief and prevention of vascular compromise. As untreated GCA can lead to sudden, irreversible loss of vision as well as other less common consequences of vasculitis, many physicians have treated GCA with immediate high-dose (≥ 1 mg/kg of prednisone or equivalent) glucocorticoid therapy *(40,51,52)*. Some controversy exists among the fields of rheumatology, ophthalmology, and neurology as to whether pulse doses of intravenous glucocorticoids as high as 1 g of methylprednisolone daily for the first 3 d are necessary for the treatment of GCA-induced vascular compromise. There have been no studies that adequately compare glucocorticoid dose regimens for patients with GCA-induced visual disturbances.

Retrospective studies have not found an advantage to the use of initial high-dose glucocorticoids *(40,51–53)*. However, excluding patients with established ocular or neurological complications, any dose of prednisone above 20 mg daily or the equivalent seems to be equipotent in preventing future visual or neurological complications. These studies found that only 2–5% of patients without visual or neurological manifestations initially, develop them after glucocorticoid treatment. Visual or neurological complications usually occurred during tapering of glucocorticoid dosage, and were mostly transient and seemingly responsive to increases in glucocorticoid dosage *(40)*.

Various glucocorticoid tapering schedules have been employed for the treatment of GCA. The data available indicate that a moderately rapid tapering schedule (to 20 mg of prednisone daily over 2 mo) is associated with more relapses but no increase in visual complications (54). Similarly, alternate day glucocorticoid dosing is associated with a greater risk of relapse than daily dosing (55). Alternate day therapy completely controlled arteritis in only 30% of patients compared to 75% on daily therapy of equal dose. However, retrospective studies have found life-threatening side effects of glucocorticoid therapy such as severe infections and major upper gastrointestinal bleeds to be twice as common in GCA patients taking 30–40 mg of prednisone as those taking lower doses (14% vs 33%) (52).

This body of literature seems to suggest that in patients with GCA without visual symptoms the equivalent of 40 mg of prednisone followed by a tapering schedule aiming to achieve a 20 mg daily dose in 2 mo will sufficiently suppress disease symptoms and prevent visual consequences while limiting glucocorticoid-related side effects. For patients with visual or neurological manifestations, 1 mg/kg initial dosage would seem reasonable to attempt to prevent further damage from vasculitis, but there is no evidence for superior efficacy of higher doses. Furthermore, it is unlikely that glucocorticoids reverse established visual loss but they may reduce the risk of further visual deterioration (56). As speed of initiation of glucocorticoid administration may be more important than overall dose, intravenous administration should be used in patients with delayed or abnormal gastrointestinal absorption.

In an effort to reduce the cumulative toxicity of glucocorticoids, the use of various immunosuppressive agents has been studied in patients with GCA. Small, open-labeled or underpowered studies of azathioprine (57), dapsone (58), cyclophosphamide (59), and cyclosporin (60) were not definitive regarding drug efficacy. Recently, two moderately sized, randomized, double-blind, placebo-controlled trials of weekly oral methotrexate as adjuvant therapy to glucocorticoids in patients with GCA were performed (61,62). The first study of 42 patients at a single center demonstrated a reduction in clinical relapses and total glucocorticoid dose in the methotrexate and prednisone group vs the prednisone alone group. In contrast, the second study of 98 patients at 16 centers showed no benefit in terms of relapse or prednisone dose sparing in the patients treated with methotrexate, although relapses of polymyalgia rheumatica symptoms were less frequent in the methotrexate group. Although there were some differences in the method of glucocorticoid tapering and disease assessment, these two studies were quite complementary. The starkly different results are difficult to understand. Until and unless other data become available, the question of the efficacy of low- to medium-dose methotrexate for GCA is not settled. There are currently plans to study newer biological agents, such as inhibitors of tumor necrosis factor-α (TNF-α), in GCA. Future collaborative studies of GCA should help refine therapy.

Prognosis for GCA

The overall prognosis for GCA is generally favorable if the disease is recognized and treated early. Only 1% of patients with GCA will die of the disease, usually due to aortic dissection (33). However, up to 15% of patients will lose vision in one eye, and 2% will suffer a stroke even with glucocorticoid therapy, leading to significant morbidity (Table 1). Although most patients can expect to be symptom free at the end of 3 yr of glucocorticoid therapy, up to half will still require a small dose of prednisone and most patients with GCA will experience the morbidity of glucocorticoid side effects *(25)*.

TAKAYASU'S ARTERITIS

History of Takayasu's Arteritis

Perhaps the earliest description of Takayasu's arteritis (TAK) was made in 1830, when Dr. Rokushu Yamamoto detailed the medical history of a 45-yr-old man with fever who lost his right radial pulse and developed a decreased left radial pulse while maintaining normal lower extremity pulsations *(63)*. In 1905, Dr. Mikito Takayasu, an ophthalmologist, described arteriovenous anastomoses of retinal vessels in a 21-yr-old woman. Although he did not describe the remainder of her vascular exam, his report is accepted as the first scientific documentation of "pulseless disease" or TAK. Dr. Kunio Ohta published the first pathologic description of the disease in 1940.

Epidemiology of TAK

TAK primarily affects young women, with a female-to-male ratio ranging from 1.6:1 to 8:1 depending on the study *(64)*. The average age at disease onset is 30, with only 15% developing the disease after age 40 *(65)*. TAK also has a higher incidence in people of Asian descent with 10% of patients with TAK in the NIH cohort being Asian, while Asians comprise only 2.9% of the US population *(65)*. The disease has a worldwide distribution with an incidence ranging from 200 per million in Japan to only 2 per million in Minnesota *(66)*.

Histology of Takayasu's Arteritis

The histological features of TAK are indistinguishable from that of GCA, with lymphocytic and plasma cell infiltrate around the vasa vasorum, medial necrosis, and neovascularization, as well as intimal proliferation *(67)*. As the acute inflammatory stage resolves, marked adventitial and medial fibrosis ensues. However, clinical signs and symptoms are frequently inaccurate in predicting histological activity. The NIH TAK series demonstrated that 44% of arterial biopsies from patients thought to be in remission exhibited active inflammation *(65)*.

Pathogenesis of Takayasu's Arteritis

Although the cause of TAK is not well understood, there may be a genetic predisposition as evidenced by HLA associations *(68)*. The disease begins with an initial inflammatory phase during which T cells are thought to be activated by an unknown antigen and infiltrate the adventitia and outer media of the aorta and/or its major branches. This phase is usually asymptomatic, but can include fever, arthralgia, and weight loss *(69)*. The activated T cells appear to be guided to particular regions in the vascular system by chemoattractant chemokines such as Regulated on Activation, Normal T Cell Expressed and Secreted (RANTES) *(70)*. Levels of RANTES correlate with disease activity, but are elevated above levels found in healthy controls even at times of apparent disease quiescence. Similarly to GCA, activated T cells are thought to produce vascular inflammation through the secretion of IL-6, which is found at high levels in aortic tissue from patients with TAK *(71)*. Serum IL-6 levels also correlate with disease activity *(70)*.

Clinical Manifestations of TAK

The initial manifestations of TAK may include constitutional symptoms of malaise, fever, and weight loss in two thirds of patients, but are frequently absent in older patients (Table 2) *(72)*. Systemic symptoms are then followed by manifestations of vascular insufficiency, which are a hallmark of this disease *(69)*. The clinical manifestations of TAK are generally related to the function of the territory supplied by diseased arteries (Fig. 3). The most common areas of disease are the subclavian arteries, with stenosis found in 54–92% of cases *(65,69,73,74)*. The aorta is the next most commonly involved site (53–80%) followed by the renal arteries (38–62%). Lower extremity arteries are affected in 17–25% of cases but rarely in isolation. For unclear reasons, left-sided carotid and upper extremity artery involvement is twice as common as right-sided disease. Aneurysms occur in 9–27% of patients and are more frequently found in the aorta compared to its branch vessels *(65)*. Furthermore, aneurysms are most commonly found in poststenotic regions with only 4% occurring in isolation.

Patients with TAK often report upper extremity claudication (29–62%), due to subclavian or axillary artery lesions, and carotodynia (32%) *(65)*. Lower extremity involvement with intermittent claudication is less common. Central nervous system symptoms including lightheadedness and headache are common *(65)*. Headache may be related to vascular insufficiency or new onset hypertension due to renal artery stenosis. Malignant hypertension can also produce volume overload, dyspnea, and orthopnea. In the NIH cohort, 17 of 20 patients with hypertension had renal artery stenosis, although not all patients with renal artery stenosis had hypertension. Dyspnea may be a manifestation of aortic insufficiency secondary to aortic root dilatation or pulmonary hypertension due to pulmonary artery involvement *(75,76)*.

Less common but potentially catastrophic arterial involvement of the coronary arteries has been reported in 9% of patients *(69)*, and may result in angina, myocardial infarction, and death. Thus, chest pain in patients with TAK must be carefully evaluated for coronary artery disease despite the young age. Similarly, TAK should be considered in young women with symptoms of angina and evidence for myocardial ischemia. Coronary lesions are mostly ostial (73%) or nonostial proximal (18.5%) and half occur in the left main coronary artery *(77,78)*. Other unusual, but lethal, manifestations of TAK include isolated pulmonary arteritis (7.5%), and isolated thoracic aortic (2.7%) and abdominal aortic aneurysms (1.4%) *(76)*.

During the physical examination, hypertension (33–72%), bruits (80–94%) and diminished pulses (53–96%) are often found *(65,69,73,74)*. Blood pressure should be taken in all four extremities, as a stenotic lesion will lower blood pressure distally. It is important to realize that not all stenotic lesions produce symptoms of claudication, as obstruction develops gradually, allowing collateral circulation to develop. Routine fundoscopic examination can detect abnormalities in 40% of patients including arterial narrowing (21%), venous dilatation (27%), microaneurysms (3%), and classic arteriovenous anastomoses (5%) as described by Dr. Takayasu himself *(79)*. Aortic regurgitation occurs in 20% of patients *(65)* with a detectable murmur in half, and an increased pulse pressure in 74%, of these patients. Cardiac examination can also show evidence of left (28%) or right (7%) heart failure *(69)*. Abdominal palpation and auscultation may reveal signs of aortic aneurysm or renal artery stenosis. Musculoskeletal examination will demonstrate synovitis in one fifth of patients, usually a nonerosive, symmetric,

Table 2
Clinical Manifestations of TAK at the Time of Diagnosis

Clinical findings	Percent of TAK patients
Fever	11–25
Malaise	30–56
Weight loss	17–22
Arthralgias	6–53
Claudication	29–62
Pulse deficit	60–100
Bruit	28–94
Vascular pain	32
ESR elevation	72–83
CRP elevation	23
Anemia	25

Data from refs. *65,69,73,74.*

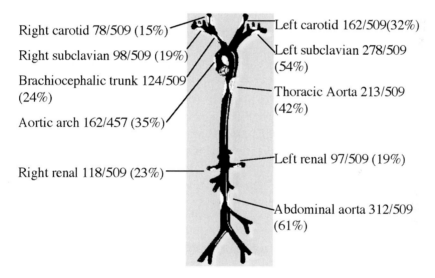

Fig. 3. Regions of arterial involvement in TAK *(65,69,73,74).*

peripheral polyarthritis of small and large joints *(74)*. Neurological evaluation may detect signs of a stroke and skin inspection identifies erythema nodosum in 8% of patients *(65)*.

Laboratory Testing in Takayasu's Arteritis

Currently used laboratory studies are of moderate value for diagnosis and treatment of TAK. ESR is elevated in 72–83% of patients with early, active disease *(69,74)* and tends to decline with disease duration *(72)*. However, even in patients thought to be in remission, 44% have ESR elevation *(65)*. Furthermore, tissue samples from four patients during bypass surgery demonstrated disease activity, but only one patient had an elevated ESR *(65)*. Many patients with active TAK have a normal ESR. Thus there are serious questions about both the sensitivity and specificity of ESR in TAK.

Other laboratory tests are even less helpful for determination of disease activity in TAK. The CRP is elevated in 23% of cases *(69)*, while anemia is present in 25–44% *(69,74)*. This may suggest a dichotomy between the systemic inflammatory response, which correlates well with acute phase reactants, and vascular inflammation, which correlates less well. There is no association of TAK with antinuclear antibodies or rheumatoid factor, and recent studies have failed to find an association with antiaortic antibodies *(80)*. Perhaps future studies will determine particular serum cytokine levels, which will be more sensitive and specific for vascular inflammation *(70)*.

Diagnosis of TAK

The diagnosis of TAK is based on findings confirming inflammation, fibrosis, and stenosis of large arterial vessels without alternative causes for these findings. In most cases these findings include the history of claudication in conjunction with systemic symptoms, bruits, and pulse deficits on examination, and radiographic evidence of large vessel stenosis. Angiography has traditionally been used to survey areas of vascular involvement, and magnetic resonance imaging (MRI) as well as ultrasound can be complementary by adding information about vessel wall thickness and inflammation. The American College of Rheumatology proposed criteria for the classification of TAK in 1990 which include (1) disease onset at age ≤40, (2) extremity claudication, (3) decreased brachial artery pulse, (4) systolic blood pressure difference > 10mmHg between arms, (5) subclavian or aortic bruit, and (6) arteriographic indication of narrowing or occlusion of the aorta or its major branches *(66)*. Meeting three or more of the six criteria provides a sensitivity of 90.5% and a specificity of 97.8% for differentiating TAK from other types of vasculitis *(66)*. Clinical criteria in conjunction with serologic studies help exclude alternative causes such as infection, other vasculitidies, and noninflammatory vasculopathy. While histological section may be consistent with the diagnosis of TAK, the large-caliber vessels involved are not easily biopsied and are rarely obtained. Owing to the low incidence and indolent nature of TAK, diagnosis is often delayed for years.

Treatment of Takayasu's Arteritis

Treatment of TAK can be subdivided into treatment of the underlying inflammatory process and treatment of the arterial narrowing that follows. Glucocorticoids remain the mainstay of treatment for vascular inflammation but, unfortunately, are not always effective. In the NIH cohort of TAK, high-dose glucocorticoids induced "clinical remission" in only 50% of patients over an average of 22 mo *(65)*. However, a study from the Mayo Clinic found that 8 of 16 patients treated with high doses (1 mg/kg) of glucocorticoids regained absent pulses *(74)*. Others have documented radiographically the regression of arterial stenosis after glucocorticoid treatment *(81)*. The chronic nature of TAK necessitates prolonged glucocorticoid use that is associated with significant toxicity.

Immunosuppressive agents are used in the treatment of TAK to both improve remission rates and provide a "steroid-sparing" effect. There are no large-scale or well-designed studies to assess the relative efficacy of various immunosuppressive agents. Cyclophosphamide (2 mg/kg) induced "remission" in 33% of patients from the NIH cohort who failed on glucocorticoids alone *(65)*. A smaller study found that methotrexate in combination with glucocorticoids could induce "remission" in 13 of 16 patients resistant to glucocorticoids alone *(82)*. Small case series of successful use of mycophenolate mofetil for TAK resistant to glucocorticoids have been reported. Cyclophosphamide, azathioprine, and mycophenolate mofetil are other therapies proposed for use in TAK *(83)*. Anecdotally, vasculitis centers appear to commonly use methotrexate and azathioprine and reserve cyclophosphamide for extreme circumstances.

Further uncertainty about the efficacy of treatment arises from disparate effects of glucocorticoids on the systemic inflammatory symptoms and on vascular stenosis. Whereas systemic symptoms and markers of inflammation such as the ESR improve within days to weeks, vascular abnormalities improve over months *(74)*. In addition, vascular compromise can progress during therapy in two thirds of cases while systemic symptoms are absent *(65)*. These data suggest that continuous, long-term therapy with an immunosuppressive agent such as methotrexate may help both taper glucocorticoid dosage, thus limiting side effects, and reduce subclinical disease progression. This strategy of prolonged therapy has yet to be proven in clinical trials. It is also important to realize that worsening vascular compromise may be due to fibrotic changes in a vessel and not active inflammation. This observation highlights the need for better measures of disease activity.

Perhaps as important as treating the inflammatory component of TAK is the treatment of disease complications. Because heart failure is the main cause of mortality in TAK, aggressive management of hypertension is vital *(84)*. Angiotensin converting enzyme inhibitors, however, should not be used unless bilateral renal artery stenosis has been ruled out. Treatment with β-blockers has been shown to effectively reduce morbidity in patients with aortic insufficiency due to TAK *(85,86)*. Furthermore, treatment of hyperlipidemia will prevent additional injury to already compromised vessels.

Interventional procedures such as bypass grafting and angioplasty play a role in relieving ischemia due to TAK, although the outcomes have been mixed. While angioplasty can be performed successfully in more than 80% of cases, the 5-yr patency rates have ranged from 33% to 60% depending on the artery *(87–89)*. Complete vessel occlusion and long segments of stenosis are negative predictors for angioplasty success. Any advantage to stent placement for vascular insufficiency of inflammatory cause is still to be determined. While a study of long-term outcome in subclavian angioplasty showed no correlation between elevated ESR and restenosis rate *(88)*, patients with active vasculitis of any artery are generally discouraged from undergoing nonemergent angioplasty. In addition, 1 of 20 patients suffered the complication of distal embolization during the procedure. Renal artery angioplasty can result in normalization of blood pressure in 50% of technically successful cases and improvement in another 30% *(65,89)*.

Bypass grafting also remains an option for treatment of inflammatory vessel stenosis. Of 60 described cases of coronary artery bypass grafting in TAK, 5 operative deaths occurred *(78)*. In the 50 bypass procedures performed during the NIH study, 24% were complicated by restenosis *(65)*. Most of these restenoses occurred in synthetic grafts, as only 1 of 11 autologous graft placements developed restenosis. The chronic, progressive nature of TAK also induces bypass graft occlusion. Therefore, postoperative glucocorticoid therapy may be warranted. Of those patients who received postoperative glucocorticoid treatment, 11 of 12 vessels were patent on short-term follow-up compared to 6 of 13 grafts in patients without postoperative glucocorticoids *(78)*. Interestingly, after adjusting for major complications, patients treated surgically do not have a statistically different survival from those who receive medical treatment alone *(90)*.

Prognosis of Takayasu's Arteritis

The mortality rate of TAK is 13% over 13 yr with 62% of deaths occurring in the first 5 yr after diagnosis *(90)*. Deaths associated with TAK result mainly from involvement of the renal and pulmonary arteries as well as from heart failure *(90)*. TAK is a chronic and often progressive disease. The NIH cohort showed that 45% of patients have disease flares over an average of 5.3 yr. Not surprisingly, 88% of patients developed new angiographic lesions during a period of "active" disease. However, even more concerning was the finding of new lesions during apparent clinical "remission" in 61% of cases *(65)*.

OTHER CAUSES OF LARGE VESSEL VASCULITIS

A number of other autoimmune diseases have been associated with large vessel inflammation including Behçet's disease, ankylosing spondylitis, relapsing polychondritis, retroperitoneal fibrosis, and Cogan's syndrome. However, as LVV is an uncommon feature of these diseases, we mention only some of them briefly.

Behçet's Disease

Behçet's disease (BD) is a systemic autoimmune disease that usually presents with recurrent oral and genital ulcers as well as uveitis *(91)*. The uveitis may be sight threatening. Arthritis, rash, vasculitis, and systemic symptoms are all part of BD. This disease is much more common in Turkey, along the silk route, and in parts of Japan than in other parts of the world. Men are at slightly greater risk (RR 1.3) than women and symptoms usually develop in young to middle-aged adults.

The prevalence of vascular involvement in patients with BD at a major hospital in Turkey was found to be 28% (of 137 patients) *(92)*. However, only 5 of 38 patients with vascular lesions or 3.6% of all patients with BD had arterial disease. Vasculitis is more common among men (RR 4.4) and in those with a positive pathergy test or eye involvement. In addition, vascular inflammation is almost never the presenting manifestation of BD but occurs an average of 7 yr after the first sign of disease *(93)*.

Arterial involvement may be occlusive and/or aneurysmal and involve the aorta and its main branches. Unlike in TAK, occlusive lesions are more frequent in the lower extremities, and usually are single lesions *(94)*. BD holds a particular predilection for the pulmonary arteries, and can also involve arteries supplying the gastrointestinal system. BD is one of the few vascular disorders to affect both the arterial and venous systems. Phlebitis and venous thrombosis are common problems in BD. Stroke is a particularly devastating problem in BD and can result from vasculitis or thrombosis.

Mucocutaneous lesions and arthritis respond to treatment with colchicine *(95)*, methotrexate *(96)*, or thalidomide *(97)*. Uveitis requires aggressive immunosuppressive therapy with azathioprine *(98)*, cyclosporin A *(99)*, clorambucil *(100)*, or other agents. Immunosuppression with clorambucil or cyclophosphamide may provide benefit over glucocorticoids alone for the vasculitis of BD *(93)*, but controlled studies have not been performed.

The tendency toward aneurysm and clot formation frequently complicates interventional procedures such as angioplasty and bypass grafting. Although postoperative glucocorticoids seem to decrease rates of restenosis, one center reported that 84% of grafts failed over 6 yr despite glucocorticoids *(93)*. A frequent cause of death in patients with aneurysms is vessel rupture *(94)*. The overall mortality rate for BD patients after 15 yr of arterial involvement is 34% *(93)*.

Relapsing Polychondritis

Relapsing polychondritis (RPC) shares many features with BD. This disorder is characterized by recurrent and progressive inflammation of cartilaginous structures and severe lesions in the eyes, ears, and upper respiratory system. RPC presents with recurrent 1- to 2-wk long episodes of painful ear swelling in one fourth of cases and as arthritis in another fourth, while almost never presenting as arteritis. The disease is most common during adulthood, does not have a sex predilection *(101)*, and has rarely been reported in non-Caucasian races *(102)*. Histological evaluation reveals perichondral inflammation, loss of basophilic staining of the cartilage matrix, and replacement of cartilage with fibrous tissue. The histology of inflamed vessels can be distinguished from that of other large vessel arteritidies by histochemical staining demonstrating the loss of glycosaminoglycans *(103)*.

The periodic inflammation commonly affects the ears (85–95%), while sparing the ear lobes, and the joints (52–85%), producing an inflammatory, nonerosive, asymmetric, oligo- or polyarthritis affecting the large and small joints. Other areas of involvement include the nasal cartilage (48–72%); the eyes (51–65%), producing an often severe scleritis, uveitis, or keratitis; the larynx and trachea (48–67%); and the cochlea and vestibular apparatus (26–53%) *(101,102,104)*.

Cardiac involvement can be manifest by conduction defects in 1–2% or valvular disease in 6–9% of cases. Valvular incompetence can be due to inflammatory dilatation of the aortic ring or, less commonly, valvulitis *(105)*.

Arterial inflammation has been reported in 10–18% of patients *(102)*, with half of these cases involving large arteries *(101)*. Unlike TAK, there is no predilection for upper extremity vessels; many cases involve only a single lesion and aneurysm formation is as common as stenosis (Fig. 4).

Treatment of RPC with glucocorticoids seems to be effective in many patients but those with resistant disease, with respiratory tract involvement, or with a vasculitic component should be treated with additional medications such as cyclophosphamide, azathioprine, methotrexate, or dapsone. Thirteen percent of deaths from RPC are a result of vasculitis or ruptured aneurysm and 50% are due to airway collapse *(101)*. The overall mortality rate has been reported to range from 30% in 4 yr *(101)* to 6% in 8 yr *(102)*. The rarity of this disease has prevented any controlled studies of immunosuppressive therapy.

Spondyloarthopathy

The seronegative spondyloarthropathies, including ankylosing spondylitis (AS), reactive arthritis, psoriatic arthritis, and arthritis associated with inflammatory bowel disease, are associated with aortitis. Most reports of aortitis concern patients with AS, an autoimmune disease causing inflammation primarily in the sacroiliac joints and spine. AS is one of the more common rheumatic diseases to cause aortitis. Proximal aortic involvement develops in about 5% of patients after an average of 15 yr resulting in aortic valve incompetence *(106)*. AS typically affects young adults with a 3:1 male predominance, causing inflammatory back pain and enthesitis.

Along with iritis and apical lung fibrosis, cardiovascular involvement is an extraskeletal manifestation of AS. Aortic insufficiency occurs due to fibrotic thickening

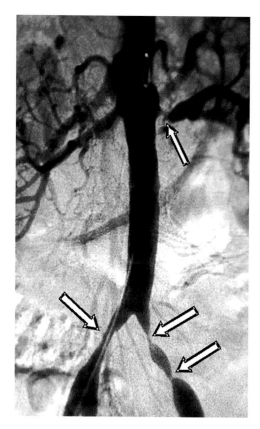

Fig. 4. Angiogram of patient with relapsing polychondritis showing renal artery and iliac stenosis (*open arrows*).

of the aortic valve cusps and the aortic wall behind and above the sinuses of Valsalva as well as below the aortic valve, forming a subvalvular ridge *(107,108)*. This characteristic subvalvular extension "bump" is characteristic of AS and can progress to thickening of the basal portion of the anterior mitral leaflet as well as conduction abnormalities (Fig. 5) *(107)*. Transesophageal echocardiography can detect this subvalvular ridge in about 80% of AS cases with mild to moderate aortic insufficiency, whereas transthoracic echocardiography is unable to visualize this pathologic structure *(109)*. On histological section, typical vasculitic involvement of the aorta can be seen.

Aortic insufficiency usually develops in long-standing disease with peripheral joint involvement *(110)*. On autopsy, 20% of patients with AS have aortic valve disease but only half of these patients have clinically detectable valvular dysfunction prior to death *(111)*. On the other hand, 7–19% of lone aortic insufficiency cases are associated with spondyloarthropathies *(112,113)*, suggesting that patients with unexplained aortic insufficiency should be evaluated for spondyloarthopathy.

Empiric treatment with glucocorticoids and cyclophosphamide for the aortitis of AS has been used but controlled trials are lacking. Similar to other inflammatory causes of aortitis, surgical treatment is complicated by aneurysm formation and leaks in prostheses *(106)*.

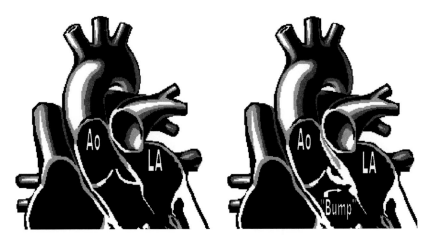

Fig. 5. Cartoon of aortic lesion due to ankylosing spondylitis with thickening of the posterior aortic wall, aortic leaflet, and mitral leaflet as well as subvalvular "bump."

RADIOLOGIC AND ULTRASOUND ASSESSMENT

Diagnostic imaging is helpful in the assessing LVV in three ways: (1) defining and localizing new symptomatic lesions, (2) screening for asymptomatic lesions, and (3) monitoring disease progression. The three main modalities to accomplish these goals include conventional angiography, magnetic resonance angiography (MRA), and duplex ultrasound. Each method offers particular advantages and drawbacks as outlined in Table 3. While there are case reports of the use of computed tomography (CT) scanning *(114)*, nuclear imaging *(115)*, and positron emission tomography (PET) scanning in the literature *(116)*, these modalities have not been well characterized for evaluation of large vessel vasculitis.

Angiography for Large Vessel Vasculitis

Angiography has long been the radiographic gold standard for evaluating vascular lesions. Angiography can evaluate any arterial vessel of large to medium caliber but has a number of disadvantages: it is invasive, requires contrast dye use, and does not evaluate vessel wall thickness. Angiographic images of vessels damaged by inflammation appear as smoothly tapering stenotic areas both at the leading and trailing ends *(117)*. This is in distinction to the irregular, coarse lesions seen in arteriosclerotic disease. In LVV, areas of stenosis alternate with segments of normal diameter and rarely involve small to medium arteries without also involving more proximal vessels. Furthermore, because the progression to stenosis is not usually acute, bridging collateral arteries may be present and help differentiate vasculitis from thrombotic, embolic, or vasospastic causes of stenosis. Angiographic imaging with sufficient contrast and prolonged filming can detect these collaterals that other imaging modalities would miss.

Angiography is excellent for evaluating the distribution of vessel involvement, and detecting diseased but asymptomatic vessels. However, there are no definitive angiographic distinctions among the various large vessel vasculitidies. Traditional contrast

Table 3
Comparison of Radiographic Modalities Useful for Evaluating LVV

Imaging modality	Invasive	Cost	Localization of established lesions	Detection of early disease	Monitoring disease activity/ therapeutic response	Operator dependence	Lumen assessment	Wall assessment
Angiography	+++	+++	+++	++	+	+	+++	0
MRA	+	++	++	+++ (Aorta)	+++ (Aorta)	++	++	++
Doppler Ultrasound	0	+	++	+++ (Periphery)	+++ (Periphery)	+++	+	+++

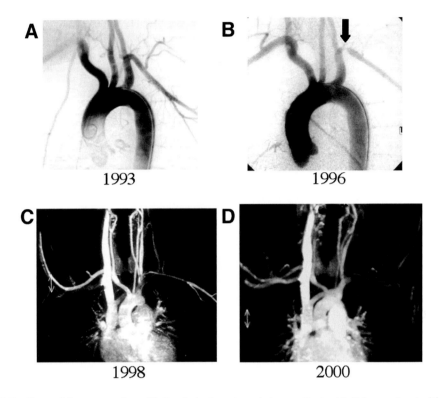

Fig. 6. Radiographic progression of left subclavian stenosis in a patient with Takayasu's arteritis using different imaging modalities. **(A)** Initial angiogram without abnormalities. **(B)** Follow-up angiogram with focal stenosis (*solid arrow*). **(C)** Gadolinium-enhanced magnetic resonance angiogram with long stenosis **(D)** Gadolinium enhanced magnetic resonance angiogram with near occlusion.

angiography can also be combined with angioplasty and stent placement for the treatment of vascular insufficiency syndromes.

Magnetic Resonance Angiography for LVV

Magnetic resonance angiography (MRA) has emerged as an alternative imaging modality for LVV owing to its noninvasive nature and avoidance of ionic contrast dye. The ability of MRA to detect changes in lumen size in medium to large arteries is close to that of angiography although it still lacks the resolution to clearly image small to medium arteries. Furthermore, owing to flow turbulence at a narrowed segment, MRA can overestimate a moderate stenosis *(118)*. Nevertheless, MRA has shown accuracy comparable to angiography in detection of vasculitic lesion in the aorta and its proximal major branches (Fig. 6).

MRA holds an advantage over conventional arteriography in its ability to detect vessel wall thickening and inflammation, which can precede stenosis (Fig. 7) *(119)*. This vessel thickness can be measured and followed over time as a marker of disease activity and response to therapy. Wall enhancement can also help differentiate new and active lesions from old, fibrotic damage *(120)*. When aortic wall enhancement equals or exceeds that of the myocardial tissue, disease activity is thought to be present.

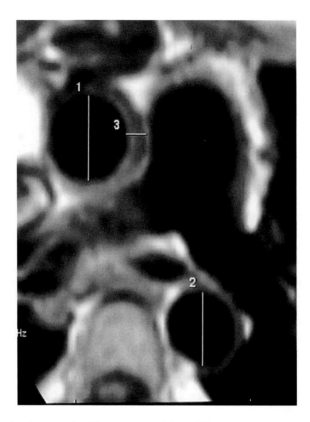

Fig. 7. MRI of aortic involvement in Takayasu's arteritis. While the vascular lumens of the ascending (1) and descending (2) aorta are near normal, the wall of the ascending aorta (3) is clearly thickened.

Unfortunately, current technology limits vessel wall evaluation to the aorta and its proximal branches, and MRA techniques have not yet become standarized.

Doppler Ultrasound for LVV

The development of high-resolution duplex ultrasound technology has led to its increased use for evaluation and monitoring of vasculitis. Like MRA, it is noninvasive and low risk. In addition, it avoids the enclosed chamber of an MRI. However, its accuracy depends heavily on the experience of the ultrasonographer in evaluating inflamed vessels. Ultrasound is also limited by overlying bony structures, and deep vessels such as the aorta can be difficult to study (118). Other shortcomings of ultrasound include failure to detect small collateral vessels and short mildly stenotic lesions.

There are a number of advantages to ultrasound evaluation. Ultrasonography reveals details of peripheral vessel wall thickness that can be monitored for change with disease activity or treatment (121). It can also detect perivascular edema, a sign of active vasculitis that may respond to glucocorticoid treatment (122,123). This edema resembles a dark, circumferential halo around an inflamed artery. In fact, one well-designed study found that duplex ultrasound of the temporal artery can diagnose temporal arteritis with 93% sensitivity and specificity (124). However, these data have not been confirmed.

The addition of Doppler to ultrasound allows for the assessment of blood flow. A change from the normal three-phase blood flow pattern is indicative of an upstream

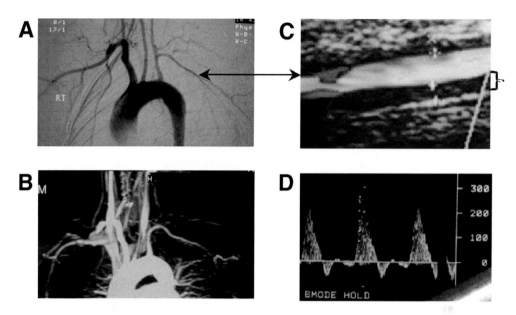

Fig. 8. Comparison of conventional angiogram, magnetic resonance angiogram and duplex ultrasound in a patient with Takayasu's arteritis. **(A)** Conventional angiogram showing distal subclavian stenosis. **(B)** Magnetic resonance angiogram demonstrating distal subclavian stenosis. **(C)** Duplex ultrasound of distal subclavian at region shown to be involved by angiogram (*solid arrow*). Bracket outlines vessel wall thickening which is not appreciable on angiogram or magnetic resonance angiogram. **(D)** B-mode Doppler waveform in thickened subclavian vessel. The normal three-phase waveform has been replaced by a single phase, suggesting loss of vascular compliance.

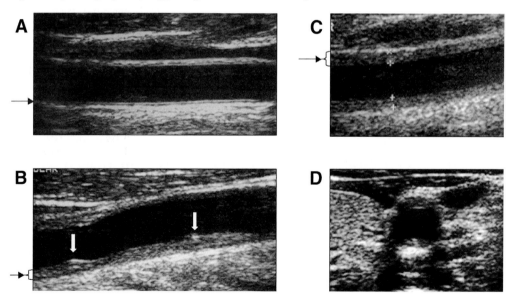

Fig. 9. Ultrasound evaluation of common carotid arteries. **(A)** Healthy 30-yr-old volunteer with normal, thin vessel wall (*solid arrow*). **(B)** A 70-yr-old patient pre-coronary artery bypass graft surgery with a thick, irregular vessel wall (*solid arrow with bracket*) and bright echogenic plaques (*open arrows*). **(C)** A 23-yr-old patient with Takayasu's arteritis causing smooth vessel wall thickening (*solid arrow with bracket*)—note absence of irregularity or plaque. **(D)** Vessel wall involved by TAK in transverse section demonstrating circumferential wall thickening but without hypoechoic wall edema.

vascular lesion. A recent study comparing color Doppler flow ultrasound plus transcranial Doppler and panaortoarteriography found a good correlation between these two techniques for brachiocephalic trunk, common carotid artery, and extracranial vertebral arteries, respectively *(118)*. Similar comparison also found good correlation between MRA, and panaorto-arteriography (118). Comparative images obtained through angiography, MRA and ultrasound from a patient with Takayasu's arteritis help highlight the differences between these techniques (Fig. 8).

Ultrasound has also been able to find common carotid artery wall thickening in vessels that appear normal on arteriography. One study found intima–media thickening in 89% of stenotic common carotid artery segments in patients with TAK *(125)*. Homogeneous, circumferential thickening can distinguish inflammatory vessel lesions from atherosclerotic disease (Fig. 9).

At this time we would recommend the initial use of conventional panaortoangiography in addition to duplex ultrasound of the carotid and vertebral vessels for diagnosis and localization of the extent of vascular injury as the initial studies of a new patient. MRA would serve well for follow-up surveillance and assessment of aortic disease, while duplex ultrasound is best suited for early detection and follow-up monitoring of peripheral lesions. The current role of ultrasound and MRA in the diagnosis and management of LVV is still being determined. As technological advances continue, angiography may become less necessary for diagnostic purposes, but it has the additional advantage of allowing for immediate treatment of vessel stenosis with angioplasty.

SUMMARY

LVV is an unusual but potentially devastating cause of arterial insufficiency. Giant cell arteritis is the most common cause of LVV and affects people over the age of 50, while TAK is a much less common condition that affects primarily young women. Other autoimmune disorders such as spondyloarthropathy, relapsing polychondritis, and Behçet's disease, although not primarily large-vessel vasculitidies, are well recognized causes of large-vessel inflammation. Despite the infrequency of these conditions, vascular insufficiency due to vasculitis should be suspected in any individual not predisposed to atherosclerotic disease (such as a young woman), with new symptoms of systemic inflammation, or with an unusual distribution of affected vessels (such as the subclavian arteries). The use of laboratory inflammatory markers, ultrasound, MRA, conventional angiography, and arterial biopsy can help establish the diagnosis. Despite the paucity of randomized, placebo-controlled, double-blinded clinical trials of therapeutic agents for causes of LVV, immunosuppressive medications such as glucocorticoids, methotrexate, cyclophosphamide, and others seem to help retard further arterial injury. However, these medications are associated with potentially serious side effects and should be used only in conjunction with vigilant clinical follow-up, laboratory measurements of inflammation, and periodic imaging studies to assess disease activity and therapeutic efficacy.

REFERENCES

 1. Hutchinson J. Diseases of the Arteries. Arch Surg 1890;1:323.
 2. Harrison C. Giant-cell or temporal arteritis: a review. J Clin Pathol 1948;1:197–211.
 3. Chakrabarty A, Franks AJ. Temporal artery biopsy: is there any value in examining biopsies at multiple levels? J Clin Pathol 2000;53:131–136.

4. Evans JM, O'Fallon WM, Hunder GG. Increased incidence of aortic aneurysm and dissection in giant cell (temporal) arteritis: a population-based study. Ann Intern Med 1995;122:502–507.

5. Brack A, Martinez-Taboada V, Stanson A, Goronzy JJ, Weyand CM. Disease pattern in cranial and large-vessel giant cell arteritis. Arthritis Rheum 1999;42:311–317.

6. Hayreh SS, Podhajsky PA, Zimmerman B. Occult giant cell arteritis: ocular manifestations. Am J Ophthalmol 1998;125:521–526.

7. Poller DN, van Wyk Q, Jeffrey MJ. The importance of skip lesions in temporal arteritis. J Clin Pathol 2000;53:137–139.

8. Gonzalez-Gay MA, Garcia-Porrua C, Llorca J, Gonzalez-Louzao C, Rodriguez-Ledo P. Biopsy-negative giant cell arteritis: clinical spectrum and predictive factors for positive temporal artery biopsy. Semin Arthritis Rheum 2001;30:249–256.

9. Ostberg G. Temporal arteritis in a large necropsy series. Ann Rheum Dis 1971;30:224–235.

10. Nordborg E. Epidemiology of biopsy-positive giant cell arteritis: an overview. Clin Exp Rheumatol 2000;18(Suppl):S15–17.

11. Hunder GG, Bloch DA, Michel BA, et al. The American College of Rheumatology 1990 criteria for the classification of giant cell arteritis. Arthritis Rheum 1990;33:1122–1128.

12. Baldursson O, Steinsson K, Bjornsson, J, Lie, JT. Giant cell arteritis in Iceland: an epidemiologic and histopathologic analysis. Arthritis Rheum 1994;37:1007–1012.

13. Smith CA, Fidler WJ, Pinals RS. The epidemiology of giant cell arteritis: report of a ten-year study in Shelby County, Tennessee. Arthritis Rheum 1983;26:1214–1219.

14. Bengtsson BA, Malmvall BE. The epidemiology of giant cell arteritis including temporal arteritis and polymyalgia rheumatica: incidences of different clinical presentations and eye complications. Arthritis Rheum 1981;24:899–904.

15. Boesen P, Sorensen SF. Giant cell arteritis, temporal arteritis, and polymyalgia rheumatica in a Danish county: a prospective investigation, 1982–1985. Arthritis Rheum 1987;30:294–299.

16. Sonnenblick M, Nesher G, Friedlander Y, Rubinow A. Giant cell arteritis in Jerusalem: a 12-year epidemiological study. Br J Rheumatol 1994;33:938–941.

17. Gonzalez E, Varnes WT, Lisse JR, Daniels JC, Hokanson JA. Giant-cell arteritis in the southern United States: an 11-year retrospective study from the Texas Gulf Coast. Arch Intern Med 1989;149:1561–1565.

18. Cimmino MA, Zaccaria A. Epidemiology of polymyalgia rheumatica. Clin Exp Rheumatol 2000;18:S9–11.

19. Hall S, Persellin S, Lie JT, O'Brien PC, Kurland LT, Hunder GG. The therapeutic impact of temporal artery biopsy. Lancet 1983;2:1217–1220.

20. Lie JT. Histopathologic specificity of systemic vasculitis. Rheum Dis Clin North Am 1995;21:883–909.

21. Lie J, Brown AL Jr, Carter ET. Spectrum of aging changes in temporal arteries. Its significance, in interpretation of biopsy of temporal artery. Arch Path Lab Med 1970;90:278–285.

22. Lie J. Histopathologic specificity of systemic vasculitis. Rheum Dis Clin North Am 1995;21:883–909.

23. Esteban MJ, Font C, Hernandez-Rodriguez J, et al. Small-vessel vasculitis surrounding a spared temporal artery: clinical and pathological findings in a series of twenty-eight patients. Arthritis Rheum 2001;44:1387–1395.

24. Gabriel SE, O'Fallon WM, Achkar AA, Lie JT, Hunder GG. The use of clinical characteristics to predict the results of temporal artery biopsy among patients with suspected giant cell arteritis. J Rheumatol 1995;22:93–96.

25. Chmelewski WL, McKnight KM, Agudelo CA, Wise CM. Presenting features and outcomes in patients undergoing temporal artery biopsy: a review of 98 patients. Arch Intern Med 1992;152:1690–1695.

26. Achkar AA, Lie JT, Hunder GG, O'Fallon WM, Gabriel SE. How does previous corticosteroid treatment affect the biopsy findings in giant cell (temporal) arteritis? Ann Intern Med 1994;120:987–992.

27. Weyand CM, Goronzy JJ. Arterial wall injury in giant cell arteritis. Arthritis Rheum 1999;42:844–853.

28. Weyand CM, Goronzy JJ. Pathogenic principles in giant cell arteritis. Int J Cardiol 2000;75(Suppl 1):S9–S15.

29. Kaiser M, Weyand CM, Bjornsson J, Goronzy JJ. Platelet-derived growth factor, intimal hyperplasia, and ischemic complications in giant cell arteritis. Arthritis Rheum 1998;41:623–633.

30. Hunder G. Giant cell arteritis and polymyalgia rheumatica. Med Clin N Am 1997;81:195–219.

31. Salvarani C, Hunder GG. Musculoskeletal manifestations in a population-based cohort of patients with giant cell arteritis. Arthritis Rheum 1999;42:1259–1266.

32. Ninet JP, Bachet P, Dumontet CM, Du Colombier PB, Stewart MD, Pasquier JH. Subclavian and axillary involvement in temporal arteritis and polymyalgia rheumatica. Am J Med 1990;88:13–20.

33. Klein RG, Hunder GG, Stanson AW, Sheps SG. Large artery involvement in giant cell (temporal) arteritis. Ann Intern Med 1975;83:806–812.

34. Liozon E, Herrmann F, Ly K, et al. Risk factors for visual loss in giant cell (temporal) arteritis: a prospective study of 174 patients. Am J Med 2001;111:211–217.

35. Gonzalez-Gay MA, Blanco R, Rodriguez-Valverde V, et al. Permanent visual loss and cerebrovascular accidents in giant cell arteritis: predictors and response to treatment. Arthritis Rheum 1998;41:1497–1504.

36. Gonzalez-Gay MA, Garcia-Porrua C, Llorca J, et al. Visual manifestations of giant cell arteritis: trends and clinical spectrum in 161 patients. Medicine (Baltimore) 2000;79:283–292.

37. Cid MC, Font C, Oristrell J, et al. Association between strong inflammatory response and low risk of developing visual loss and other cranial ischemic complications in giant cell (temporal) arteritis. Arthritis Rheum 1998;41:26–32.

38. Nesher G. Neurologic manifestations of giant cell arteritis. Clin Exp Rheumatol 2000;18:S24–26.

39. Hayreh SS, Podhajsky PA, Zimmerman B. Ocular manifestations of giant cell arteritis. Am J Ophthalmol 1998;125:509–520.

40. Myles AB. Steroid treatment in giant cell arteritis. Br J Rheumatol 1992;31:787.

41. Wilkinson IM, Russell RW. Arthritis of the head and neck in giant cell arteritis. Arch Neurol 1972;27:378–391.

42. Font C, Cid MC, Coll-Vinent B, Lopez-Soto A, Grau JM. Clinical features in patients with permanent visual loss due to biopsy-proven giant cell arteritis. Br J Rheumatol 1997;36:251–254.

43. Le Hello C, Levesque H, Jeanton M, et al. Lower limb giant cell arteritis and temporal arteritis: followup of 8 cases. J Rheumatol 2001;28:1407–1412.

44. Rasmussen TE, Hallett JW, Metzger RL, et al. Genetic risk factors in inflammatory abdominal aortic aneurysms: polymorphic residue 70 in the HLA-DR B1 gene as a key genetic element. J Vasc Surg 1997;25:356–364.

45. Salvarani C, Hunder GG. Giant cell arteritis with low erythrocyte sedimentation rate: frequency of occurrence in a population-based study. Arthritis Rheum 2001; 45:140-5.

46. Kyle V, Cawston, TE, Hazleman, BL. Erythrocyte sedimentation rate and C reactive protein in the assessment of polymyalgia rheumatica/giant cell arteritis on presentation and during follow up. Ann Rheum Dis 1989;48:667–671.

47. Hayreh SS, Podhajsky PA, Zimmerman B. Occult giant cell arteritis: ocular manifestations. Am J Ophthalmol 1998;125:521–526.

48. Salvarani C, Macchioni P, Boiardi L, et al. Soluble interleukin 2 receptors in polymyalgia rheumatica/giant cell arteritis: clinical and laboratory correlations. J Rheumatol 1992;19:1100–1106.

49. Salvarani C, Boiardi L, Macchioni P, et al. Role of peripheral CD8 lymphocytes and soluble IL-2 receptor in predicting the duration of corticosteroid treatment in polymyalgia rheumatica and giant cell arteritis. Ann Rheum Dis 1995;54:640–644.

50. Weyand CM, Fulbright JW, Hunder GG, Evans JM, Goronzy JJ. Treatment of giant cell arteritis: interleukin-6 as a biologic marker of disease activity. Arthritis Rheum 2000;43:1041–1048.

51. Delecoeuillerie G, Joly P, Cohen de Lara A, Paolaggi JB. Polymyalgia rheumatica and temporal arteritis: a retrospective analysis of prognostic features and different corticosteroid regimens (11 year survey of 210 patients). Ann Rheum Dis 1988;47:733–739.

52. Nesher G, Rubinow A, Sonnenblick M. Efficacy and adverse effects of different corticosteroid dose regimens in temporal arteritis: a retrospective study. Clin Exp Rheumatol 1997;15:3033-#306.

53. Lundberg I, Hedfors E. Restricted dose and duration of corticosteroid treatment in patients with polymyalgia rheumatica and temporal arteritis. J Rheumatol 1990;17:1340–1345.

54. Kyle V, Hazleman BL. Treatment of polymyalgia rheumatica and giant cell arteritis. I. Steroid regimens in the first two months. Ann Rheum Dis 1989;48:658–661.

55. Hunder GG, Sheps SG, Allen GL, Joyce JW. Daily and alternate-day corticosteroid regimens in treatment of giant cell arteritis: comparison in a prospective study. Ann Intern Med 1975;82: 613–618.

56. Hayreh SS. Steroid therapy for visual loss in patients with giant-cell arteritis. Lancet 2000;355:1572–1573.

57. De Silva M, Hazleman BL. Azathioprine in giant cell arteritis/polymyalgia rheumatica: a double-blind study. Ann Rheum Dis 1986;45:136–138.

58. Doury P, Pattin S, Eulry F, Thabaut A. The use of dapsone in the treatment of giant cell arteritis and polymyalgia rheumatica. Arthritis Rheum 1983;26:689–690.

59. de Vita S, Tavoni A, Jeracitano G, Gemignani G, Dolcher MP, Bombardieri S. Treatment of giant cell arteritis with cyclophosphamide pulses. J Intern Med 1992;232:373–375.

60. Schaufelberger C, Andersson R, Nordborg E. No additive effect of cyclosporin A compared with glucocorticoid treatment alone in giant cell arteritis: results of an open, controlled, randomized study. Br J Rheumatol 1998; 37:464-5.

61. Jover JH-G, C. Morado, IC. Vargas, E. Banares, A. Fernandez-Gutierrez, B. Combined treatment of giant-cell arteritis with methotrexate and prednisone. a randomized, double-blind, placebo-controlled trial. Ann Intern Med 2001;134:106–114.

62. Hoffman G, Cid M, Hellmann D, et al. A multicenter, randomized, double-blind, placebo-controlled study of adjuvant methotrexate treatment for giant cell arteritis. Arthritis Rheum, in press.

63. Numano F, Kakuta T. Takayasu arteritis: five doctors in the history of Takayasu arteritis. Int J Cardiol 1996;54(Suppl):S1–10.

64. Numano F, Okawara M, Inomata H, Kobayashi Y. Takayasu's arteritis. Lancet 2000;356:1023–1025.

65. Kerr GS, Hallahan CW, Giordano J, et al. Takayasu arteritis. Ann Intern Med 1994;120:919–929.

66. Arend WP, Michel BA, Bloch DA, et al. The American College of Rheumatology 1990 criteria for the classification of Takayasu arteritis. Arthritis Rheum 1990;33:1129–1134.

67. Sharma BK, Jain S, Radotra BD. An autopsy study of Takayasu arteritis in India. Int J Cardiol 1998; 66(Suppl 1):S85–90.

68. Gravanis M. Giant cell arteritis and Takayasu aortitis: morphologic, pathogenetic and etiologic factors. Int J Cardiol 2000;75(Suppl 1):S21–33.

69. Lupi-Herrera E, Sanchez-Torres G, Marcushamer J, Mispireta J, Horwitz S, Vela JE. Takayasu's arteritis: clinical study of 107 cases. Am Heart J 1977;93:94–103.

70. Noris M, Daina E, Gamba S, Bonazzola S, Remuzzi G. Interleukin-6 and RANTES in Takayasu arteritis: a guide for therapeutic decisions? Circulation 1999;100:55–60.

71. Seko Y. Takayasu arteritis: insights into immunopathology. Jpn Heart J 2000; 41:15-26.

72. Nakao K, Ikeda M, Kimata S, Niitani H, Niyahara M. Takayasu's arteritis: clinical report of eighty-four cases and immunological studies of seven cases. Circulation 1967;35:1141–1155.

73. Canas CA, Jimenez CA, Ramirez LA, et al. Takayasu arteritis in Colombia. Int J Cardiol 1998;66 (Suppl 1):S73–79.

74. Hall S, Barr W, Lie JT, Stanson AW, Kazmier FJ, Hunder GG. Takayasu arteritis: a study of 32 North American patients. Medicine (Baltimore) 1985;64:89–99.

75. Deyu Z, Guozhang L. Clinical study of aortic regurgitation with aortoarteritis. Int J Cardiol 2000; 75(Suppl 1):S141–S145.

76. Lie JT. Pathology of isolated nonclassical and catastrophic manifestations of Takayasu arteritis. Int J Cardiol 1998;66(Suppl 1):S11–21.

77. Kihara M, Kimura K, Yakuwa H, et al. Isolated left coronary ostial stenosis as the sole arterial involvement in Takayasu's disease. J Intern Med 1992;232:353–355.

78. Amano J, Suzuki A. Coronary artery involvement in Takayasu's arteritis: collective review and guideline for surgical treatment. J Thorac Cardiovasc Surg 1991;102:554–560.

79. Kiyosawa M, Baba T. Ophthalmological findings in patients with Takayasu disease. Int J Cardiol 1998; 66(Suppl 1):S141–147.

80. Baltazares M, Mendoza F, Dabague J, Reyes PA. Antiaorta antibodies and Takayasu arteritis. Int J Cardiol 1998;66(Suppl 1):S183–187; discussion S189.

81. Tanigawa K, Eguchi K, Kitamura Y, et al. Magnetic resonance imaging detection of aortic and pulmonary artery wall thickening in the acute stage of Takayasu arteritis: improvement of clinical and radiologic findings after steroid therapy. Arthritis Rheum 1992;35:476–480.

82. Hoffman GS, Leavitt RY, Kerr GS, Rottem M, Sneller MC, Fauci AS. Treatment of glucocorticoid-resistant or relapsing Takayasu arteritis with methotrexate. Arthritis Rheum 1994;37:578–582.

83. Daina E, Schieppati A, Remuzzi G. Mycophenolate mofetil for the treatment of Takayasu arteritis: report of three cases. Ann Intern Med 1999;130:422–426.

84. Hoffman G. Treatment of resistant Takayasu's arteritis. Rheum Dis Clin N Am 1995;21:73–80.

85. Moncada GA, Hashimoto Y, Kobayashi Y, Maruyama Y, Numano F. Usefulness of beta blocker therapy in patients with Takayasu arteritis and moderate or severe aortic regurgitation. Jpn Heart J 2000;41:325–337.

86. Hashimoto Y, Tanaka M, Hata A, Kakuta T, Maruyama Y, Numano F. Four years follow-up study in patients with Takayasu arteritis and severe aortic regurgitation; assessment by echocardiography. Int J Cardiol 1996;54(Suppl):S173–176.

87. Fava MP, Foradori GB, Garcia CB, et al. Percutaneous transluminal angioplasty in patients with Takayasu arteritis: five-year experience. J Vasc Interv Radiol 1993;4:649-52.

88. Joseph S, Mandalam KR, Rao VR, et al. Percutaneous transluminal angioplasty of the subclavian artery in nonspecific aortoarteritis: results of long-term follow-up. J Vasc Interv Radiol 1994;5: 573–580.

89. Sharma BK, Jain S, Bali HK, Jain A, Kumari S. A follow-up study of balloon angioplasty and de-novo stenting in Takayasu arteritis. Int J Cardiol 2000;75(Suppl 1):S147–152.

90. Ishikawa K, Maetani S. Peripheral arterial and aortic diseases: long-term outcome for 120 Japanese patients with Takayasu's disease: clinical and statistical analyses of related prognostic factors. Circulation 1994;90:1855–1860.

91. Sakane T, Takeno M, Suzuki N, Inaba G. Behcet's disease. N Engl J Med 1999;341:1284–1291.

92. Koc Y, Gullu I, Akpek G, et al. Vascular involvement in Behcet's disease. J Rheumatol 1992;19: 402–410.

93. Le Thi Huong D, Wechsler B, Papo T, et al. Arterial lesions in Behcet's disease. A study in 25 patients. J Rheumatol 1995;22:2103–2113.

94. Hamza M. Large artery involvement in Behcet's disease. J Rheumatol 1987;14:554–559.

95. Yurdakul S, Mat C, Tuzun Y, et al. A double-blind trial of colchicine in Behcet's syndrome. Arthritis Rheum 2001;44:2686–2692.

96. Jorizzo JL, White WL, Wise CM, Zanolli MD, Sherertz EF. Low-dose weekly methotrexate for unusual neutrophilic vascular reactions: cutaneous polyarteritis nodosa and Behcet's disease. J Am Acad Dermatol 1991;24:973–978.

97. Hamuryudan V, Mat C, Saip S, et al. Thalidomide in the treatment of the mucocutaneous lesions of the Behcet syndrome: a randomized, double-blind, placebo-controlled trial. Ann Intern Med 1998;128: 443–450.

98. Hamuryudan V, Ozyazgan Y, Hizli N, et al. Azathioprine in Behcet's syndrome: effects on long-term prognosis. Arthritis Rheum 1997;40:769–774.

99. Sullu Y, Oge I, Erkan D, Ariturk N, Mohajeri F. Cyclosporin-A therapy in severe uveitis of Behcet's disease. Acta Ophthalmol Scand 1998;76:96–99.

100. Smulders FM, Oosterhuis JA. Treatment of Behcet's disease with chlorambucil. Ophthalmologica 1975;171:347–352.

101. McAdam LP, O'Hanlan MA, Bluestone R, Pearson CM. Relapsing polychondritis: prospective study of 23 patients and a review of the literature. Medicine (Baltimore) 1976;55:193–215.

102. Trentham DE, Le CH. Relapsing polychondritis. Ann Intern Med 1998;129:114–122.

103. Cipriano PR, Alonso DR, Baltaxe HA, Gay WA, Jr, Smith JP. Multiple aortic aneurysms in relapsing polychondritis. Am J Cardiol 1976;37:1097–1102.

104. Michet CJ, Jr, McKenna CH, Luthra HS, O'Fallon WM. Relapsing polychondritis. Survival and predictive role of early disease manifestations. Ann Intern Med 1986;104:74–78.

105. Esdaile J, Hawkins D, Gold P, Freedman SO, Duguid WP. Vascular involvement in relapsing polychondritis. Can Med Assoc J 1977;116:1019–1022.

106. Stewart SR, Robbins DL, Castles JJ. Acute fulminant aortic and mitral insufficiency in ankylosing spondylitis. N Engl J Med 1978;299:1448–1449.

107. Bulkley BH, Roberts WC. Ankylosing spondylitis and aortic regurgitation: description of the characteristic cardiovascular lesion from study of eight necropsy patients. Circulation 1973;48:1014–1027.

108. Ansell BB, Bywaters EGL, Doniach, I. The aortic lesion of ankylosing spondylitis. Br Heart J 1958;20: 507.

109. Arnason JA, Patel AK, Rahko PS, Sundstrom WR. Transthoracic and transesophageal echocardiographic evaluation of the aortic root and subvalvular structures in ankylosing spondylitis. J Rheumatol 1996;23:120–123.

110. O'Neill TW, Bresnihan B. The heart in ankylosing spondylitis. Ann Rheum Dis 1992;51:705–706.

111. Davidson PB, Baggenstoss AH, Slocumb CH, Daugherty GW. Cardiac and aortic lesions in rheumatoid spondylitis. Mayo Clin Proc 1963;36:427–435.

112. Bergfeldt L, Insulander P, Lindblom D, Moller E, Edhag O. HLA-B27: an important genetic risk factor for lone aortic regurgitation and severe conduction system abnormalities. Am J Med 1988;85: 12–18.

113. Townend JN, Emery P, Davies MK, Littler WA. Acute aortitis and aortic incompetence due to systemic rheumatological disorders. Int J Cardiol 1991;33:253–258.

114. Park JH, Chung JW, Im JG, Kim SK, Park YB, Han MC. Takayasu arteritis: evaluation of mural changes in the aorta and pulmonary artery with CT angiography. Radiology 1995;196:89–93.
115. Miller JH, Gunarta H, Stanley P. Gallium scintigraphic demonstration of arteritis in Takayasu disease. Clin Nucl Med 1996;21:882–883.
116. Hoffmann M, Corr P, Robbs J. Cerebrovascular findings in Takayasu disease. J Neuroimaging 2000;10:84–90.
117. Stanson AW, Klein RG, Hunder GG. Extracranial angiographic findings in giant cell (temporal) arteritis. Am J Roentgenol 1976;127:957–963.
118. Cantu C, Pineda C, Barinagarrementeria F, et al. Noninvasive cerebrovascular assessment of Takayasu arteritis. Stroke 2000;31:2197–2202.
119. Atalay MK, Bluemke DA. Magnetic resonance imaging of large vessel vasculitis. Curr Opin Rheumatol 2001;13:41–47.
120. Choe YH, Kim DK, Koh EM, Do YS, Lee WR. Takayasu arteritis: diagnosis with MR imaging and MR angiography in acute and chronic active stages. J Magn Reson Imaging 1999;10:751–757.
121. Park SH, Chung JW, Lee JW, Han MH, Park JH. Carotid artery involvement in Takayasu's arteritis: evaluation of the activity by ultrasonography. J Ultrasound Med 2001;20:371–378.
122. Schmidt WA, Kraft HE, Borkowski A, Gromnica-Ihle EJ. Color duplex ultrasonography in large-vessel giant cell arteritis. Scand J Rheumatol 1999;28:374–376.
123. Schmidt WA. Doppler ultrasonography in the diagnosis of giant cell arteritis. Clin Exp Rheumatol 2000;18(Suppl 20):S40–42.
124. Schmidt WA, Kraft HE, Vorpahl K, Volker L, Gromnica-Ihle EJ. Color duplex ultrasonography in the diagnosis of temporal arteritis. N Engl J Med 1997;337:1336–1342.
125. Sun Y, Yip PK, Jeng JS, Hwang BS, Lin WH. Ultrasonographic study and long-term follow-up of Takayasu's arteritis. Stroke 1996;27:2178–2182.

INDEX